Non-invasive respiratory support
A practical handbook

Second edition

Edited by

ANITA K SIMONDS MD FRCP
Consultant in Respiratory Medicine,
Royal Brompton and Harefield NHS Trust,
London, UK

A member of the Hodder Headline Group
LONDON
Distributed in the USA by
Oxford University Press Inc., New York

First published in Great Britain in 2001 by
Arnold, a member of the Hodder Headline Group,
338 Euston Road, London NWI 3BH

http://www.arnoldpublishers.com

Distributed in the United States of America by
Oxford University Press Inc.,
198 Madison Avenue, New York, NY10016
Oxford is a registered trademark of Oxford University Press

Whilst the advice and information in this book are believed to be true and
accurate at the date of going to press, neither the authors nor the publisher
can accept any legal responsibility or liability for any errors or omissions
that may be made. In particular (but without limiting the generality of the
preceding disclaimer) every effort has been made to check drug dosages;
however, it is still possible that errors have been missed. Furthermore,
dosage schedules are constantly being revised and new side-effects
recognized. For these reasons the reader is strongly urged to consult the
drug companies' printed instructions before administering any of the drugs
recommended in this book.

British Library Cataloguing in Publication Data
A catalogue record for this book is available from the British Library

Library of Congress Cataloging-in-Publication Data
A catalog record for this book is available from the Library of Congress

ISBN 0 340 76259 4 (pb)

3 4 5 6 7 8 9 10

Typeset in 10/12 pt Minion by
Scribe Design, Gillingham, Kent, UK
Printed and bound in India

What do you think about this book? Or any other Arnold title?
Please send your comments to feedback.arnold@hodder.co.uk

Contents

Contributors

Mrs Penny Agent
Physiotherapist, Royal Brompton and Harefield NHS Trust, London UK

Dr Nicolino Ambrosino
Chief, Lung Function Unit, Fondazione Salvatore Maugeri, Medical Centre of Gussago, Gussago, Italy

Ms Julia Bott
Physiotherapist, London, UK

Dr MA Branthwaite
Barrister, formerly Consultant Physician and Consultant Anaesthetist, Royal Brompton and Harefield NHS Trust, London, UK

Ms Susan Callaghan
Senior Nurse, Royal Brompton and Harefield NHS Trust, London, UK

Dr Marco Confalonieri
Unit of Pneumology, Trieste General Hospital, Italy

Dr Mark W Elliott
Consultant Physician, St James's University Hospital, Leeds, UK

Mr Stephen Heather
Chief Respiratory Support Technician, Respiratory Support Service, Royal Brompton and Harefield NHS Trust, London, UK

Professor Nicolas S Hill
Professor of Medicine, Brown University, Director, Critical Care Services, Rhode Island Hospital, Providence, Rhode Island, USA

Dr Patrick Leger
Affaires Medicales, Association Française contre les Myopathies, France

Dr Stefano Nava
Respiratory Unit, I.R.C.C.S. Fondazione Salvatore Maugeri, Instituto Scientifico di Pavia, Pavia, Italy

Dr Anita K Simonds
Consultant in Respiratory Medicine, Royal Brompton and Harefield NHS Trust, London, UK

Mrs Sarah Ward
Senior Respiratory Support Technician, Respiratory Support Service, Royal Brompton and Harefield NHS Trust, London, UK

Foreword

Few areas in respiratory medicine have advanced as rapidly as non-invasive ventilation in the last 5 years. Not only has nasal intermittent positive pressure ventilation (NIPPV) been confirmed as effective therapy in acute hypercapnic exacerbations of COPD, it has an increasing role in acute respiratory failure due to non-COPD causes. The application of NIPPV in chronic ventilatory failure has been extended from conventional indications in chest wall and stable neuromuscular disease, to progressive neuromuscular disorders and paediatric neuromusculo-skeletal disease. NIPPV is now widely used in the Intensive Care Unit, Emergency Room and in general respiratory wards, so that medical staff, nurses, therapists and technicians in all these areas need to be familiar with the technique. In some countries the prevalence of domiciliary NIPPV has increased five-fold in as many years. To highlight these developments this edition has been extended to include new or expanded chapters on NIPPV in acute respiratory failure, NIPPV in the Intensive Care Unit and High Dependency Unit, paediatric non-invasive ventilation, and problem solving; with contributions from leading exponents in Europe and the USA. The risk-management of the home ventilator-dependent patient, together with ethical and medico-legal aspects of assisted ventilation are now covered in detail.

It is evident however, that many dilemmas and controversies remain – does long term NIPPV confer benefit in patients with chronic ventilatory failure due to COPD? When should therapy be initiated? What are the key mechanisms of action? What are the effects of NIPPV on quality of life in rapidly progressive disorders? In the field of sleep medicine, nasal continuous positive airway pressure (CPAP) therapy has been shown to reduce somnolence and improve the quality of life in moderate and severe obstructive sleep apnoea (OSA), but its role in mild OSA and heart failure and impact on vascular disease is not yet clear.

The aim of this book is to explain not only how to apply NIPPV, but why it works, and when to use it. In addition to step-by-step practical guidance on how to set up a ventilator, information is provided on the outcome of non-invasive ventilation in acute and chronic situations, so that those applying the technique can justify their decision-making. The advice given is in line with recently published guidelines and consensus conferences on non-invasive ventilation, and these are indicated clearly where relevant. I am grateful to Paul Hyett and C. Wim Witjens for contributions to the illustrations.

A.K. Simonds

Preface

The increasing use of non-invasive respiratory support (i.e. the provision of mechanical ventilatory assistance without the need for an invasive airway) is one of the most remarkable developments in the field of mechanical ventilation over the past dozen years. This transformation and the decreasing use of invasive mechanical ventilation, particularly in the home, has been driven by the many potential advantages of non-invasive over invasive ventilation. These include greater patient comfort and ease of administration (at least in chronic settings), reduced morbidity and mortality, and more economical administration. However, as is emphasized in the text, these advantages can be realized only if appropriate patients are selected and the technology is administered properly.

The earliest forms of non-invasive ventilators were negative pressure ventilators including the 'iron lung'. These so-called tank ventilators were first described during the 1800s, but saw their greatest use during the first half of the 20th century, when the polio epidemics created a great need for ventilatory assist devices and the wide availability of electricity provided a readily available power source.[1] The polio epidemics also stimulated the development of alternative non-invasive 'body' ventilators, so-called because they functioned by alternating pressure on various parts of the body. These included more portable versions of negative pressure ventilators such as the jacket ventilator[2] or chest cuirass and the so-called abdominal displacement ventilators.[3] These consisted of devices such as the rocking bed or intermittent abdominal pressure respirator (pneumobelt) that assisted ventilation by effecting diaphragmatic motion via displacement of the abdominal viscera.

By the late 1950s and 1960s, however, the obvious advantages of invasive positive pressure ventilation over 'body' ventilators for the support of patients with acute respiratory failure led to the virtual replacement of traditional non-invasive techniques by invasive positive pressure ventilation. Non-invasive techniques continued to be used long-term for survivors of the polio epidemics as well as for others with chronic respiratory failure due to neuromuscular disease or chest wall deformities.[4,5] However, surveys during the mid-1980s in the US revealed that only a minority of muscular dystrophy clinics were using such techniques, and most individuals with progressive neuromuscular illnesses were either ventilated via tracheostomies or permitted to expire peacefully without attempts at ventilatory assistance.[6]

Interest in non-invasive ventilation began to resurface during the mid 1980s, after the development of the nasal continuous positive airway pressure (CPAP) mask for the therapy of obstructive sleep apnoea.[7] Investigators learned that when nasal masks were attached to portable positive pressure ventilators and used intermittently in patients with restrictive thoracic disorders, day-time hypoventilation and symptoms of chronic respiratory failure reversed.[8,9,10] Soon after, reports began emerging of the successful use of non-invasive positive pressure techniques, either by nasal or oronasal mask, to support patients with various kinds of acute respiratory failure.[11,12] The past decade has seen a rapid evolution of these techniques so that non-invasive positive pressure ventilation has assumed a central role in the management of patients with chronic respiratory failure due to restrictive thoracic disorders and in patients with acute respiratory failure due to COPD.

The current volume on non-invasive respiratory support, edited by Dr Anita Simonds, provides a comprehensive perspective on the current status of non-invasive ventilatory techniques. Starting with practical aspects of non-invasive ventilation, including a discussion of ventilator modes and equipment used, the text describes applications of non-invasive ventilation in the acute setting, including initiation and problem solving. Topics related to use in different hospital settings, including the Intensive Care Unit, High Dependency Unit and Emergency Room are next discussed, and a considerable emphasis is placed on applications of non-invasive ventilation in the home, both for the well-accepted restrictive thoracic disorder indications, but also the more controversial applications in patients with chronic obstructive disorders. The volume covers not only non-invasive positive pressure ventilation that is used most often currently, but also applications of negative pressure ventilators as well as continuous positive airway pressure and physiotherapy. Chapters are devoted to the important topic of delivery of non-invasive ventilation to children as well as the organization of home ventilator networks in Europe. The ethical and medico-legal issues raised by non-invasive ventilatory support are discussed in the final chapter.

In order to provide a more consistent and readable text, Dr Simonds has written many of the chapters herself. She has also invited contributions from prominent colleagues in the UK, including Dr Mark Elliott, who has contributed seminal work in the area of non-invasive applications to patients with COPD; Julia Bott, an accomplished chest physiotherapist highly skilled in the application of non-invasive ventilation; and Dr Margaret Branthwaite, a long-recognized authority in the field. Prominent workers from France and Italy have also contributed, including Dr Patrick Leger, who has extensive experience working in the well-organized French home ventilator network, and Drs Stefano Nava, Marco Confalonieri and Nico Ambrosino, who have made numerous contributions with regard to physiologic consequences of non-invasive ventilation as well as expanding clinical applications. Dr Simonds and her contributors make for a highly accomplished and experienced group of authors who provide a thorough coverage of the topic. The practical and user-friendly approach should render this volume an extremely valuable one for all students, trainees, and respiratory clinicians interested in mechanical ventilation. I anticipate that it will be frequently used and cited and, despite the rapid advances that will undoubtedly continue within this expanding field, the book will occupy a prominent place on bookshelves for years to come.

Nicholas S. Hill, MD
Professor of Medicine, Brown University
Director, Critical Care Services, Rhode Island Hospital
Providence, Rhode Island, USA

REFERENCES

1. Wilson JL. Acute anterior poliomyelitis. *N Engl J Med* 1932; **206**: 887–93.
2. Spalding JMK, Opie L. Artificial respiration with the Tunnicliffe breathing-jacket. *Lancet* 1958; **1**; 613–15.
3. Hill NS. Use of the rocking bed, pneumobelt, and other noninvasive aids to ventilation. In: Tobin MJ (ed.) *Principles and practice of mechanical ventilation*. London: McGraw-Hill, 1994.
4. Curran FJ. Night ventilation by body respirators for patients in chronic respiratory failure due to late stage Duchenne muscular dystrophy. *Arch Phys Med Rehabil* 1981; **62**: 270–74.
5. Garay SM, Turino GM, Goldring RM. Sustained reversal of chronic hypercapnia in patients with alveolar hypoventilation syndromes. Long-term maintenance with noninvasive nocturnal mechanical ventilation. *Am J Med* 1981; **62**: 270–74.
6. Colbert AP, Schock NC. Respirator use in progressive neuromuscular diseases. *Arch Phys Med Rehabil* 1985; **66**: 760–62.
7. Sullivan CE, Issa FG, Berthon-Jones M, *et al*. Reversal of obstructive sleep apnoea by continuous positive airway pressure applied through the nares. *Lancet* 1981; **1**: 862–65.
8. Elliott MW, Simonds AK. Nocturnal assisted ventilation using bilevel positive airway pressure: the effect of expiratory positive airway pressure. *Eur Respir J* 1995; **8**: 436–40.
9. Bach JR, Alba A, Mosher, *et al*. Intermittent positive pressure ventilation via nasal access in the management of respiratory insufficiency. *Chest* 1987; **94**: 168–70.
10. Kerby GR, Mayer LS, Pingleton SK. Nocturnal positive pressure ventilation via nasal mask. *Am Rev Respir Dis* 1987; **135**: 738–40.
11. Meduri GU, Conoscenti CC, Menashe P, *et al*. Noninvasive face mask ventilation in patients with acute respiratory failure. *Chest* 1989; **96**: 865–70.
12. Elliott MW, Steven MH, Phillips GD, *et al*. Non-invasive mechanical ventilation for acute respiratory failure. *BMJ* 1990; **300**: 358–60.

1

Modes of non-invasive ventilatory support

A K SIMONDS

INTRODUCTION

Spontaneous ventilation can be assisted or replaced by delivering intermittent positive pressure to the airway or applying intermittent negative pressure to the chest wall. The physiological and clinical aims of mechanical ventilation are shown in Table 1.1. Ventilatory methods are described as invasive if the airway is intubated, or internal placement of electrodes is required, as in diaphragm pacing. Non-invasive modes avoid airway intubation and are therefore not suitable in individuals with impaired airway reflexes, excessive bronchial secretions, or complete ventilatory dependence. The various methods are listed below. Non-invasive modes form the subject of this book, but these are compared and

Table 1.1 *Aims of mechanical ventilation*

Physiological	Clinical
To improve gas exchange	To correct hypoxaemia
To optimize lung volumes	To correct respiratory acidosis
To reduce the work of breathing	To reverse atelectasis
	To reduce myocardial oxygen consumption
	To stabilize the chest wall
	To reduce intracranial pressure
	To buy time for therapies to work/recovery

contrasted with invasive ventilation, where appropriate, in acute and chronic clinical situations.

1   Non-invasive
(a) Positive pressure via:
  • nasal mask
  • facemask
  • nasal plugs
  • mouthpiece.
(b) Negative pressure via:
  • iron lung/tank ventilator
  • cuirass
  • pneumojacket/pneumosuit
  • combined with high frequency oscillation: Hayek oscillator.
2   Invasive via:
  • tracheostomy
  • diaphragm pacing.
3   Ventilatory adjuncts
  • pneumobelt
  • rocking bed.

The concept of applying ventilatory support non-invasively has always been attractive, and because of their relative simplicity the development of these techniques preceded that of airway intubation and intermittent positive pressure ventilation. The initial stimulus for experimentation with both mask ventilation and negative pressure ventilation was to resuscitate infants and those saved from drowning. Expired air ventilation to resuscitate the newborn has been traced back to records from 1472,[1] and subsequently Fothergill reported successful mouth to mouth ventilation in 1744. Glass nasal masks to facilitate resuscitation were available as early as 1760, but presumably were fragile and very uncomfortable. From a more invasive point of view, Versalius in the 16th century was aware that positive pressure applied to the trachea would inflate the lungs,[2] and in 1667 Hooke demonstrated that it was possible to keep a dog alive by applying a pair of bellows to the upper airway. From the early 19th to mid 20th centuries developments in negative pressure ventilation predominated both for acute and chronic applications.

HISTORICAL DEVELOPMENT OF NEGATIVE PRESSURE VENTILATION (NPV)

Woollam[3] cites the Scotsman John Dalziel as the first to construct a tank ventilator (or 'iron lung') in 1832. Similar ideas flourished elsewhere in Europe and the USA, with Hauke describing a cabinet type ventilator in Austria in 1874. Dr Alfred Jones of Kentucky patented the first American tank ventilator in 1864. These early workers advocated the use of negative pressure respiration in a myriad of conditions including asphyxia, atelectasis, croup, diphtheria, bronchitis, seminal weakness and paralysis! It is interesting to note that Hauke and his coworker,

Waldenburg were also among the first to use continuous positive airway pressure via a facemask to treat pneumonia and atelectasis. Earlier, in 1854 Woillez in France had outlined the principles of artificial ventilation. In 1876 he produced the Spiropore, a tank ventilator with a remarkable resemblance to 20th century models. Bellows were used to evacuate air from a metal cylinder which encased the patient's body. Sporadic developments continued over the next 50 years, but it was not until the 1930s that negative pressure ventilation was put to extensive use.

Drinker and colleagues reported an improved iron lung system in 1929.[4] This had an effective airtight seal and portholes to observe the patient and incorporate a sphygmomanometer and stethoscope. According to Woollam[5] this equipment was first demonstrated in the UK in 1931, prompting brisk correspondence in *The Lancet* of that year.[6] Subsequent versions include the Both wooden cabinet respirator, and a rotating model designed by Kelleher to facilitate physiotherapy and postural drainage (Figure 1.1).

Parallel to the evolution of the iron lung, more portable negative pressure devices were being developed. Hauke used a metal cuirass to enclose the anterior part of the chest in adults and children in the 1870s. Stimulated by the death of his infant son, the brilliant innovator Alexander Graham Bell devised a negative pressure jacket with the aim of supporting ventilation in premature infants in 1881. Experimentally, he used the jacket with apparent success to resuscitate drowned cats, but its potential was not recognized by the scientific community. Early versions of the cuirass were evacuated with a foot-powered bellows pump. Eisenmenger in Hungary devised a motorized fan extraction system in 1927. Further practical modifications, the Sahlin–Stille cuirass and Burstall jacket appeared in the 1930s.[5] These models were made of metal and therefore cumbersome and inflexible. This deficiency was overcome with the introduction of plastic or polyurethane shells and jacket devices comprising a nylon garment secured over a lightweight frame (e.g. Tunnicliffe jacket, Emerson wrap and pneumosuit).

1938 saw a major poliomelitis outbreak in the UK. The pressing need for widely available ventilatory support for patients with respiratory muscle paralysis was recognized by the Medical Research Council. As a result negative pressure tank

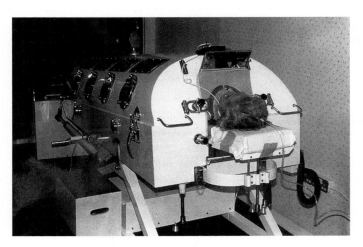

Figure 1.1 *Iron lung constructed c. 1950.*

ventilators were distributed throughout the UK and the Empire, the equipment being financed by Lord Nuffield. Serious polio epidemics continued in Europe and the USA throughout the 1940s and 1950s. In their observations on the use of respirators in poliomyelitis, Plum and Wolff[7] found the tank ventilator to be the safest device for managing ventilatory insufficiency, but cautioned against overventilation. They found that the cuirass used in the acute phase of the illness was too inefficient.

The American Council on Physical Medicine in 1947 examined the efficiency of the negative pressure ventilatory equipment then available and issued an outline of requirements for future cuirass systems. Many of the problems identified by this report and other studies that followed[8] are familiar to recent workers in the field and were re-investigated in the 1980s.

Although the use of negative pressure ventilation undoubtedly saved many lives, mortality from acute poliomyelitis remained high, even after the introduction of tracheostomy for bulbar paralysis in 1943 and the modification of tank ventilators to incorporate tracheostomized cases. Larssen and Ibsen introduced manual intermittent positive pressure ventilation during an overwhelming polio epidemic in Copenhagen in 1952.[1] This development halved previous mortality rates and saw the rapid replacement of negative pressure by positive pressure techniques. These trends ushered in the concept of the Intensive Care Unit, with the aim of providing life support, particularly mechanical ventilation.

With the wane in use of negative pressure ventilation (apart from the use in some convalescent polio patients), indications for its application changed to more chronic respiratory disorders. Bourteline-Young and Whittenberger[9] in 1951 describe the use of the tank ventilator in two patients with end stage emphysema. One patient experienced a rapid correction of arterial blood gas tensions after a short period of negative pressure ventilation and improvement was maintained a year later. Success was attributed to the resetting of respiratory drive following correction of hypercapnia. No benefit was seen in the second patient who, notably, had a history of bronchiectasis and recurrent wheeze. In 1963 the short-term effects of NPV using a body suit (Emerson wrap) were studied in a further group of patients with emphysema and CO_2 retention.[10] Synchronization of the negative pressure pump was achieved by sensing a drop in intranasal or tracheostomy pressure. In stable patients the use of NPV resulted in a fall in $PaCO_2$ and correction of acidosis. Less marked changes were seen in patients with an acute exacerbation of chronic obstructive lung disease. Trials of NPV in chronic obstructive pulmonary disease (COPD) in the 1960s and 1970s produced mixed results.[11,12]

RECENT APPLICATIONS OF NPV

With the recognition of the influence of respiratory muscle weakness and physiological changes during sleep on the pathogenesis of ventilatory failure negative pressure techniques were re-explored in the 1970s and early 1980s.[13–15] Pneumosuits or negative pressure jackets were favoured for home use by many centres, although tailor made cuirasses and more portable iron lungs continued to be employed in patients with chest wall and neuromuscular disease. Use of NPV in the home fell substantially following the introduction of NIPPV and a series of randomized controlled trials showing that domiciliary NPV was ineffective in COPD,[16–18] although a number of exponents continue to use acute and chronic NPV intensively. The outcome of these techniques in restrictive and obstructive ventilatory disorders is described in detail in Chapters 9,11 and 12.

POSITIVE PRESSURE VENTILATION

Invasive techniques

Following Hooke's pioneering work with tracheal insufflation, Kite described oral and nasal intubation for resuscitation purposes in 1788,[19] and Trendelenberg should probably be credited with using the first cuffed tracheostomy in humans in 1871. Further developments in intubation arose with the need to prevent aspiration during surgery to the upper airway, to deliver anaesthetic gases, and as treatment for laryngeal diphtheria. Franz Kuhn invented a metal guide for oral intubation in 1901 and a year later described nasotracheal intubation for inhalational anaesthesia. Patients breathed spontaneously during these procedures. By the end of the 19th century it had been shown that life could be sustained without respiratory movement 'apnoeic ventilation' using gaseous insufflation.

Manually powered bellows were the only means of applying positive pressure to the airways until the development of automatic artificial ventilators. Draeger, a company specializing in mine rescue apparatus was one of the first companies to manufacture a positive pressure ventilator in 1907.[29] The need for intermittent positive pressure ventilation these was prompted by rapid advances in thoracic surgery necessitating a controlled surgical field and prevention of paradoxical respiration and mediastinal shift.[1] In 1940 Crafoord[21] reported the successful use of the spiropulsator developed by Frenckner of Stockholm in 100 thoracic surgery cases. The Danish poliomyelitis epidemic in 1952 saw the further intensive use of intermittent positive pressure ventilation (IPPV) via tracheostomy. Bjork and Engstrom described the use of IPPV for postoperative respiratory failure in 1955.[2]

Non-invasive positive pressure ventilation

Until the late 20th century the only techniques suitable for long-term respiratory support in the home were tracheostomy ventilation or NPV. Despite the fact that nasal masks had been used for acute respiratory failure as early as the 1760s, and rubber facemasks have been used to deliver gaseous anaesthetics for many years, the re-emergence of mask ventilation depended on the development of vinyl and subsequently silicone interfaces which are user friendly and can be manufactured commercially. Continuous positive airway pressure (CPAP) used via a facemask has a role in treating hypoxaemia due to acute conditions such as pulmonary oedema, pneumonia and atelectasis, and may also reduce the work of breathing[22] and sleep disordered breathing[23] in patients with respiratory insufficiency due to COPD.

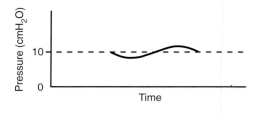

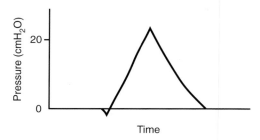

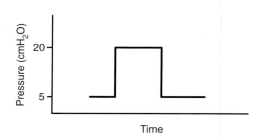

Figure 1.2 *Pressure profiles of continuous positive airway pressure (CPAP) (top), triggered nasal ventilation (middle) and bilevel positive pressure support ventilation (bottom).*

Sullivan and colleagues[24] in 1981 recognized the value of nasal CPAP in the treatment of obstructive sleep apnoea (OSA) (Chapter 16). Mask CPAP therapy for OSA was the springboard to development of nasal intermittent positive pressure ventilation (NIPPV) for patients with chronic ventilatory failure. The technique of CPAP and NIPPV are, of course, different despite the fact that similar facemasks or nasal masks can be employed. During CPAP patients continue to breathe spontaneously at their own rate and depth, whereas during NIPPV minute ventilation is augmented with gas flow being determined predominantly by the ventilator. Bi-level pressure support can also be delivered by mask. Airway pressure profiles for CPAP, NIPPV and bilevel pressure support ventilation are displayed in Figure 1.2.

Since its introduction in the 1980s there has been a very rapid uptake of NIPPV in Europe and the USA for patients requiring home ventilatory support. Figure 1.3 shows the growth in number of patients in France using NIPPV in comparison to other methods of ventilatory support, including tracheostomy-IPPV. NIPPV was first applied to patients with neuromuscular disorders and chest wall disease and use has now extended to some subgroups with chronic obstructive lung disease. It is interesting to reflect that the wheel has turned full circle and NIPPV is now used extensively in acute respiratory failure echoing its pioneering role in individuals requiring resuscitation, centuries ago.

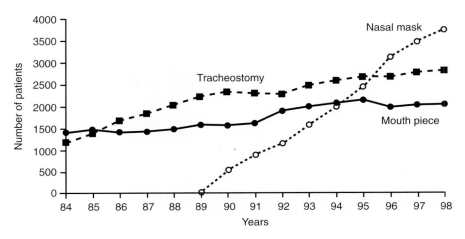

Figure 1.3 *Trends in domiciliary assisted ventilation in France 1984–1998 (Data from ANTADIR with permission).*

Mouth ventilation

Intermittent positive pressure breathing (IPPB) delivered by small pressure cycled machines was used widely as a therapy for COPD several decades ago, but declined in use when benefit over and above standard nebulized bronchodilator use could not be confirmed. Mouth intermittent positive pressure ventilation (MIPPV) is used for some patients with COPD particularly in France,[25] but has a more closely defined role in neuromuscular patients with minimal ventilatory capacity.[26–28]

Ventilatory adjuncts

These devices have a limited application for partial respiratory support and may be combined with other modes. For example, a patient with Duchenne muscular dystrophy may use NIPPV at night, but utilize the pneumobelt for support for short periods while in a wheelchair during the day. The rocking bed is occasionally used in selected patients with diaphragm weakness, but is inappropriate in those with severe ventilatory failure or abnormal lung mechanics. Further details on these ventilatory adjuncts are given in the next chapter.

Pneumobelt (Figure 1.4)

The original version of the pneumobelt, the Bragg–Paul pulsator was devised by the physicist Willian Bragg in 1938. He is said to have created the system from several rubber football bladders which were placed around the abdomen and lower thorax and inflated to aid expiration.[5] Current models can be used with high pressure NIPPV ventilators such as the Nippy (B&D Electromedical). The Pneumobelt is unsuitable in patients with a severe scoliosis, but may prove helpful

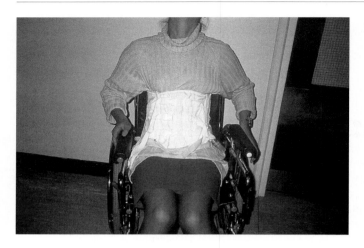

Figure 1.4 *The Pneumobelt.*

in providing partial daytime ventilatory support in wheel chair bound individuals, e.g. with Duchenne muscular dystrophy.

The rocking bed

The novel employment of a rocking bed to facilitate diaphragm excursion was described by Eve[29] in an article titled 'Actuation of the inert diaphragm by gravity method' in 1932. Here gravity assisted movement of the abdominal contents is used to displace the diaphragm. In poliomyelitis outbreaks a fast rocking bed was used at rates of up to 24 oscillations a minute, rotating through an arc of 20 degrees from the horizontal. It was found to be of most value in the recovery phase of the disease. However, in some patients the rocking bed was able to delay the need for more intensive ventilation and aid weaning.[7]

REFERENCES

1   Young JD, Sykes MK. Artificial ventilation: history, equipment, techniques. In: Moxham J, Goldstone J (eds). *Assisted ventilation*, 1st edn. London: BMJ Publishing Group, 1994: 1–17.

2   Atkinson RS, Rushman GB, Lee JA. The history of anaesthesia. In: Atkinson RS, Rushman GB, Lee JA (eds). *A synopsis of anaesthesia*, 8th edn. Bristol: John Wright, 1979: 1–30.

3   Woollam CHM. The development of apparatus for intermittent negative pressure respiration (1) 1832–1918. *Anaesthesia* 1976; **31**: 537–47.

4   Drinker P, McKhann CF. The use of a new apparatus for prolonged administration of artificial respiration. *JAMA* 1929; **92**: 1658–61.

5   Woollam CHM. The development of apparatus for intermittent negative pressure respiration (2) 1919–1976. *Anaesthesia* 1976; **31**: 666–85.

6   Drinker P. Prolonged administration of artificial respiration. *Lancet* 1931; **2**: 1186–8.

7   Plum F, Wolff HG. Observations on acute poliomyelitis with respiratory insufficiency. *JAMA* 1951; **146**: 442–6.

8   Bryce-Smith R, Davis HS. Tidal exchange in respirators. *Curr Res Anaes Analges* 1954; **33**: 73–85.

9   Bourteline-Young HG, Whittenberger JL. The use of artificial respiration in pulmonary emphysema accompanied by high carbon dioxide levels. *J Clin Invest* 1951; **30**: 838–46.

10 Marks A, Bocles J, Morganti L. A new ventilatory assistor for patients with respiratory acidosis. *N Engl J Med* 1963; **268**: 61–8.

11 McClement JH, Christianson LC, Hubayton RT, Simpson DG. The body type respirator in the treatment of chronic obstructive pulmonary disease. *Ann NY Acad Sci* 1965; **121**: 746–50.

12 Fountain FF, Reynolds LB, Tickle SM. Use of extrathoracic assisted breathing in the management of chronic obstructive lung disease. *Am J Phys Med* 1973; **52**: 277–88.

13 Rochester DF, Braun NM, Laine S. Diaphragmatic energy expenditure in chronic respiratory failure. *Am J Med* 1977; **63**: 223–31.

14 Braun NM, Marino WD. Effect of daily intermittent rest of respiratory muscles in patients with severe chronic airflow limitation (CAL). *Chest* 1984; **85**: 59s–60s. (Abstract).

15 Garay SM, Turino GM, Goldring RM. Sustained reversal of chronic hypercapnia in patients with alveolar hypoventilation syndromes. *Am J Med* 1981; **70**: 269–74.

16 Zibrak JD, Hill NS, Federman EC, Kwa SL, O'Donnell C. Evaluation of intermittent long term negative-pressure ventilation in patients with severe COPD. *Am Rev Respir Dis* 1988; **138**: 1515–18.

17 Celli B, Lee H, Criner G, *et al*. Controlled trial of external negative pressure ventilation in patients with severe chronic airflow limitation. *Am Rev Respir Dis* 1989; **140**: 1251–6.

18 Shapiro SH, Ernst P, Gray-Donald K, *et al*. Effect of negative pressure ventilation in severe chronic obstructive pulmonary disease. *Lancet* 1992; **340**: 1425–9.

19 Kite C. *An essay on the recovery of the apparently dead*. London: Dilly, 1788.

20 Rendell-Baker L, Pettis JL. The development of positive pressure ventilators. In: Atkinson RS, Boulton TB (eds). *The history of anaesthesia*, 1st edn. London: The Royal Society of Medicine, 1987: 402–21.

21 Crafoord C. Pulmonary ventilation and anesthesia in major chest surgery. *J Thoracic Surg* 1940; **9**: 237–53.

22 Petrof BJ, Legare M, Goldberg P, Milic-Emili J, Gottfried SW. Continuous positive airway pressure reduces work of breathing and dyspnea during weaning from mechanical ventilation in severe chronic obstructive pulmonary disease. *Am Rev Respir Dis* 1990; **141**: 281–9.

23 Petrof BJ, Kimoff RJ, Levy RD, Cosio MG, Gottfried SB. Nasal continuous positive airway pressure facilitates respiratory muscle function during sleep in severe chronic obstructive pulmonary disease. *Am Rev Respir Dis* 1991; **143**: 928–35.

24 Sullivan CE, Issa FG, Berthon-Jones M, Eves L. Reversal of obstructive sleep apnea by continuous positive pressure applied through the nares. *Lancet* 1981; **1**: 862–5.

25 Muir J-F. Intermittent positive pressure ventilation (IPPV) in patients with chronic obstructive pulmonary disease (COPD). *Eur Respir Rev* 1992; **2**(10): 335–45.

26 Bach JR, Alba AS, Bohatiuk G, Saporito L, Lee M. Mouth intermittent positive pressure

ventilation in the management of postpolio respiratory insufficiency. *Chest* 1987; **91**: 859–64.

27 Bach JR, Alba AS, Saporito LR. Intermittent positive pressure ventilation via the mouth as an alternative to tracheostomy for 257 ventilator users. *Chest* 1993; **103**: 174–82.

28 Sortor S. Pulmonary issues in quadriplegia. *Eur Respir Rev* 1992; **2**(10): 330–4.

29 Eve FG. Actuation of inert diaphragm by gravity method. *Lancet* 1932; **2**: 995–7.

2

Equipment for NIPPV: ventilators, interfaces and accessories

A K SIMONDS

INTRODUCTION

The choice of appropriate ventilatory equipment depends on a number of crucial factors:

- The degree of ventilator dependency
- Underlying pathophysiology and likelihood of progression
- Level of general mobility/dexterity/muscle strength
- Staff familiarity with equipment
- Patient and family choice
- Cost.

THE IDEAL VENTILATOR

Ventilators for home use have developed via two main evolutionary pathways. Original positive pressure home ventilators were derived from volume preset ICU-type ventilators, e.g. the PLV 100 and 102. Models such as the Monnal D utilize a large black rebreathing bag reminiscent of anaesthetic type ventilators, and most incorporate standard alarms thereby retaining the trappings of ICU functionality and appearance. Conversely, most of the pressure preset bilevel ventilators such as the BiPAP S and S/T (Respironics Inc.) were designed to treat adults with the obstructive sleep hypopnoea syndrome in the home, and therefore do not contain alarms and are simpler to set up. So far there have been very few ventilators designed specifically for paediatric home use.

The ideal ventilator for domiciliary use would combine the following characteristics:

- User-friendly
- Portable and quiet
- Operates in assist/assist control and control modes
- Can appply CPAP
- Sensitive trigger
- Battery option
- Low pressure, high pressure and power failure alarms
- Versatile
- Dual voltage 110/240 v
- Reliable and robust
- Low cost/low maintenance
- Provides compliance data for downloading via modem or during clinic visits.

As expected no such model exists, but a number now come close to meeting these optimum requirements.

VOLUME OR PRESSURE VENTILATORS

There is some confusion in terminology with some authors using the terms volume and pressure *targeted* ventilation, others using the term volume and pressure *triggered* ventilation. These terms are often used interchangeably, but strictly speaking some pressure ventilators are triggered in response to changes in flow and some ventilators do not reach preset target levels e.g. due to leak. In the interests of clarity, in this book the terms pressure preset and volume preset will be used to describe the fundamental steps that are required to set up the machine (i.e. determine tidal volume or flow/rate in a volume preset machine, and inspiratory +/– expiratory pressure in a pressure preset model). Pressure preset machines include those which deliver bilevel pressure support. In the last year or two, models which incorporate both volume and pressure preset modes have been brought onto the market.

It is interesting to note that virtually all of the long term outcome studies of NIPPV in patients with neuromuscular and chest wall disease used volume preset machines as these were the most suitable models for home use in the 1980s, whereas more recent trials of NIPPV in acute exacerbations of COPD almost exclusively employed pressure preset ventilators such as BiPAP (Respironics, Inc.) and VPAP. In theory, the performance of volume and pressure preset ventilators will differ in several important ways as listed below (Table 2.1), and these differences may be more significant depending on whether patients are ventilated invasively or non-

Table 2.1   *Differences between volume preset and pressure preset ventilators*

Characteristic	Volume preset ventilator	Pressure preset ventilator
Delivery	Delivers a constant tidal volume in the face of changing airways resistance and lung compliance	Delivered tidal volume will fall with increasing airways resistance or fall in lung compliance
Leak compensation	Poor leak compensation	Good leak compensation
Addition of PEEP/EPAP	Can add PEEP, but many models do not incorporate this	EPAP available on bilevel pressure support machines
Peak airway pressure	Difficult to limit peak airway pressure	Can preset maximum IPAP which can be advantageous in patients with previous pneumothorax, bullous lung disease, hyperinflation or gastic distension
Size	Ventilators tend to be bulky	Usually smaller than volume preset models

invasively. In practice, few comparative studies have been carried out, and the majority of these have used lung models which do not necessarily accurately represent lung and chest wall mechanics *in vivo*.

Comparisons in patients with chronic ventilatory failure

Short-term comparisons of the effects of pressure and volume preset ventilators on arterial blood gas tension have shown little difference between modes. After 2 hours use of non-invasive ventilation using two pressure preset machines (BiPAP, Respironics Inc., and Nippy, B&D Electromedical) and two volume preset models (Monnal D, Deva Medical, and BromptonPAC, PneuPAC Co.) Meecham Jones *et al.*[1] showed an average improvement in PaO_2 of 1.57 kPa with the pressure preset machines and 1.33 kPa with the volume preset devices. $PaCO_2$ fell by an average of 1.07 kPa and 1.16 kPa respectively (P = NS).

A further study[2] has assessed the effects of various home ventilators on ventilatory pattern and the work of breathing in chronic stable restrictive and obstructive patients with respiratory failure. Compared to spontaneous ventilation, inspiratory pressure support, bilevel pressure support and volume preset ventilation all produced a significant improvement in tidal volume (V_T) and minute ventilation, a fall in respiratory rate and reduction in inspiratory effort activity; whereas CPAP did not diminish inspiratory workload (Figure 2.1).

As an overnight comparison is more representative of changes in gases during nocturnal hypoventilation, Restrick and colleagues[3] carried out a three night study of patients with chronic ventilatory failure randomized to spontaneous ventilation, volume preset ventilation or bilevel pressure support. Both modes significantly improved nocturnal oxygen saturation, but there was no difference in mean SaO_2

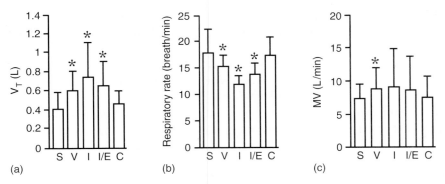

Figure 2.1 *Comparison of the effects of different modes of NIPPV and continuous positive airway pressure on mean (SD) (a) tidal volume (V_T); (b) respiratory rate; and (c) minute ventilation for spontaneous ventilation (S), NIPPV with volume preset ventilator (V), inspiratory pressure support without EPAP (I) and bilevel positive pressure support (I/E) and continuous positive airway pressure (C). *p < 0.05 (compared with S).*

or time spent at SaO_2 values less than 90% in subjects requiring inspiratory pressures of less than 25 cmH_2O. However, patients requiring an inflation pressure of more than 25 cmH_2O were less well served using the standard BiPAP S model which offers a maximum IPAP of 24 cmH_2O. These individuals, who tend to have either low chest wall/lung compliance or severe airflow obstruction, are likely to benefit form either a pressure preset machine that can offer higher inspiratory pressure or a volume preset ventilator.

To establish the most suitable mode for long term domiciliary use Schonhofer *et al.*[4] swapped a group of 30 patients from volume preset to pressure preset ventilation after a month of volume controlled nocturnal therapy. After a month of pressure ventilation 18 patients demonstrated stability in arterial blood gas tensions, while 10 showed an increase in mean (SD) $PaCO_2$ from 5.7 (0.4) to 6.6 (0.5) kPa. Patients in whom CO_2 control deteriorated on pressure preset therapy had a lower mean SaO_2 and higher $PaCO_2$ before starting NIPPV which suggests that in patients at the severe end of the chronic ventilatory failure spectrum, volume preset ventilation may offer advantages if adequate control is not achieved with a pressure preset ventilator. However, in a smaller open study 10 patients who were deteriorating using the Monnal D volume preset ventilator were transferred to the Nippy pressure preset ventilator. Overall, a sustained improvement in PaO_2 and $PaCO_2$ was seen in all but one patient. It is possible that this result was due to adverse trigger characteristics of the Monnal machine.

Comparison in patients with acute on chronic ventilatory failure

These trials are much more difficult to conduct as patients are not steady state, parity in ventilator setting is difficult to achieve, and frequent changes in ventilatory equipment may reduce compliance, confuse patients and lead to suboptimal progress. However, in a short term physiological study of four modes (inspiratory pressure support, bilevel pressure support, CPAP and volume preset ventilation) in patients with an acute exacerbation of COPD (mean Pao_2 5.1 kPa, mean $Paco_2$ 9.3 kPa, mean FEV_1 0.59 L) all modes improved Pao_2 to a similar extent, but there was no siginificant change in $Paco_2$. Studies of a longer duration are required to assess CO_2 control in detail. It is notable that in this acute trial the addition of EPAP to inspiratory pressure support did not offer any advantage over inspiratory pressure support alone, although it is arguable whether the settings were truly comparable.

Use of expiratory positive pressure

There are theoretical advantages to the addition of expiratory positive airway pressure (EPAP). Indeed, in bilevel pressure support models the application of positive pressure during expiration is essential to flush deadspace CO_2 and prevent rebreathing when used with expiratory ports such as the whisper swivel valve. A minimum EPAP level of 4 cmH_2O is recommended with BiPAP (Respironics) models. Benefits associated with EPAP are listed below.

EPAP may:

• Prevent rebreathing of CO_2
• Stabilize the upper airway during sleep
• Recruit alveoli and thereby increase functional residual capacity
• Decrease a tendency to mico- or macroatelectasis
• Reduce the inspiratory work required to trigger inspiration in patients with intrinsic PEEP.

To investigate these potential benefits 15 patients with obstructive and restrictive disorders were studied with polysomnography while receiving IPAP only on one night and IPAP plus EPAP on the other night in random order.[5] Seven patients had neuromusculoskeletal disorders and eight COPD. IPAP was set at near maximum tolerated (mean 19 cmH_2O). End expiratory oesophageal pressure (EEPoes) was measured in 12 subjects and EPAP matched to EEPoes value. In subjects with EEPoes of zero EPAP was set at 5 cmH_2O. Nocturnal mean and minimum Sao_2 and maximum transcutaneous PCO_2 improved with the IPAP/EPAP combination compared to IPAP alone in the neuromusculoskeletal group (Figure 2.2). Contrary to expectation there was no advantage to the addition of EPAP in the COPD patients overall although 3/8 patients did show an improvement in minimum Sao_2, transcutaneous CO_2 or both with the application of EPAP. All patients receiving an EPAP of 5 cmH_2O ($n = 10$) demonstrated benefit, whereas the five subjects receiving higher levels of EPAP (6–12 cmH_2O) showed no significant change. The results indicate that EPAP can be helpful in patients with neuromusculoskeletal disorders and in selected patients with COPD. High levels of EPAP (>6 cmH_2O) appear to offset any beneficial effects on alveolar recruitment and upper airway function by either increasing expiratory muscle load and/or reducing effective IPAP especially in patients with severe airflow obstruction. A further concern is that the application of EPAP could result in haemodynamic compromise. Ambrosino et al.[6] measured

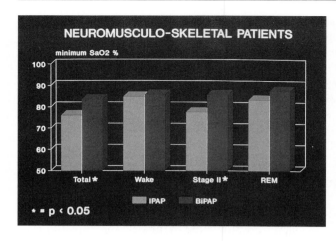

Figure 2.2 *Effect of IPAP and IPAP/EPAP (Bilevel) on minimum Sao_2 during sleep in patients with neuromusculoskeletal disease. Mean minimum Sao_2 is increased by the addition of EPAP for total sleep time and during stage 2 non-REM sleep.*

pulmonary artery pressure (PAP) and cardiac output in stable COPD patients requiring IPAP and IPAP/EPAP over a 10-minute period.

Compared with values breathing spontaneously PAP rose and cardiac output plus oxygen delivery fell with the addition of EPAP. These changes were small and it is difficult to know whether they are clinically significant and/or whether adaptive mechanisms would come into play when IPAP/EPAP is used over a longer period e.g. overnight. A note of caution is indicated as Mehta et al.[7] showed increased morbidity in patients with cardiogenic pulmonary oedema using bilevel pressure support compared to CPAP therapy which may have been related to the hypotensive effffects of EPAP. However, selection of patients may have played a part here (see Chapter 4). Taking this information into account EPAP levels of 4–5 cmH$_2$O are indicated in most patients. Higher levels should be used with caution and haemodynamic effects monitored carefully. EPAP level should be kept at minimum in patients with bullous lung disease and pneumothorax. It should also be remembered that each additional cmH$_2$O of EPAP reduces the level of pressure support by one cmH$_2$O, so IPAP and EPAP levels should be considered together.

LABORATORY LUNG MODEL STUDIES

Comparison of non-invasive ventilators with an ICU ventilator

As non-invasive ventilators originally designed for home use are now being increasingly applied in acute respiratory failure, comparisons with ICU-designed ventilators are important. Bunburaphong et al.[8] have examined the performance of nine commonly used bilevel pressure support ventilators (the BiPAP S/T 30, and S/T 20 (Respironics Inc), VPAP (ResMed), DP90 (Taema), PB335 (Nellcor Puritan Bennett), O'NYX (Pierre Medical), Ventil+ (SEFAM), Quantum PSV (Healthdyne), and Companion 320I/E (Nellcor Puritan Bennett), and compared their ability to respond to inspiratory demand with the Nellcor Puritan Bennett 7200ae adult critical care ventilator. The effects of three levels of pressure support (5, 10 and 15 cmH$_2$O) at two lung compliance values (50 and 80 mL/cm H$_2$O) and four peak inspiratory flow demands (20, 40, 60, 80 L/min) on the key variables: *inspiratory delay time, inspiratory trigger pressure, inspiratory area per cent, expiratory delay time, expiratory area* and *ventilator peak flow* were assessed using a bellows in a box lung model. Nearly all models performed at least as well as the ICU ventilator and were not adversely affected by changes in compliance. This suggests that they are capable of meeting the ventilatory demands of patients with acute respiratory failure. Only the DP90 and VPAP did not out perform the ICU model in all areas. As the authors point out, the study is limited by the fact that no *in vivo* corroboration has been attempted, and the design is based on the assumption that the Nellcor Puritan Bennett ICU ventilator has near optimal performance characteristics. In addition, it must be remembered that non-invasive ventilators do not have the ability to deliver precisely measured FiO_2, have little in the way of alarms, and serious rebreathing may occur in models without true expiratory valves.

The extent of rebreathing and expiratory workload generated by home ventilators compared with ICU ventilators has been measured in another artificial lung model study by Lofaso *et al.*[9] This showed significant rebreathing in bilevel models with a common inspiratory/expiratory tubing, which fell as EPAP levels were increased. The work performed by the ventilator during inspiratory pressure support was similar, but peak flows varied more widely. Helpfully the authors extended the comparison to patients, but all were intubated. No difference in $PaCO_2$, minute ventilation, tidal volume and respiratory rate was seen, but trigger sensitivity and initial flow rate acceleration varied between the home and ICU device. Importantly, the work of breathing (measured by the oesophageal pressure time product) was 30% higher with the home model.

Comparison of volume and pressure preset home ventilators

Changes in tidal volume, peak airway pressure and mean airway pressure in response to variation in leak and patient effort were assessed using the pressure preset Nippy (B&D Electromedical), and BiPAP (Respironics Inc.) ventilators, and volume preset Monnal D (Taema) and Companion 280 Puritan Bennett models.[10] At a similar tidal volume, the peak airway pressure generated by the Monnal D and Nippy was up to 100% greater than the Companion 2801 and BiPAP. When a leak was added to the circuit the tidal volume generated by the Companion 2801 and Monnal D fell by >50% whereas with the Nippy and BiPAP, tidal volume was maintained by an increase in flow. Minute volume adaptation to increasing patient-simulated effort differed between machines, but tended to respond more closely with the Nippy and BiPAP.

Accuracy of tidal volume delivery in volume preset home ventilators

One disadvantage of pressure preset ventilators is that they are less able to compensate for changes in resistance than volume preset models. This may become clinically significant in the acute and chronic respiratory failure patient on an hour by hour or even minute by minute basis as airway resistance may be altered dynamically by nasal blockage, bronchospasm, airway secretions and fall in pharyngeal tone during sleep. It is constructive to categorize volume preset ventilators into those with a:

- Piston chamber (e.g. PLV 100, Respironics; PV 501, Breas Medical)
- Rotary piston (e.g. Companion 2801, Puritan Bennett)
- Compressor blower (O'NYX +, Mallikrodt; Airox Home 1, Bio MS)
- Standard compressor (Monnal D, DCC, Taema; Ecole 3, 3-XL, 2-A, Saime).

Lofaso and colleagues[11] tested a series of these ventilators with each set to deliver a tidal volume of 300, 500 and 800 mL over a range of simulated respiratory resistance (increased to create a peak airway pressure of 40–60 cmH$_2$O). For each ventilator the difference between the desired tidal volume and actual delivered volume was recorded. The results showed major discrepancies between the preset and delivered tidal volumes. Overall, the rotary piston ventilators were most accurate in their delivery, but a fall in tidal volume with increasing pressure was seen in nearly all ventilators. As might be expected discrepancies were most marked with low preset tidal volumes in the presence of high peak airway pressure.

TRIGGERED, ASSIST/CONTROL OR CONTROLLED MODE VENTILATION?

In triggered or assist mode the user is required to make a respiratory effort to generate a breath, whereas in assist/control mode (also known as spontaneous/timed mode) breaths can be triggered, but there is a back-up controlled automatic cycling rate which operates if the patient fails to trigger the machine for a predetermined period of time. Ventilators set in control mode deliver breaths regardless of patient effort. In most patients breathing is most comfortably and safely augmented using assist/control mode. Patients will usually trigger the ventilator during wakefulness, but many with neuromuscular and chest wall disorders are reliant on the ventilator working in control mode during sleep. Some centres advocate controlled ventilation in order to maximally rest the respiratory muscles and reduce the work of breathing. There are disadvantages to this approach in that some patients become desynchronized with the imposed respiratory rate, and there is a distinct possibility of overventilation particularly in neuromuscular patients with low minute ventilation requirements. The resulting fall in Paco$_2$ can provoke dysrhythmias, vasoconstriction and cerebral hypoperfusion. Active glottic closure characterized by stridor may occur as protective mechanism in this situation. In general most authorities favour assist control (spontaneous timed) mode, but assist mode alone may be suitable in patients with well preserved ventilatory drive, e.g. cystic fibrosis and some COPD patients. Control mode may be helpful when there are major problems in reducing the Paco$_2$ level, or the patient suffers from primary alveolar hypoventilation syndrome.

VENTILATOR MODELS

Descriptions of several ventilators are given below. In general they outline principles of action of the major types of ventilator and it should be recognized that a number of different models possess similar performance characteristics. These characteristics should always be checked rather than assumed, however.

Pressure preset ventilators

BIPAP (Respironics Inc., Murrysville, USA)

Models BiPAP S, BiPAP S/T 20, BiPAP ST30. Designed for home, not life support use. Add-in alarm modules available for in hospital applications.

ST30

Dimensions 20 × 23 × 39 cm.
Weight 8 kg.
Modes: Spontaneous (S), Spontaneous/Timed (S/T), Timed (T).
IPAP range 4–30 cmH$_2$O (4–24 cmH$_2$O in other BiPAP models).
EPAP range 4–30 cmH$_2$O.
Operator settings: IPAP, EPAP, breaths per minute, % IPAP time (operates only in Timed mode).
Advantages: Portable, robust, reliable, simple to operate. Equipment and parts widely available throughout the world.
Disadvantages: Relatively expensive. Risk of CO$_2$ rebreathing at low IPAP/EPAP levels.

HARMONY S/T (Respironics Inc.) (Figure 2.3)

The Harmony is a bilevel pressure support device similar to the BiPAP (but smaller) and designed to ultimately replace the BiPAP range. Suitable for home and non-life support hospital use. IPAP and EPAP are set by slider switches with maximum

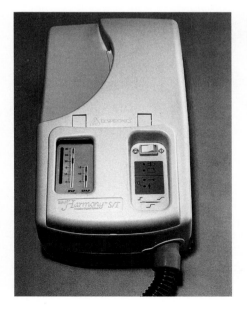

Figure 2.3 *Harmony ventilator (Respironics Inc.).*

IPAP of 30 cmH$_2$O available. A battery pack can be purchased as an optional extra. System and patient alarms are fitted; patient alarms include power failure, disconnection and low battery power.

Dimensions: 31.75 × 18.4 × 14.6 cm.

Weight: 2.9 kg.

Advantages: Small and lightweight (for other advantages and disadvantages see BiPAP).

VPAP II ST (ResMed, Abingdon, UK) (Figure 2.4)

Designed for home and hospital use, but not as life support ventilator.

Modes: CPAP, Spontaneous, Spontaneous/Timed, Timed. Default mode S/T.

Dimensions: 14.2 × 24 × 35 cm.

Weight: 3.5 kg.

Power supply 110/240 V.

IPAP range 2–25 cmH$_2$O.

EPAP range 2–IPAP level.

Set breaths per minute: 5–30.

Operator settings: IPAP, EPAP, IPAP max, breaths per minute, Start pressure, IPAP min, Smartstart option, set rise time, delay time.

Advantages: Lightweight, robust, reliable, simple to operate. Smartstart and compliance download facility. Increasingly available worldwide.

Disadvantage: Maximum IPAP of only 25 cmH$_2$O. No external battery system as yet, but this may be available in future.

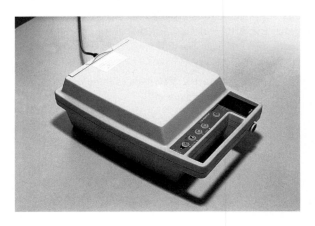

Figure 2.4 *VPAP II ST ventilator (ResMed).*

BREAS PV 401

Pressure preset offering pressure controlled mode (PCV) and pressure support (PSV) option designed for home and non-life support hospital use.

In PCV mode ventilation is controlled by the ventilator. The patient's breathing rate is controlled by the rate setting, but if the trigger function is used the patient can trigger additional breaths. The duration of inspiration is determined by the inspiratory time setting.

In PSV mode the ventilator is controlled by the patient with inspiration determined by trigger function and exhalation by expiratory sensing. If triggering does not occur, set rate takes over.

IPAP 6–40 cmH$_2$O.

EPAP not available on this model. A PEEP adapter can be added to expiratory port.

Alarms: Power failure, low pressure, low delivered volume.

Voltage: 115 or 230 V AC.

External battery port 24 V DC. Optional internal battery.

Operator settings: Pressure, rate, inspiratory trigger, plateau, inspiratory time (only in PCV mode), expiratory trigger (only in PSV mode).

Advantages: Portable, quiet, external and internal battery options.

Disadvantage: No EPAP in this model.

NIPPY VENTILATOR (B&D Electromedical, Warwicks, UK) (Figure 5.6)

Pressure preset system designed for home use. Basic model does not provide expiratory positive pressure, but this is available in Nippy II machine. Neither version provides pressure support.

Voltage 115/230.

Maximum inspiratory pressure 35 cmH$_2$O.

Dimensions:
  Length 370 mm
  Width 230 mm, height 230 mm
  Weight 7.3 kg.

Operator settings: Inspiratory pressure, inspiratory time, expiratory time, trigger sensitivity.

Alarms: Low pressure, high pressure, power failure.

Advantages: Ease of set-up. Convenience for carrying. Users like the fact it doesn't *look* like a ventilator. Quiet operation. Reliable.

Disadvantages: No pressure support option. Limited availability of equipment and parts outside the UK.

Puritan Bennett PB 335

Pressure preset ventilator designed for home use, IPAP/EPAP mode for use primarily in patients with obstructive sleep apnoea.

Modes: CPAP, IPAP/EPAP, Assist/Control mode.

IPAP 3–35 cmH$_2$O.

EPAP 3–20 cmH$_2$O.

Settings IPAP and EPAP sensitivity, ramp, I:E ratio, rate, delay time.

OTHER EXAMPLES OF PRESSURE PRESET VENTILATORS

DP 90 (Taema), Quantum PSV, Silenzio delta, Ventil+.

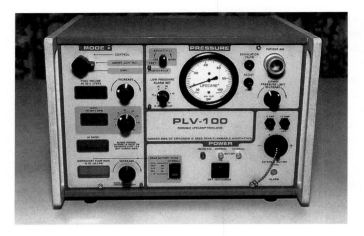

Figure 2.5 *PLV 100 ventilator (Respironics Inc.).*

Volume preset ventilators

LIFECARE PLV 100 (Figure 2.5)

Volume preset ventilator, designed for long-term home use, but usable in hospital/ HDU environment. Can be used in paediatric and adult patients.
Dimensions: 22.9 × 31.1 × 31.1 cm.
Weight: 12.8 kg.
Modes: Control, Assist-Control, SIMV.
Operator settings: Mode, tidal volume, rate, I:E ratio, inspiratory flow rate, sensitivity, low pressure alarm, airway pressure limit.
Tidal volume range 0.05 to 3.0 litres.
Inspiratory flow rate 10 to 120 L/min.
Rate (BPM): 2–40.
220/110 volts. 12 V Internal and external battery.
Alarms: Apnoea, low pressure, high pressure, power.
Advantages: Reliable. Can be used in adults and children. Suitable for ITU/HDU/ward and home use. Good range of alarms. Internal battery, so can be easily used for transportation. Widely available worldwide.
Disadvantages: Expensive. Fairly bulky. No EPAP, but can add PEEP valve.

BROMPTONPAC (PneuPAC Ltd., Luton)

Volume preset assist/control ventilator consisting of control module and separate compressor; built for home use. Can be used powered by oxygen cylinder or wall oxygen supply using Adapter PAC, or TransPAC.
Dimensions:
  Control module 22 × 23 × 10.5 cm. Weight 2.9 kg.
  Compressor 28 × 39 × 39 cm. Weight 17 kg.
Operator settings: Flow, inspiratory time, expiratory time.

Advantages: Very powerful ventilator, can be used in patients with high thoracic impedence requiring high inflation pressures. Sensitive trigger, designed to avoid breath stacking.

Disadvantages: Very bulky and heavy. Not suitable for patients with low minute ventilation requirements. Only available in UK. Requires twice yearly servicing.

OTHER EXAMPLES OF VOLUME PRESET VENTILATORS

Companion 2801, PV 501, Eole 1, 2, Monnal D, DCC, EV 800.

Combination mode ventilators

VISION (Respironics Inc., Murrysville, USA)

Specifically designed for High Dependency Unit use, the Vision provides pressure support ventilation, CPAP, and can incorporate proportional assist ventilation (PAV) mode.

IPAP range 4–40 cmH$_2$O.

EPAP range 4–20 cmH$_2$O.

Rate 4 to 40 bpm.

Timed inspiration 0.5 to 0.40 s.

Alarms: low pressure, high pressure, apnoea, low minute ventilation.

Optional oxygen module: control range 21–100% O$_2$.

PAV mode: Obstructive, restrictive, mixed, normal lung: quick start menu settings.

ACHIEVA (Puritan Bennett)

Portable volume ventilator with pressure support facility, suitable for use in adults and children. ICU and home applications.

Modes: Assist control, SIMV, Spontaneous.

Operator settings: Volume, sensitivity, breath rate, pressure, PEEP.

Dimensions: 27.3 × 33.8 × 39.6 cm.

Weight: 14.5 kg.

Batteries:

External – approximately 20 hours' operation under normal load.

Internal (back-up use only) – approximately 4 hours.

Alarms: Low pressure/apnoea, high pressure, setting error, power switch over, low power, O$_2$ failure.

Advantages: Potentially useful combination of modes for in-hospital use.

Disadvantages: Expensive and limited indications for home use.

BREAS PV 403 (Breas Medical, Farnham, Surrey) (see Figure 5.7)

Portable pressure support and volume control ventilator, suitable for use with tracheostomy and mask ventilation.

Modes: Pressure control ventilation (PCV), pressure support ventilation (PSV), volume control ventilation (VCV), and SIMV.

Dimensions: 35 × 17.5 × 26 cm.

Weight: 5.5 kg.

Settings: pressure 6–50 cmH$_2$O.

Rate 4–40/min, inspiratory time 0.5 to 5 s, Trigger −2 to 8 cmH$_2$O, tidal volume 0.3 to 1.8 L, minute volume 2 to 50 L/min, max peak flow 120 L/min.

Alarms: Low pressure/leak, low tidal volume, power failure.

Battery: Internal and external options.

Accessories: PEEP adapter, remote alarm, calendar compliance software, oxygen adapter.

PULMONETIC LTV1000 (Pulmonetic Systems, Colton, USA)

Volume and pressure controlled ventilator intended for invasive and non-invasive ventilation in adults and children.

Modes:

   Volume: assist/control, SIMV.

   Pressure: PSV – assist control and spont, CPAP.

Dimensions: 8 × 23 × 30 cm.

Weight: 5.75 kg.

Operator settings: Tidal volume 50–2000 mL, breath rate 0–80, inspiratory time 0.3 to 9.9 s, pressure control 1 to 99 cmH$_2$O, pressure support 1 to 60 cmH$_2$O, PEEP/CPAP 0–20 cmH$_2$O.

Alarms: Disconnect, low power, high pressure, low pressure, low minute volume, apnoea, battery.

Batteries:

   External 3–9 hours' use.

   Internal 60 minutes.

Programmable in English, French, German, Spanish, Italian, Swedish, Danish and Japanese.

Advantages: Small size. Useful for HDU/ITU use and transportation.

Disadvantages: Add on PEEP valve. Expensive and too complex for home non-invasive application.

NON-INVASIVE POSITIVE PRESSURE INTERFACES

These take the form of either nasal masks, full facemasks, or nasal plug type devices (Figures 2.6 and 2.7). Use in individual circumstances is outlined in Table 2.2, but it is important where possible, to allow patients choice in the matter. An uncomfortable mask will not only reduce compliance but also the efficiency of the technique. Newer masks on the market include the Profile and Contour deluxe (Respironics Inc.) range, the Mirage mask system and Sullivan Bubble Cushion mask (ResMed). Improved design allows the mask to fit the contour of the face better, thereby reducing leak (Figure 2.6) The Mirage (ResMed) and Profile (Respironics Inc.) series are latex-free. Several series are now designed to be used with either CPAP or NIPPV. The CPAP version of the mask is vented, but the nasal ventilation version is unvented

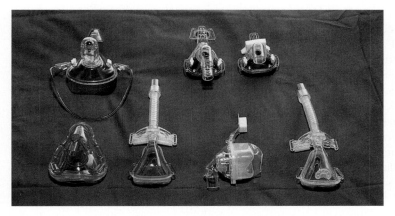

Figure 2.6 *Nasal and full facemasks. From left to right: Top: Full facemask (Respironics), Profile LN and MS mask (Respironics Inc.). Bottom: Mirage full facemask, Mirage nasal mask (CPAP) (ResMed), Sullivan Bubble Cushion mask and Mirage nasal mask (ResMed).*

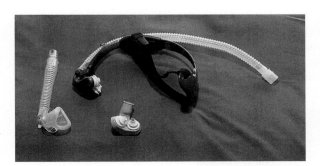

Figure 2.7 *Small nasal interfaces. Left to right: Simplicity nasal mask (Respironics Inc.), Breeze (overhead) circuit (Mallinkrodt), Adams circuit nasal plugs (Puritan Bennett).*

Table 2.2 *Advantages and disadvantages of nasal mask interfaces*

Interface	Advantages	Disadvantages
Nasal mask	Good for long term use in adults	Problems in patients with mouth leaks, or nasal pathology
Full facemask	Can solve problems with mouth leak. Useful in confused patients and children	Can be claustrophobic. Theoretical risk of aspiration after vomiting
Nasal plugs	No pressure over nasal bridge. Helpful for claustrophobic individuals. Can be used easily by patients wearing spectacles	Can be unstable and slip off face. Not available in small enough sizes for young children
Customized	Improved fit. Some patients may be impossible to fit with a standard 'off the peg' mask. Reduced deadspace	Need time to construct. Some variants may not last as long as commercial masks, therefore may cost more

and designed to be used in a circuit containing an exhalation port. It is important not to muddle the two. To differentiate the mask types in the Mirage series, the vented CPAP masks are clear and colourless, and the nasal ventilation masks blue. Similarly there are a variety of vented and unvented full facemasks for use with CPAP and NIPPV. Some have a quick release mechanism to remove the mask rapidly if vomiting or aspiration occurs, although in practice this is rarely required. The Mirage full facemask (Resmed) has an anti-asphyxia valve which automatically opens to reduce rebreathing if pressure from the flow generator falls, e.g. in a power cut or following disconnection of circuit. Smaller interfaces which may be helpful in claustrophobic patients include the Adams Circuit nasal plugs (Puritan Bennett), Breeze circuit (Mallinkrodt) and Simplicity mask (Respironics Inc.) (Figure 2.7). Appropriate selection of mask may affect outcome. In a short-term study Navalesi *et al.*[12] showed that nasal masks were better tolerated than nasal plugs or the full facemask, but minute ventilation was greater with the facemask. However, the importance of patient preference may often override these considerations.

While some long-term NIPPV patients may require customized masks due to atypical facial configuration, jaw contractures etc., it is possible to fit most acute patients with standard commercial masks. Semi-customized masks are now becoming available. These include models which are mouldable after heating, and the Topmask system (Weinmann). In the latter the mask is held to the patient's face and quick drying cement injected into the mask rim which then configures the mask to the patient's face. Customized masks may produce more effective ventilation as a result of reduced deadspace and less air leak,[13] and may also prove helpful in individuals who experience recurrent nasal bridge sores with standard commercial masks (Figure 2.8).

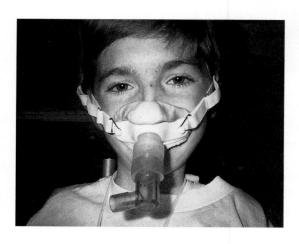

Figure 2.8 *Customizing a mask: creation of initial mould.*

HEATED HUMIDIFIERS (Figure 2.9)

HC100 Fisher Paykel: Can be used with CPAP and mask ventilation. Heater control scale of 1–9 corresponds to heater plate temperature of approximately 47–65°C. An initial setting of 5 is recommended.
Dimensions: 6.5 × 13.5 × 15 cm.
Weight 0.8 kg.

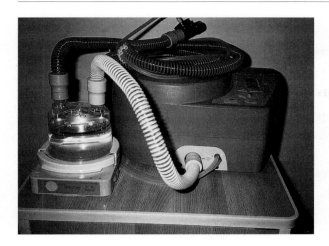

Figure 2.9 *PV 401 ventilator (Breas Medical) with humidifier.*

Examples of negative pressure systems

EMERSON NEGATIVE PRESSURE PUMP 33-CR

For use with custom cuirasses, pneumosuits or portable iron lung systems.
Maximum negative pressure -90 cmH$_2$O.
Respiratory rate: 0–49/min.
Inspiratory time: 0–5 s.
Can set a background constant negative pressure (CNEP) upon which negative
    pressure inspiratory swings can be imposed, i.e. CNEP is equivalent to CPAP in
    a positive pressure system.
Weight: 11 kg.
Dimensions: 40 $\times$ 27.5 $\times$ 30 cm.
An assist mode is also available which allows the patient to trigger breaths through
    a nasal cannula or breaths can be triggered remotely by a manual squeeze bulb.

HAYEK OSCILLATOR (Breasy Medical Equipment Ltd., London, UK) (Figure 2.10)

Non-invasive negative pressure ventilator combining negative pressure via cuirass
    with high frequency oscillation and positive pressure expiration. Neonatal,
    paediatric and adult applications in ICU/HDU/ward.
Operator settings: rate (ventilation) 8 to 60 cycles/min, secretion clearance 8 to 999
    cycles/min, inspiratory pressure 0 to -49 cmH$_2$O, expiratory pressure 0 to
    49 cmH$_2$O.
I : E ratio 6 : 1 to 1 : 6. Triggering : time.
Alarms: High/low expiratory pressure, high/low inspiratory pressure, major part
    failure, high temperature.

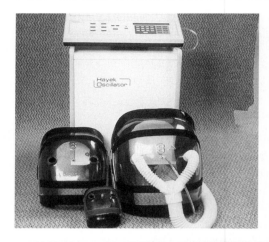

Figure 2.10 *Hayek oscillator.*

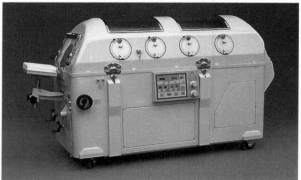

Figure 2.11 *Contemporary iron lung (Coppo Biella).*

TANK VENTILATOR (POLMONE D'ACCIAIO) MODEL C 900 COPPA BIELLA (Figure 2.11)

Modern iron lung.

Negative pressure range up to 80 cmH$_2$O.

Positive pressure up to 80 cmH$_2$O.

Duration inspiration 0.4 to 6 s.

Duration expiration 0.4 to 6 s.

Inspiratory pause 0.2 to 1.9 s. Expiratory pause 0.3 to 1.9 s.

Temperature control. Porthole capability for introducing catheters and monitoring lines.

Microprocessor controls, liquid crystal display panel.

REFERENCES

1   Meecham Jones DJ, Wedzicha JA. Comparison of pressure and volume preset nasal ventilator systems in stable chronic respiratory failure. *Eur Respir J* 1993; **6**: 1060–4.

2   Elliott MW, Aquilina R, Green M, Moxham J, Simonds AK. A comparison of different modes of non-invasive ventilatory support: effects on ventilation and inspiratory muscle effort. *Anaesthesia* 1994; **49**: 279–83.

3   Restrick LJ, Fox NC, Ward EM, Paul EA, Wedzicha JA. Comparison of pressure support ventilation with nasal intermittent positive pressure ventilation in patients with nocturnal hypoventilation. *Eur Respir J* 1993; **6**: 364–70.

4   Schonhofer B, Sonneborn M, Haidl P, Bohrer B, Kohler D. Comparison of two different modes for noninvasive mechanical ventilation in chronic respiratory failure: volume versus pressure controlled device. *Eur Respir J* 1997; **10**: 184–91.

5   Elliott MW, Simonds AK. Nocturnal assisted ventilation using bilevel positive airway pressure: the effect of expiratory positive airway pressure. *Eur Respir J* 1995; **8**: 436–40.

6   Ambrosino N, Nava S, Torbicki A, *et al*. Haemodynamic effects of pressure support and PEEP ventilation by nasal route in patients with stable chronic obstructive pulmonary disease. *Thorax* 1993; **48**: 523–8.

7   Mehta S, Jay GD, Woolard RH, *et al*. Randomized prospective trial of bilevel versus continuous positive airway pressure in acute pulmonary edema. *Crit Care Med* 1997; **25**: 620–8.

8   Bunburaphong T, Imanaka H, Nishimura M, *et al*. Performance characteristics of bilevel pressure ventilators: a lung model study. *Chest* 1997; **111**: 1050–60.

9   Lofaso F, Brochard L, Hang T, Lorino H, Harf A, Isabey D. Home versus intensive care pressure support devices. Experimental and clinical comparison. *Am J Respir Crit Care Med* 1996; **153**: 1591–9.

10   Smith IE, Shneerson JM. A laboratory comparison of four positive pressure ventilators used in the home. *Eur Respir J* 1996; **9**: 2410–15.

11   Lofaso F, Fodil R, Lorino H, *et al*. Inaccuracy of tidal volume delivered by home mechanical ventilators. *Eur Respir J* 2000; **15**: 338–41.

12   Navalesi P, Fanfilla F, Frigerio P, Gregoretti C, Nava S. Physiologic evaluation of noninvasive mechanical ventilation delivered with three types of masks in patients with chronic hypercapnic respiratory failure. *Crit Care Med* 2000; **28**: 1785–90.

13   Tsuboi T, Ohi M, Otsuka N, *et al*. The efficacy of a custom-fabricated nasal mask on gas exchange during nasal intermittent positive pressure ventilation. *Eur Respir J* 1999; **13**: 152–6.

3

Non-invasive ventilation in acute exacerbations of chronic obstructive pulmonary disease

MW ELLIOTT

KEYPOINTS

- Non-invasive ventilation reduces the need for intubation in selected patients with an acute exacerbation of COPD.
- Complications, particularly pneumonia, are reduced.
- Staff expertise is more important than location.
- Non-invasive ventilation should be seen as a means of preventing endotracheal intubation rather than as an alternative.

INTRODUCTION (Table 3.1)

An exacerbation of chronic obstructive airway disease (COPD) of sufficient severity to necessitate hospital admission indicates a poor prognosis, carrying a 6 to 26%

Table 3.1   *Background against which NIPPV used in acute exacerbations of COPD*

- acute exacerbations cause significant mortality
- risk of complications, particularly VAP, following intubation
- intubated patients, with COPD, may subsequently prove difficult to wean

mortality.[1–3] An 11% hospital mortality has been reported, increasing over the next 2 months, 6 months and 2 years of follow-up to 20%, 33% and 49% respectively.[2] Another study found 5-year survival rates of 45% after hospital discharge and this decreased to 28% with any further episode of hospitalization.[4] The outcome of invasive mechanical ventilation (IMV) in patients with COPD is disappointing, with reported survivals of between 20% and 50%.[5] In two large European multi-centre studies[6,7] 20% of patients who had been intubated and mechanically ventilated subsequently proved difficult to wean, with a diagnosis of COPD being the best predictor of weaning difficulty.[7] Endotracheal intubation (ETI) is associated with a range of complications of which the most important is ventilator associated pneumonia (VAP). For every day intubated there is a 1% risk of developing VAP, which results in a high morbidity and mortality.[8,9]

There is currently great interest in the use of non-invasive positive pressure ventilation (NIPPV) in the management of acute exacerbations of COPD. It has a number of potential advantages compared with IMV. Physiologically NIPPV is little different from IMV; positive pressure is delivered to the lungs, but because of difficulties in getting a perfect seal with the mask it is theoretically less efficient than invasive ventilation. However this may also be to its advantage. Barotrauma, such as pneumothorax, is not uncommon with ventilation after intubation but it has not been reported in any of the major studies of NIPPV, perhaps because the lack of a complete seal between the mask and the face acts as a safety valve, preventing high pressures being transmitted to the lungs. NIPPV decreases inspiratory muscle effort and respiratory rate and increases tidal volumes and oxygen saturation in patients with COPD both when stable[10] and during an acute exacerbation.[11] Arterial PaO_2 increases and $PaCO_2$ decreases with NIPPV.[12,13] In a study by Celikel *et al.*[14] NIPPV significantly improved PaO_2, $PaCO_2$, pH and respiratory rate while medical treatment achieved only an improvement in respiratory rate. For the same FiO_2 the $A–aO_2$ increases due to a rise in clearance of CO_2 and hence increased respiratory exchange ratio.[13] There is a fall in cardiac output leading to a slight decrease in systemic oxygen delivery, but this is not accompanied by a change in oxygen delivery. There appears to be no improvement in VA/Q ratio with NIPPV.[13]

The obvious attraction of NIPPV is the avoidance of intubation and its attendant complications. Its use opens up new opportunities in the management of patients with ventilatory failure, particularly with regard to location and the timing of intervention. With NIPPV, paralysis and sedation are not needed and ventilation outside the Intensive Care Unit (ICU) is an option. Given the considerable pressure on ICU beds in some countries, the high costs and the fact that for some patients admission to ICU is a distressing experience,[15] this is an attractive option. Patients with severe COPD are often functioning close to the point at which the respiratory muscle pump can no longer maintain effective ventilation. With NIPPV ventilatory support can be introduced at an earlier stage in the evolution of ventilatory failure than would be usual when a patient is intubated, and it is possible with NIPPV to give very short periods of ventilatory support, which in some cases may be sufficient to reverse the downward spiral into life-threatening ventilatory failure. Patients can co-operate with physiotherapy and eat normally.[16] Intermittent ventilatory support is possible, patients can start mobilizing at an early stage and can communicate with medical and nursing staff and with their family; this is likely to reduce feelings of power-lessness and anxiety associated with ventilatory support.[17] However NIPPV does have its limitations. Concerns have been voiced that it may delay ETI and mechan-ical ventilation, resulting in a worse outcome.[18–20] NIPPV is time consuming for medical and nursing staff.[21] The nasal or facemask is uncomfortable and some patients find it very claustrophobic and unpleasant. Facial pressure sores occur in 2% of patients[22] and with NIPPV the upper airway is not protected and the lower airway cannot be accessed. This therefore limits the technique's applicability in those who are unconscious or have significant secretion retention (see Table 3.2).

Table 3.2 *Advantages and disadvantages of NIPPV*

Advantages	Disadvantages
• Intermittent ventilation possible	• ?Less effective
• 'Early' ventilatory support an option	• Mask uncomfortable/claustrophobic
• Ventilation outside the ICU possible	• Time consuming for medical and
• Patients can co-operate with	nursing staff
physiotherapy	• Facial pressure sores
• Patients can eat and drink normally	• Airway not protected
• Communication with family and staff	• No direct access to bronchial tree for
possible	suctioning if secretions excessive

EVIDENCE FOR USE OF NIPPV IN ACUTE EXACERBATIONS OF COPD

There have been eight prospective randomized controlled trials (RCT) of NIPPV mostly in acute exacerbations of COPD published, both within and outside of the ICU. Brochard *et al.*[22] showed that NIPPV for patients with exacerbations of COPD in the ICU reduced the intubation (11/43 v 31/42, $p < 0.001$) and mortality rates (4/43 v 12/42, $p = 0.02$) compared with conventional medical therapy. NIPPV also improved pH, PaO_2, respiratory rate and encephalopathy score at 1 hour and was associated with a shorter hospital stay (23 days v 35 days, $p = 0.005$) and a lower complication rate (16% v 48%, $p = 0.001$). Most of the excess mortality and compli-cations, particularly pneumonia, were attributed to ETI. These data suggest that NIPPV may be superior to IMV, but importantly this was a highly selected group of patients with the majority (70%) of potentially eligible patients excluded from the study. In a smaller study ($n = 31$) in two North American ICUs Kramer *et al.*[23] showed a marked reduction in intubation rate, particularly in the subgroup with COPD ($n = 23$) (all patients 31% v 73%, $p < 0.05$; COPD 67% v 9% $p < 0.05$). However mortality, hospital stay and charges were unaffected. Those enrolled had a severe exacerbation, as evidenced by a mean pH of 7.28. In a further ICU study

Celikel[14] showed a more rapid improvement in various physiological parameters and a trend towards a reduction in the need for ventilatory support, but there was no difference in intubation rate or survival.

Martin et al.[24] have recently reported a prospective RCT comparing NIPPV with usual medical care in 61 patients including 23 with COPD. The mean pH at entry was 7.27 and respiratory rate 28 breaths per minute. In common with other studies there was a significant reduction in intubation rate (6.4 v 21.3 intubations per 100 ICU days, $p = 0.002$) but no difference in mortality (2.4 v 4.3 deaths per 100 ICU days, $p = 0.21$). Although the intubation rate was lower in the COPD subgroup (5.3 v 15.6 intubations per 100 ICU days, $p = 0.12$) this did not reach statistical significance; this may simply reflect the small sample size. The median time from admission to randomization was 2 days; 52% of the control group were intubated by day 2 after study entry as compared with only 16% of the NIPPV group. Three patients in the NIPPV group and one in the control group required ETI to maximize the safety of other procedures (e.g. bronchoscopy) and two patients in the NIPPV group required ETI because of haemodynamic compromise related to massive gastrointestinal bleeding. All other patients required ETI because of progressive ventilatory failure; in other words only four of the intubations in the NIPPV group were because of a failure to control respiratory failure compared with 16 in the control group. The median duration of NIPPV was 2 days and mean IPAP 11.4 + 3.8 cmH$_2$O and EPAP 5.7 + 1.6 cmH$_2$O. Eighteen of 32 patients in the NIPPV group used nasal masks, 12 an oronasal interface, one nasal pillows and one a full facemask.

It is important to note that there is no direct comparison between IMV and NIPPV and the two techniques should be viewed as complementary, with NIPPV considered a means of obviating the need for ETI rather than as a direct alternative. These studies performed on ICUs show that NIPPV is possible and that the prevention of ETI is advantageous. However the generalizability of these results from the wards into everyday clinical practice is uncertain; results achieved in enthusiastic units as part of a clinical trial may not be achievable in other units lacking the same skill levels or commitment to making NIPPV work.

There have been four prospective RCTs of NIPPV outside the ICU, which have shown less clear-cut results. Bott et al.[25] randomized 60 patients to either conventional treatment or NIPPV. NIPPV was initiated by research staff who spent 15 minutes to 4 hours initiating it (average 90 min) and led to a more rapid correction of pH and Pa$_{CO_2}$. Nine out of 30 of the conventional treatment group died compared with 3/30 of the NIPPV group. On an intention to treat analysis these figures were not statistically significant, but when those unable to tolerate NIPPV were excluded a significant survival benefit was seen (9/30 v 1/26, $p = 0.014$). Generalizabilty from this study, although performed on general wards, to routine practice is again difficult given that staff additional to the normal ward complement set up NIPPV. The high mortality rate (30%) in the control group was surprising considering that the mean pH was only 7.34. In addition the low intubation rate, while reflecting UK practice, has been criticized.

Barbe et al.[26] initiated NIPPV in the emergency department and continued it on a general medical ward. To ease some of the problems of workload and compliance NIPPV was administered for 3 hours twice a day. In this small study ($n = 24$) there were no intubations or deaths in either group and arterial blood gas tensions improved equally in both the NIPPV group and in the controls. However the mean pH at entry in each group was 7.33 and at this level of acidosis significant mortality is not expected; in other words it was unlikely that such a small study would show an improved outcome when recovery would be expected anyway.[3]

Wood et al.[20] randomized 27 patients with acute respiratory distress to conventional treatment or NIPPV in the emergency department. Intubation rates were similar (7/16 v 5/11) but there was a non-significant trend towards increased mortality in those given NIPPV (4/16 v 0/11, $p = 0.123$), attributed to a delay in intubation as conventional patients requiring invasive ventilation were intubated after a mean of 4.8 hours compared with 26 hours in those on NIPPV ($p = 0.055$). It is difficult to draw many conclusions from this study since the two groups were not well matched, with more patients with pneumonia, which is associated with a reduced likelihood of success for NIPPV,[18] in the NIPPV group and the level of ventilatory support was very modest (inspiratory positive airway pressure 8 cm H_2O).

We have recently reported a multicentre RCT of NIPPV in acute exacerbations of COPD ($n = 236$) on general respiratory wards in 13 centres.[27] NIPPV was applied by the usual ward staff according to a simple protocol. 'Treatment failure', a surrogate for the need for intubation, defined by a priori criteria was reduced from 27% to 15% by NIPPV ($p < 0.05$). In-hospital mortality was also reduced from 20% to 10% ($p < 0.05$). Subgroup analysis suggested that the outcome in patients with pH < 7.30 after initial treatment was inferior to that in the studies performed in the ICU; these patients are probably best managed in a higher dependency setting with individually tailored ventilation. Staff training and support are crucial wherever NIPPV is performed and operator expertise more than any other factor is likely to determine the success or otherwise of NIPPV.

LONGER TERM EFFECTS OF NIPPV IN ACUTE EXACERBATIONS OF COPD

In another study 24 patients treated with NIPPV showed more rapid improvement in blood gases and a better pH and respiratory rate at discharge as compared with matched historical controls.[28] Only two patients receiving NIPPV required intubation compared with nine controls. Hospital stays were also shorter in the survivors in the NIPPV group but the in-hospital survival rates were no different. However, long-term survival at 12 months was significantly better in the patients receiving NIPPV (71% v 50%). Vitacca et al.[29] also found no difference in hospital mortality in patients receiving NIPPV compared with historical controls who were intubated and ventilated (20% v 26%), however a survival advantage to NIPPV became apparent at three (77% v 52%) and 12 (70% v 37%) months. Bardi et al.[30] in a prospective controlled study, though with the allocation to the control group or ventilatory support determined by availability of personnel and equipment rather than randomly, of 30 patients found no significant difference in within hospital events, though there was a trend towards an advantage with NIPPV. Patients allocated to NIPPV had a further four (50% received NIPPV) and to the control group six (16% received NIPPV) subsequent exacerbations and there was a statistically significant difference in long-term survival, with a marked advantage to the NIPPV group. The reasons for this were not clear, but it was postulated that this may have included greater improvements in pH, tidal volume and FEV_1, compared with admission, in the NIPPV group. However the FEV_1 at discharge in the NIPPV group was 50% predicted compared with 40% predicted in the control group, suggesting more severe obstructive airways disease in the controls. The fact that fewer patients in the control group received NIPPV for subsequent exacerbations may also have been relevant.

The possible longer term survival advantage when NIPPV is given during an acute exacerbation is intriguing. It has been suggested that it is due to imperfect matching of the control and patient groups.[31] However there are other possible explanations. If ICU care has been prolonged, and weaning difficult, there may be reluctance, on the part of either medical staff or the patients themselves, to consider IMV for a subsequent exacerbation. Secondly it is possible that IMV has adverse effects which may be significant later; electrophysiological and biopsy evidence of muscle dysfunction has been shown after as little as one week of invasive ventilation.[32,33] Such dysfunction of the respiratory muscles will reduce the capacity of the respiratory muscle pump, which may increase the risk of ventilatory failure in subsequent exacerbation. These observations however are speculative and need to be substantiated in further prospective randomized studies with larger numbers of patients.

THE ROLE OF NIPPV AFTER IMV

Some patients require intubation from the outset and others after a failed trial of NIPPV. Patients with COPD may be difficult to wean from IMV[34] and NIPPV has been used successfully in weaning.[35,36] Nava et al.[37] performed a prospective multi-centre randomized controlled trial of the use of NIPPV as a means of weaning patients with COPD, who had failed a T-piece weaning trial after 48 hours of ETI, controlled mechanical ventilation and aggressive suctioning to clear secretions. A total of 56% of the patients had required ETI on presentation and 44% after a failed trial of NIPPV (mean pH at presentation = 7.18). If patients failed the weaning trial they were randomized to further intubation and mechanical ventilation or NIPPV. NIPPV was associated with a shorter duration of ventilatory support (10.2 days v 16.6 days), a shorter ITU stay (15.1 days v 24 days), less nosocomial pneumonia (0/25 v 7/25) and an improved 60-day survival (92% v 72%). Girault et al.[38] in a further RCT involving 33 patients showed a reduction in the duration of IMV (4.6 ± 1.9 v 7.7 ± 3.8 days) and a reduced mean daily ventilatory support, but an increased total duration (11.5 ± 5.2 v 3.5 ± 1.4 days) of ventilatory support when the non-invasive approach was used. There was no difference in percentage of patients successfully weaned or in complication rates. In patients not suitable for NIPPV from the outset or those who fail, ETI for 24 to 48 hours to gain control and then early extubation on to NIPPV has significant advantages over prolonged endotracheal intubation.

A proportion of patients weaned from invasive ventilation subsequently deteriorate and require further ventilatory support. Hilbert et al.[39] reported 30 patients with COPD who developed hypercapnic respiratory distress within 72 hours of extubation. They were treated with mask bilevel pressure support ventilation. Only six of these 30 patients as compared with 20 of 30 historical controls required reintubation. Although in-hospital mortality was not significantly different, the mean duration of ventilatory assistance and length of intensive care stay related to the event were significantly shortened by non-invasive ventilation.

STAFFING AND COSTS

In an early report of the use of NIPPV in six patients Chevrolet et al.[21] found that, particularly in patients with obstructive lung disease, the technique was very time consuming for the nurses and this was largely wasted since all patients eventually had to be intubated. As with any new technique there is a learning curve and the same group have subsequently published more encouraging results.[40] In the ICU, in which there are high nurse to patient ratios, any additional work associated with NIPPV is unlikely to have a major effect, but the issue of medical and nursing time is very relevant if the technique is to be performed in the ward environment. Nurses and therapists will have responsibility for a much larger number of patients and any extra work associated with NIPPV may mean that other tasks and patients are neglected.

In their RCT comparing standard treatment with or without NIPPV in a general ward setting Bott et al.[25] found no difference in nursing care requirements, recorded on a daily basis by asking the senior nurse to record the amount of care needed using a simple visual analogue scale. This may have underestimated the care requirements associated with NIPPV because ventilation was initiated and maintained by staff supernumerary to the normal ward complement. In another study, with more detailed analysis of nursing and therapist activity, Kramer et al.[23] found that the Respiratory Therapist spent more time with patients in the NIPPV group, compared with the standard treatment group in the first 8 hours, but this difference did not reach statistical significance. The time required in the NIPPV group dropped significantly in the second 8-hour period. The time demands on the nurses did not differ in the two groups throughout the measurement period and neither the respiratory therapist nor the nurses considered caring for patients on NIPPV as being any more difficult than the control patients. Nava et al.[41] found that in the first 48 hours of assisted ventilation NIPPV was no more time consuming or demanding for staff than invasive mechanical ventilation. However, after the first few days of ventilation NIPPV was significantly less time consuming for both medical and nursing personnel.

Since most studies report a shorter period of ventilation and ICU and hospital stay it is has been suggested that NIPPV should be cheaper than invasive mechanical ventilation.[42,43] However patients treated with NIPPV do incur substantial financial cost during their hospitalization.[44] Nava et al.[41] found that the total cost per day was comparable for invasive and non-invasive ventilation, when NIPPV was performed on a respiratory ICU. In the study of Kramer et al.[23] the total hospital charges were 37.6 ± 7.9 (in thousands of dollars) in patients receiving NIPPV v 33.9 ± 6.9 in control patients not receiving NIPPV, which was not statistically different.[23] In a recent multicentre study from the UK the incremental cost of

NIPPV per patient avoiding the 'need for intubation' was £2829 (4639 Euros). However, the incremental savings per death avoided was £4114 (6747 Euros), by way of decreased ICU usage thus providing a strong economic argument for use of NIPPV outside the ICU.[45]

WHAT TYPE OF VENTILATOR SHOULD BE USED?

Ventilators usually used for NIPPV are either volume or pressure targeted. There are theoretical advantages to each mode, but broadly speaking they are comparable in efficacy. Volume targeted ventilators have been shown to produce more complete offloading of the respiratory muscles, but at the expense of comfort.[46] In intubated patients, however, assist pressure controlled ventilation has been shown to be more effective than assist control volume ventilation at reducing various parameters of respiratory muscle effort, though this difference was only seen at moderate tidal volumes and low flow rates.[47] In stable patients little difference in gas exchange was seen with different types of ventilator.[10,48] In terms of outcome Vitacca et al.[49] found that there was no difference whether volume targeted or pressure targeted machines were used, but pressure targeted machines were better tolerated by patients. A new mode of proportional assist ventilation (PAV) improves gas exchange and dyspnoea in stable COPD[50] and has been used successfully in the treatment of acute respiratory failure of various aetiologies.[51] PAV delivers ventilation according to patient demand, which should theoretically be more comfortable, but makes the assumption that the patient with respiratory failure knows best what he needs in terms of ventilatory support. PAV using flow assistance and PEEP achieved greatest improvement in minute ventilation, dyspnoea and reduction in pressure time product per breath of the respiratory muscles and diaphragm in patients of COPD with acute respiratory failure.[52] It has been shown to decrease patient effort and work of breathing and neuromuscular drive (P0.1) in patients with COPD being weaned off invasive mechanical ventilation.[53,54] Further data are needed comparing PAV with conventional modes of ventilation. Pressure cycled machines are usually cheaper than volume cycled flow generators and this together the fact that they tend to be better tolerated makes them the machines of first choice.

PEEP can be added during NIPPV and has beneficial effects, offloading the respiratory muscles, probably by counterbalancing the inspiratory threshold load imposed by intrinsic PEEP[55] and lavaging carbon dioxide from the mask.[56] In a short-term study in stable patients the addition of PEEP has been shown to reduce oxygen delivery despite an adequate SaO_2.[57] Mask continuous positive airway pressure (CPAP) has also been shown to significantly decrease respiratory rate and the subjective sensation of dyspnoea, decrease $PaCO_2$, increase PaO_2,[58] significantly improve ventilation[59] and avoid intubation and mechanical ventilation[60] in exacerbations of COPD. In stable patients the degree of unloading with CPAP is less than with NIPPV[10] and given the lack of randomized controlled trial data on the use of CPAP in acute exacerbation of COPD, in contrast to NIPPV (see above), its use should be confined to centres in which NIPPV is not available.

The use of other modes of non-invasive ventilation have been reported in patients with COPD exacerbation. In a retrospective uncontrolled study, 105 patients were successfully weaned and 93 were eventually discharged from hospital after intermittent negative pressure ventilation by means of an iron lung.[61] Of these 105 patients 62 were in coma and 43 had a deteriorating level of consciousness at presentation. All patients were initially ventilated continuously for 12–48 hours and subsequently received intermittent daytime ventilation till weaned. Any subsequent exacerbation was also treated with negative pressure ventilation. Survival was 92 and 37% at 1 and 5 years respectively. A more recent study by the same group was carried out in 150 patients with hypoxic hypercapnic coma (including 79% patients with COPD).[62] Of the 74 patients with only exacerbation of COPD as the cause of coma, treatment failed only in 19 (26%) patients including 14 (19%) who died. However negative pressure ventilation is only available in a few centres, which have particular expertise in the technique, and in the absence of a formal controlled trial NIPPV remains the non invasive mode of choice.

WHEN SHOULD NIPPV BE STARTED?

One of the theoretical advantages of NIPPV is that it can be started at an earlier stage in the evolution of ventilatory failure before invasive ventilation would normally be considered appropriate. It has been suggested that NIPPV should be started when the pH is < 7.35 and the respiratory rate > 30.[63,64] The data from the Yorkshire non-invasive ventilation (YONIV) trial[27] support these criteria suggesting it be instituted at an even lower respiratory rate (> 23 breaths per minute), but after a period during which the effect of drug treatment, adjustment of oxygen therapy etc. can be evaluated. Reversing ventilatory failure is likely to be easier at an early stage when theoretically lower pressures used for shorter periods may improve tolerance.[63,64] NIPPV is less likely to be effective in patients with more severe physiological disturbances at the outset, suggesting that once decompensation has been well established, the cycle of deterioration may not be broken with the use of NIPPV.[18,22] However not all patients presenting to hospital acidotic from an exacerbation of COPD require NIPPV. In a one-year period prevalence study[65] of patients with acute exacerbations of COPD of 954 patients admitted through the A&E departments in Leeds, 25% were acidotic on arrival in the Department and of these 25% had completely corrected their pH by the time of arrival on the ward. This included patients with a pH < 7.25. There was a weak relationship between the PaO_2 on arrival at hospital and the presence of acidosis, suggesting that in at least some patients, respiratory acidosis had been precipitated by high flow oxygen therapy administered in the ambulance.

WHICH FACTORS PREDICT LIKELY FAILURE OF NIPPV IN PATIENTS WITH ACUTE EXACERBATIONS OF COPD? (Table 3.3)

If NIPPV does not improve pH and respiratory rate within the first hour or two, intubation should be considered.[18,22,66] Patients with high APACHE II scores, inability to minimize the amount of mouth leak (because of lack of teeth, secretions, or

Table 3.3 *Conditions in which NIPPV is less likely to be successful*

- pH and respiratory rate do not improve within the first 30 minutes[68] to 2 hours of NIPPV[18,22,66]
- High APACHE II scores[18,67]
- Inability to minimize leak[67]
- Excessive secretions[67]
- Inability to co-ordinate with NIPPV[18,67]
- Pneumonia[18]
- Patient underweight[18]
- Greater level of neurological compromise[18]
- Low pH prior to starting NIPPV[18]

breathing pattern) or inability to co-ordinate with NIPPV are less likely to improve with NIPPV[67] and there should be a low threshold for intubation and mechanical ventilation. In another study patients who failed on NIPPV had a significantly higher incidence of pneumonia (38.5% v 8.7%), were underweight, had greater level of neurological deterioration, a higher APACHE II score and reduced compliance with ventilation as assessed by the physician in charge, compared with those who were successfully treated.[18] Although both groups had similar PaO_2/FiO_2 ratio, patients failing on NIPPV had a significantly more abnormal $PaCO_2$ and pH before starting NIPPV. Only baseline pH was found by logistic regression analysis to be able to predict success or failure of NIPPV (mean 7.28 in the successful group v 7.22 in the failure group) with a sensitivity of 97% and specificity of 71%. Poponick *et al.*[68] however found no relationship between baseline parameters and the likelihood of success of NIPPV delivered in the Emergency Room with the lack of change in blood gases after a 30-minute trial being the best predictor of the need for ETI. One problem with all these studies is that failure criteria are likely to be something of a self-fulfilling prophecy. If it is decided that the patient will be intubated if arterial blood gas tensions do not improve after 30 minutes or if there is severe acidosis, and that the patient will only be given a very limited trial of NIPPV, these will then become failure criteria, even though with persistence, adjustment of settings, change of interface etc. a different outcome might have been achieved.

Coma or confusion, upper gastrointestinal bleeding, high risk of aspiration, haemodynamic instability or uncontrolled arrhythmia have been suggested as contraindications to NIPPV.[69] These are primarily for theoretical reasons and because these patients have been excluded from previous studies, not because there is any evidence that IMV is superior in these situations.

WHERE SHOULD NIPPV BE PERFORMED? (Table 3.4)

There have been randomized controlled trials of the use of NIPPV in the Accident and Emergency Department, in the ICU and on a general ward. Two studies[20,26] in which NIPPV was initiated in the A&E have both failed to show any advantage to NIPPV over conventional therapy. There are a number of possible explanations for this, but these include the fact that patients are usually admitted to ICU when other

Table 3.4 *Factors to be considered in deciding location for NIPPV for patients with acute exacerbations of COPD**

- Staff with training and expertise in non-invasive ventilation
- Adequate staff available throughout 24-hour period (will depend upon nursing needs of other patients – for instance one nurse responsible for two very ill patients may have less time than one nurse responsible for four less severely ill patients)
- Rapid access to endotracheal intubation and invasive mechanical ventilation
- Likelihood of a successful outcome from NIPPV
- Severity of respiratory failure
- Facilities for monitoring

*In decreasing importance, i.e. most important first.

therapies have failed, whereas most of those presenting to A&E have not received any treatment; a proportion are going to improve after initiation of bronchodilator therapy, steroids etc. There are some patients who present to A&E *in extremis* and require immediate ventilatory support and for whom intubation is not considered appropriate, because the patient's previous history is well known, but for whom a trial of non-invasive ventilation would be considered. In this situation it would be reasonable to start non-invasive ventilation in A&E to stabilize the patient for transfer to the ward on which NIPPV is normally performed. In others the clinical findings suggest that intubation would not be appropriate, but the medical notes or a family member are not available to corroborate this. NIPPV may be useful in this situation to buy time in which to obtain further information or to allow the patient to recover to the point at which they can give a history. However if there is no improvement the patient should be intubated and transferred to the ICU.

NIPPV is a time consuming procedure and there is little doubt that it is more likely to be successful with higher staffing ratios, particularly when NIPPV is initi-

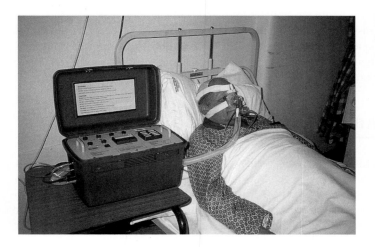

Figure 3.1 *NIPPV on a general respiratory ward.*

ated.[23] The YONIV study suggests that, with adequate staff training, NIPPV can be applied with benefit outside the ICU and that the early introduction of NIPPV on a general ward (Figure 3.1) results in a better outcome, and with cost savings, than providing no ventilatory support for acidotic patients outside the ICU. There have been no direct comparisons of NIPPV in the ICU and on a general ward and it is unlikely that there will ever be such a trial. It should be appreciated that while there is some overlap, the skills needed for non-invasive ventilation are different from those required for invasive ventilation. The outcome from NIPPV is likely to be better on a general ward where the staff have a lot of experience of NIPPV than on an ICU where there are high nurse, therapist and doctor to patient ratios and a high level of monitoring, but little experience of NIPPV. The patient's perspective is also important; many find their experience of ICU to be unpleasant[15] and the less intensive atmosphere of a non-invasive unit may be less distressing, though there is no evidence to support this assertion.

The best location for an NIPPV service will depend critically upon local factors, particularly the skill levels of doctors, nurses and therapists in looking after patients receiving NIPPV. Patient throughput is an important factor which affects the development, and retention, of the particular skills needed for NIPPV. In a recent study from the UK it has been suggested that for the average General Hospital, serving a population of 250,000 and with a standardized mortality rate for COPD of 100, six patients per month with an acute exacerbation of COPD will require NIPPV, assuming that ventilation is initiated in patients with a pH < 7.35 after initial treatment.[65] This number excludes patients with other conditions requiring NIPPV and those who require it later in their hospital stay, e.g. for weaning etc. With relatively small numbers of patients per month NIPPV is best performed in a single location, to facilitate staff training and to maximize throughput and skill retention. A proportion of patients will fail with NIPPV, requiring intubation and invasive ventilation; it is important that personnel and the facility for intubation be rapidly available if needed, if the trend to increased mortality with NIPPV, as reported by Wood et al. is to be avoided.[20] It could be argued that for patients with a high likelihood of failing, NIPPV should be initiated on the ICU and once stabilized the patient could be transferred to the ward normally providing NIPPV. In any discussion about location of an NIPPV service it is important to note that the model of hospital care differs from country to country and that 'ICU', 'high dependency unit (HDU)' and 'general ward' will have different levels of staffing, facilities for monitoring etc. Care must therefore be taken in the extrapolation of results obtained in one environment to other hospitals and countries.

In summary, staff training and experience are more important than location, and adequate numbers of staff, skilled in NIPPV, must be available throughout the 24-hour period. Because of the demands of looking after these acutely ill patients, and to aid training and skill retention, NIPPV is usually best carried out in one single sex location with one nurse, experienced in non-invasive ventilation, responsible for no more than three to four patients in total. Whether this is called an ICU, a HDU or is part of a general ward is largely irrelevant. Further studies are needed to determine the optimal threshold for initiating NIPPV, to assess the feasibility, safety and effectiveness in lower intensity settings, and to determine the cost-effectiveness both in the short and long-term.

CONCLUSION

There is now a robust evidence base for the use of NIPPV in acute respiratory disease, particularly in patients with COPD. NIPPV should be considered as a means of preventing, rather than a direct alternative to ETI and mechanical ventilation. When ETI is deemed necessary a strategy of early extubation on to NIPPV should be considered. The reduction in complications, particularly pneumonia, is a consistent and important finding.[22,37,70] The location in which NIPPV is performed depends critically upon local factors, particularly staff training and expertise. In many institutions all NIPPV should be performed on the ICU/HDU, but in others the general ward is a realistic alternative for some patients.

REFERENCES

1   Martin TR, Lewis SW, Albert RK. The prognosis of patients with chronic obstructive pulmonary disease after hospitalization for acute respiratory failure. *Chest* 1982; **82**: 310–14.
2   Connors AF, Jr., Dawson NV, Thomas C, *et al*. Outcomes following acute exacerbation of severe chronic obstructive lung disease. The SUPPORT investigators (Study to Understand Prognoses and Preferences for Outcomes and Risks of Treatments). *Am J Respir Crit Care Med* 1996; **154**: 959–67.
3   Jeffrey AA, Warren PM, Flenley DC. Acute hypercapnic respiratory failure in patients with chronic obstructive lung disease: risk factors and use of guidelines for management. *Thorax* 1992; **47**: 34–40.
4   Vestbo J, Prescott E, Lange P, Schnohr P, Jenson G. Vital prognosis after hospitalization for COPD: a study of a random population sample. *Resp Med* 1998; **92**: 772–6.
5   Hudson LD. Survival data in patients with acute and chronic lung disease requiring mechanical ventilation. *Am Rev Respir Dis* 1989; **140**: S19–S24.
6   Esteban A, Frutos F, Tobin MJ, *et al*. A comparison of four methods of weaning patients from mechanical ventilation. Spanish Lung Failure Collaborative Group. *N Engl J Med* 1995; **332**: 345–50.
7   Brochard L, Rauss A, Benito S, *et al*. Comparison of three methods of gradual withdrawal from ventilatory support during weaning from mechanical ventilation. *Am J Respir Crit Care Med* 1994; **150**: 896–903.
8   Torres A, Aznar R, Gatell JM. Incidence, risk and prognosis factors of nosocomial pneumonia in mechanically ventilated patients. *Am Rev Respir Dis* 1990; **142**: 523–8.
9   Fagon JY, Chastre J, Hance A, Montravers P, Novara A, Gibert C. Nosocomial pneumonia in ventilated patients: a cohort study evaluating attributable mortality and hospital stay. *Am J Med* 1993; **94**: 281–7.
10 Elliott MW, Aquilina R, Green M, Moxham J, Simonds AK. A comparison of different modes of noninvasive ventilatory support: effects on ventilation and inspiratory muscle effort. *Anaesthesia* 1994; **49**: 279–83.
11 Girault C, Richard J, Chevron V, *et al*. Comparative physiological effects of noninvasive assist-control and pressure support ventilation in acute hypercapnic respiratory failure. *Chest* 1997; **111**: 1639–48.

12   Brochard L, Isabey D, Piquet J, *et al*. Reversal of acute exacerbations of chronic obstructive lung disease by inspiratory assistance with a face mask. *N Engl J Med* 1990; **323**: 1523–30.

13   Diaz O, Iglesia R, Ferrer M, *et al*. Effects of noninvasive ventilation on pulmonary gas exchange and hemodynamics during acute hypercapnic exacerbations of chronic obstructive pulmonary disease. *Am J Respir Crit Care Med* 1997; **156**: 1840–5.

14   Celikel T, Sungur M, Ceyhan B, Karakurt S. Comparison of noninvasive positive pressure ventilation with standard medical therapy in hypercapnic acute respiratory failure. *Chest* 1998; **114**: 1636–42.

15   Easton C, MacKenzie F. Sensory-perceptual alterations: delirium in the intensive care unit. *Heart Lung* 1988; **17**: 229–37.

16   Pingleton SK. Complications of acute respiratory failure. *Am Rev Respir Dis* 1988; **137**: 1463–93.

17   Seneff MG, Wagner DP, Wagner RP, Zimmerman JE, Knaus WA. Hospital and 1-year survival of patients admitted to intensive care units with acute exacerbation of chronic obstructive pulmonary disease. *JAMA* 1995; **274**: 1852–7.

18   Ambrosino N, Foglio K, Rubini F, Clini E, Nava S, Vitacca M. Non-invasive mechanical ventilation in acute respiratory failure due to chronic obstructive airways disease: correlates for success. *Thorax* 1995; **50**: 755–7.

19   Ambrosino N. Noninvasive mechanical ventilation in acute respiratory failure. *Eur Respir J* 1996; **9**: 795–807.

20   Wood KA, Lewis L, Von Harz B, Kollef MH. The use of noninvasive positive pressure ventilation in the Emergency Department. *Chest* 1998; **113**: 1339–46.

21   Chevrolet JC, Jolliet P, Abajo B, Toussi A, Louis M. Nasal positive pressure ventilation in patients with acute respiratory failure. *Chest* 1991; **100**: 775–82.

22   Brochard L, Mancebo J, Wysocki M, *et al*. Noninvasive ventilation for acute exacerbations of chronic obstructive pulmonary disease. *N Engl J Med* 1995; **333**: 817–22.

23   Kramer N, Meyer TJ, Meharg J, Cece RD, Hill NS. Randomized, prospective trial of noninvasive positive pressure ventilation in acute respiratory failure. *Am J Respir Crit Care Med* 1995; **151**: 1799–1806.

24   Martin TJ, Hovis JD, Costantino JP, *et al*. A randomized, prospective evaluation of noninvasive ventilation for acute respiratory failure. *Am J Respir Crit Care Med* 2000; **161**: 807–13.

25   Bott J, Carroll MP, Conway JH, *et al*. Randomised controlled trial of nasal ventilation in acute ventilatory failure due to chronic obstructive airways disease. *Lancet* 1993; **341**: 1555–7.

26   Barbe F, Togores B, Rubi M, Pons S, Maimo A, Agusti AGN. Noninvasive ventilatory support does not facilitate recovery from acute respiratory failure in chronic obstructive pulmonary disease. *Eur Respir J* 1996; **9**: 1240–5.

27   Plant PK, Owen JL, Elliott MW. A multicentre randomised controlled trial of the early use of non-invasive ventilation for acute exacerbations of chronic obstructive pulmonary disease on general respiratory wards. *Lancet* 2000; **355**: 1931–5.

28   Confalonieri M, Parigi P, Scartabellati A, *et al*. Noninvasive mechanical ventilation improves the immediate and long-term outcome of COPD patients with acute respiratory failure. *Eur Respir J* 1996; **9**: 422–30.

29 Vitacca M, Clini E, Rubini F, Nava S, Foglio K, Ambrosino N. Non-invasive mechanical ventilation in severe chronic obstructive lung disease and acute respiratory failure: short- and long-term prognosis. *Intensive Care Med* 1996; **22**: 94–100.
30 Bardi G, Pierotello R, Desideri M, Valdisseri L, Bottai M, Palla A. Nasal ventilation in COPD exacerbations: early and late results of a prospective, controlled study. *Eur Respir J* 2000; **15**: 98–104.
31 Shneerson JM. The changing role of mechanical ventilation in COPD. *Eur Respir J* 1996; **9**: 393–8.
32 Coakley JH, Nagendran K, Honavar M, Hinds CJ. Preliminary observations on the neuromuscular abnormalities in patients with organ failure and sepsis. *Intensive Care Med* 1993; **19**: 323–8.
33 Coakley JH, Nagendran K, Ormerod IE, Ferguson CN, Hinds CJ. Prolonged neurogenic weakness in patients requiring mechanical ventilation for acute airflow limitation. *Chest* 1992; **101**: 1413–16.
34 Grassino A, Comtois N, Galdiz HJ, Sinderby C. The unweanable patient. *Monaldi Arch Chest Dis* 1994; **49**: 522–6.
35 Udwadia ZF, Santis GK, Steven MH, Simonds AK. Nasal ventilation to facilitate weaning in patients with chronic respiratory insufficiency. *Thorax* 1992; **47**: 715–18.
36 Restrick LJ, Scott AD, Ward EM, Feneck RO, Cornwell WE, Wedzicha JA. Nasal intermittent positive-pressure ventilation in weaning intubated patients with chronic respiratory disease from assisted positive-pressure ventilation. *Respir Med* 1993; **87**: 199–204.
37 Nava S, Ambrosino N, Clini E, *et al.* Noninvasive mechanical ventilation in the weaning of patients with respiratory failure due to chronic obstructive pulmonary disease. A randomized, controlled trial. *Ann Intern Med* 1998; **128**: 721–8.
38 Girault C, Daudenthun I, Chevron V, Tamion F, Leroy J, Bonmarchand G. Noninvasive ventilation as a systematic extubation and weaning technique in acute-on-chronic respiratory failure. A prospective, randomized controlled study. *Am J Respir Crit Care Med* 1999; **160**: 86–92.
39 Hilbert G, Gruson D, Porel L, Gbikpi-Benissan G, Cardinaud JP. Noninvasive pressure support ventilation in COPD patients with post extubation hypercapnic respiratory insufficiency. *Eur Respir J* 1998; **11**: 1349–53.
40 Chevrolet JC, Jolliet P. Workload on non-invasive ventilation in acute respiratory failure. In: Vincent JL (ed.) *Yearbook of intensive and emergency medicine.* Berlin: Springer, 1997: 505–13.
41 Nava S, Evangelisti I, Rampulla C, Compagnoni ML, Fracchia C, Rubini F. Human and financial costs of noninvasive mechanical ventilation in patients affected by COPD and acute respiratory failure. *Chest* 1997; **111**: 1631–8.
42 Vitacca M, Clini E, Porta R, Sereni D, Ambrosino N. Experience of an intermediate respiratory intensive therapy in the treatment of prolonged weaning from mechanical ventilation. *Minerva Anestesiol* 1996; **62**: 57–64.
43 Anderer W, Kunzle C, Dhein Y, Worth H. [Noninvasive ventilation in the acute care hospital – a cost factor?]. [German]. *Med Klin* 1997; **92** Suppl 1: 119–22.
44 Criner GJ, Kreimer DT, Tomaselli M, Pierson W, Evans D. Financial implications of noninvasive positive pressure ventilation (NIPPV). *Chest* 1995; **108**: 475–81.
45 Plant PK, Owen J, Elliott MW. A cost effectiveness analysis of non-invasive ventilation (NIV) in acute exacerbations of COPD. *Thorax* 1999; **54**: A11(abstract).

46 Girault C, Richard JC, Chevron V, *et al*. Comparative physiologic effects of noninvasive assist-control and pressure support ventilation in acute hypercapnic respiratory failure. *Chest* 1998; **111**: 1639–48.

47 Cinnella G, Conti G, Lofaso F, *et al*. Effects of assisted ventilation on the work of breathing: volume-controlled versus pressure-controlled ventilation. *Am J Respir Crit Care Med* 1996; **153**: 1025–33.

48 Meecham Jones DJ, Wedzicha JA. Comparison of pressure and volume preset nasal ventilator systems in stable chronic respiratory failure. *Eur Respir J* 1993; **6**: 1060–4.

49 Vitacca M, Rubini F, Foglio K, Scalvini S, Nava S, Ambrosino N. Non-invasive modalities of positive pressure ventilation improve the outcome of acute exacerbations in COLD patients. *Intensive Care Med* 1993; **19**: 450–5.

50 Ambrosino N, Vitacca M, Polese G, Pagani M, Foglio K, Rossi A. Short-term effects of nasal proportional assist ventilation in patients with chronic hypercapnic respiratory insufficiency. *Eur Respir J* 1997; **10**: 2829–34.

51 Patrick W, Webster K, Ludwig L, Roberts D, Wiebe P, Younes M. Non-invasive positive-pressure ventilation in acute respiratory distress without prior respiratory failure. *Am J Respir Crit Care Med* 1996; **153**: 1005–11.

52 Ranieri VM, Grasso S, Mascia L, *et al*. Effects of proportional assist ventilation on inspiratory muscle effort in patients with chronic obstructive pulmonary disease and acute respiratory failure. *Anaesthesiology* 1997; **86**: 79–91.

53 Wrigge H, Golisch W, Zinserling J, Sydow M, Almeling G, Burchardi H. Proportional assist versus pressure support ventilation: effects on breathing pattern and respiratory work of patients with chronic obstructive pulmonary disease. *Intensive Care Med* 1999; **25**: 790–8.

54 Appendini L, Purro A, Gudjonsdottir M, *et al*. Physiological response of ventilator-dependent patients with chronic obstructive pulmonary disease to proportional assist ventilation and continuous positive airway pressure. *Am J Respir Crit Care Med* 1999; **159**: 1510–17.

55 Appendini L, Patessio A, Zanaboni S, *et al*. Physiologic effects of positive end-expiratory pressure and mask pressure support during exacerbations of chronic obstructive pulmonary disease. *Am J Respir Crit Care Med* 1994; **149**: 1069–76.

56 Ferguson GT, Gilmartin M. CO_2 rebreathing during BiPAP ventilatory assistance. *Am J Respir Crit Care Med* 1995; **151**: 1126–35.

57 Ambrosino N, Nava S, Torbicki A, *et al*. Haemodynamic effects of pressure support and PEEP ventilation by nasal route in patients with stable chronic obstructive pulmonary disease. *Thorax* 1993; **48**: 523–8.

58 de Lucas P, Tarancon C, Puente L, Rodriguez C, Tatay E, Monturiol JM. Nasal continuous positive airway pressure in patients with COPD in acute respiratory failure. A study of the immediate effects. *Chest* 1993; **104**: 1694–7.

59 Potgieter PD, Rosenthal E, Benatar SR. Immediate and long-term survival in patients admitted to a respiratory ICU. *Crit Care Med* 1985; **13**: 798–802.

60 Miro AM, Shivaram U, Hertig I. Continuous positive airway pressure in COPD patients in acute hypercapnic respiratory failure. *Chest* 1993; **103**: 266–8.

61 Corrado A, Bruscoli G, Messori A, *et al*. Iron lung treatment of subjects with COPD in acute respiratory failure. Evaluation of short- and long-term prognosis. *Chest* 1992; **101**: 692–6.

62 Corrado A, De Paola E, Gorini M, *et al*. Intermittent negative pressure ventilation in the treatment of hypoxic hypercapnic coma in chronic respiratory insufficiency. *Thorax* 1996; **51**: 1077–82.
63 Elliott MW. Noninvasive ventilation in chronic obstructive pulmonary disease. *N Engl J Med* 1995; **333**: 870–1.
64 Baldwin DR, Allen MB. Non-invasive ventilation for acute exacerbations of chronic obstructive pulmonary disease. *BMJ* 1997; **314**: 163–4.
65 Plant PK, Owen J, Elliott MW. One year period prevalance study of respiratory acidosis in acute exacerbation of COPD; implications for the provision of non-invasive ventilation and oxygen administration. *Thorax* 2000; **55**: 550–4.
66 Meduri GU, Turner RE, Abou-Shala N, Wunderink R, Tolley E. Noninvasive positive pressure ventilation via face mask. First-line intervention in patients with acute hypercapnic and hypoxemic respiratory failure. *Chest* 1996; **109**: 179–93.
67 Soo Hoo GW, Santiago S, Williams AJ. Nasal mechanical ventilation for hypercapnic respiratory failure in chronic obstructive pulmonary disease: determinants of success and failure. *Crit Care Med* 1994; **22**: 1253–61.
68 Poponick JM, Renston JP, Bennett RP, Emerman CL. Use of a ventilatory support system (BiPAP) for acute respiratory failure in the emergency department. *Chest* 1999; **116**: 166–71.
69 Ambrosino N. Noninvasive mechanical ventilation in acute on chronic respiratory failure: determinants of success and failure. *Monaldi Arch Chest Dis* 1997; **52**: 73–5.
70 Antonelli M, Conti G, Rocco M, *et al*. A comparison of noninvasive positive-pressure ventilation and conventional mechanical ventilation in patients with acute respiratory failure. *N Engl J Med* 1998; **339**: 429–35.

4

NIPPV in acute respiratory failure due to non-COPD disorders

A K SIMONDS

GENERAL

Having established that the use of NIPPV reduces the need for intubation and mortality in acute exacerbations of COPD, attention has been focused on the use of NIPPV in acute respiratory failure (ARF) due to other causes such as cardiogenic pulmonary oedema, post-operative respiratory insufficiency, ARDS, pneumonia, asthma, bronchiectasis and neuromusculoskeletal disease. Patients with some of these disorders were included in early uncontrolled studies of NIPPV with positive results,[1–3] but numbers in each category are too small to draw generalizable conclusions. Kramer et al.[4] in a randomized study of NIPPV versus standard therapy showed that intubation rate with NIPPV was reduced and physiological indices improved more rapidly in a group with non-COPD disease including congestive cardiac failure, pneumonia, asthma and pulmonary embolus compared with those receiving conventional therapy. However in COPD patients the reduction in need for intubation was more marked than in the smaller non-COPD group.

In the first randomized comparison of NIPPV with conventional therapy in exclusively non-COPD patients Wysocki et al.[5] found no difference in the rate of endotracheal intubation, length of ICU stay and mortality (33% v 50%) in patients treated with non-invasive pressure support and those conventionally managed. The majority of recruits had post-operative surgical complications, pulmonary oedema or pneumonia. However, post hoc analysis of results showed that in hypercapnic patients, NIPPV produced a reduction in intubation rate (36% v 100%, $p = 0.02$), and ICU stay (13 v 32 days, $p = 0.04$). Numbers in the study were relatively small (20 in each limb) and there was a trend to higher SAPS (Simpified Acute Physiological Score) values on admission in the NIPPV group.

Investigating this area further, a multicentre Italian group has conducted a prospective, randomized controlled ICU-based trial of facemask NIPPV versus conventional mechanical ventilation in ARF patients who had failed to respond to intensive medical therapy ($n = 64$). Entry criteria were:

- ARF with deterioration despite aggressive medical management
- $PaO_2:FiO_2$ ratio < 200 on oxygen therapy
- Respiratory rate > 35/min
- Use of accessory muscles or abdominal paradox.

COPD, status asthmaticus and immunocompromised patients were excluded, as were those with more than two organ system failure. Patients were treated with either intubation and conventional ventilation with PEEP 5 cmH$_2$O, or pressure support ventilation via a facemask. Settings were adjusted until FiO$_2$ requirement was 0.6 or less. Primary endpoints were acute physiological indices and the frequency of complications. PaO$_2$:FiO$_2$ ratio improved similarly in both groups, but there was a marked reduction in complications particularly related to intubation (e.g. ventilator associated pneumonia and sinusitis) in the NIPPV group (38 v 66%, $p < 0.002$). Survival to discharge was higher in NIPPV patients with a SAPS value of < 16, compared with those with higher scores where no difference was seen between ventilatory approaches. Additional preliminary work from the group suggests that patients with ARDS are likely to do less well with NIPPV than those with other causes of ARF, which is not surprising in view of the associated profound gas exchange difficulties and multisystem nature of the syndrome.

NIPPV IN ARF DUE TO COMMUNITY ACQUIRED PNEUMONIA

Early studies comprising a heterogeneous group of patients with ARF suggested that community acquired pneumonia was a poor prognostic factor.[5,6] As an illustration, in one study all patients with pneumonia randomized to NIPPV failed therapy, compared to a success rate of nearly 60% in those in whom respiratory distress which was not attributable to pneumonia. The authors speculated that the higher failure rate in pneumonia patients was due to difficulty clearing secretions, reduced pulmonary compliance and inhomogenous gas exchange. Relatively small numbers of patients with pneumonia were recruited in the Antonelli study[7] described above and so it is difficult to draw firm conclusions. By contrast to previous discouraging results, Confalonieri and colleagues[8] have recently published findings from a prospective randomized trial in patients with ARF due to severe community acquired pneumonia (CAP). Patients ($n = 56$) on entry to a respiratory intermediate care unit were randomized to either NIPPV, or standard therapy with oxygen applied via Venturi mask. Entry criteria are shown in Box 4.1.

Box 4.1 *Criteria for diagnosing severe pneumonia*

Chest radiograph showing multilobar involvement at admission or increase in infiltrate size by 50% or more within 48 hours of admission, systolic BP less than 90 mmHg or diastolic BP less than 60 mmHg, the necessity for vasopressors for more than 4 hours or urine output less than 80 mL in 4 hours.
ARF was defined by presence of two or more of the following: severe dyspnoea and respiratory rate > 35/min and/or active contraction of abdominal muscles, Pao_2 < 68 mmHg on Fio_2 > 0.4 or $Pao_2:Fio_2$ ratio < 250 with Fio_2 > 0.5, $Paco_2$ > 50 mmHg, pH < 7.33.

Patients with an urgent requirement for endotracheal intubation, severe encephalopathy or haemodynamic instability; and those receiving long-term oxygen therapy or home ventilation were excluded.

In this study NIPPV resulted in a better outcome than in previous work.[5] For the NIPPV group there was a significant early fall in respiratory rate and the need for intubation was reduced compared with the group receiving standard treatment (21% intubation rate in NIPPV v 50% intubation rate in the standard group, $p = 0.03$). Moreover, the duration of stay in the ICU was significantly decreased (1.8 days NIPPV v six days' standard therapy). Overall hospital mortality and length of hospital stay did not differ between groups, but at 2 months more patients with pneumonia and underlying COPD were alive.

Microbiological diagnoses were reached in 57% of patients with most prevalent pathogens being *Streptococcus pneumoniae* and *Staphylococcus aureus*. Just under half the patients in each group had COPD, and in those receiving NIPPV, nursing workload was recorded as less demanding than in COPD patients with pneumonia treated conservatively. There was no evidence that use of NIPPV delayed intubation unduly in those who failed non-invasive ventilation, compared with those requiring intubation in the control group (44 v 42 hours). It should be noted that the study was carried out in a high dependency type unit with ready access to intubation if required.

This large trial is therefore reassuring in indicating that NIPPV is reasonable first line therapy in patients with severe community acquired pneumonia who fulfill the above criteria, whether they have COPD or not. This conclusion is supported by the fact that a meta-analysis of non-invasive ventilation in ARF[9] did not show pneumonia to be a significant risk factor.

NIPPV IN IMMUNOSUPPRESSED PATIENTS WITH ARF

Patients with ARF following transplantation pose difficult management problems. Antonelli *et al.*[10] found that in a group of 238 patients who received solid organ transplantation over a two-year period, 51 (21%) developed ARF. To examine the impact of NIPPV on outcome, 40 of these patients were randomized to either NIPPV or standard therapy with supplemental oxygen. Endpoints were the need for endotracheal intubation and mechanical ventilation, duration of ventilatory assistance, complications not present on admission to study, length of ICU stay and ICU mortality. After the first hour of treatment 70% of the NIPPV group had improved their PaO_2/FiO_2 ratio, compared with 25% in the standard group. Sustained improvements in gas exchange occurred in 60% of the NIPPV patients and 25% of those receiving standard treatment ($p = 0.03$). NIPPV was associated with a significant reduction in the need for intubation (20% NIPPV v 70% standard treatment, $p = 0.002$), rate of fatal complications (20% v 50%, $p = 0.05$), length of stay in ICU (mean, SD 5.5 (3) v 9 (4) days, $p = 0.03$), and ICU mortality (20% v 50%, $p = 0.05$). Overall hospital mortality did not differ between the groups.

More recently Hilbert and colleagues[11] have carried out a randomized study of early NIPPV versus standard therapy in patients with immunosuppression, pulmonary infiltrates, fever and ARF. Causes for immunosuppression included bone marrow transplantation, haematological malignancies, chemotherapy, corticosteroid therapy, and the acquired immunodeficiency syndrome. NIPPV improved arterial blood gas tensions (Figure 4.1), reduced the need for endotracheal intubation ($p = 0.03$), serious complications ($p = 0.02$), ITU death ($p = 0.03$) and hospital mortality ($p = 0.02$) compared with standard therapy. Prognosis was very poor in patients who failed NIPPV leading Hill[12] to pose the question in an accompanying editorial of whether endotracheal intubation following failed NIPPV is futile.

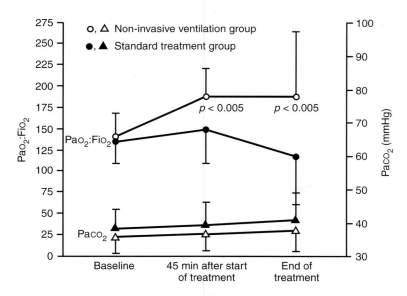

Figure 4.1 *Pao_2:Fio_2 ratio and $Paco_2$ before and after standard therapy or NIPPV in immunocompromised patients. End of treatment refers to last arterial blood gas result obtained before intubation or discharge from ICU. From Ref. 11 with permission.*

These results certainly suggest that NIPPV should be included in management protocols for immunocompromised patients. The timing is crucial, and early application is advisable. It is not clear, however, whether NIPPV offers advantages over CPAP in transplant or HIV patients, as this comparison has not been carried out.

NIPPV IN ACUTE CARDIOGENIC PULMONARY OEDEMA

There have been several open prospective studies of NIPPV in patients with ARF due to cardiogenic pulmonary oedema. Most have used bilevel positive pressure via facemask. In the study of Hoffman and Welte[13] only one of the 29 patients required intubation, mean arterial oxygen saturation increased from 73% to 90.3% on a reduced FiO_2, and pH and $PaCO_2$ decreased significantly. Haemodynamic variables remained stable. Rusterholz et al.[14] showed similar improvements in SaO_2 and pH. Patients who succeeded with NIPPV differed from those who failed the technique by having a higher $PaCO_2$ and lower creatinine phosphokinase (CPK) level at the initiation of NIPPV. These positive results should be set carefully against those from a randomized trial[15] of CPAP versus bilevel NIPPV in acute pulmonary oedema. This study was discontinued prematurely due to a worse outcome in the NIPPV group. A higher rate of myocardial infaction occurred in NIPPV patients compared with those receiving CPAP (71% NIPPV, 31% CPAP). At first sight this outcome is difficult to explain, although it might be attributable to a larger suppressant effect of NIPPV on BP, greater variation in intrathoracic pressure and decreased venous return, leading to reduced myocardial perfusion. On further analysis there was shown to be a higher CPK level before entry into the study in the patients receiving NIPPV suggesting results could have been biased by a greater number of patients with evolving myocardial infarction being randomized to NIPPV. This impression is strengthened by the fact that adverse haemodynamic changes with NIPPV were not seen in the open studies, and that successful outcome with NIPPV in acute pulmonary oedema has been demonstrated in other trials. In addition, more recently NIPPV has been compared with oxygen therapy in a randomized trial in acute cardiogenic pulmonary oedema patients.[16] Patients receiving NIPPV compared with oxygen therapy were less likely to require intubation ($p = 0.037$) and resolution of pulmonary oedema (defined as clinical improvement with $SaO_2 > 96\%$ and respiratory rate < 30/min) was quicker. No concurrent comparison with CPAP therapy was made in this study. Therefore, in the absence of definitive randomized data showing that NIPPV is as effective, or more effective than CPAP, caution should be exercised when using NIPPV in patients with an evolving myocardial infarction. CPAP should probably be the treatment of choice here unless $PaCO_2$ is markedly elevated.

NIPPV IN ACUTE SEVERE ASTHMA

Acute severe asthma associated with exhaustion and respiratory muscle fatigue is a classical indication for intubation and ventilation. However, conventional mechanical ventilation in severe asthma has a high complication rate, including the risks of barotrauma and haemodynamic collapse. The role of mask ventilation as first line therapy in ARF due to status asthmaticus has been explored in an uncontrolled study[17] of 17 patients who presented with a pH of 7.25 and $PaCO_2$ 8.6 (1.5) kPa. Facemask pressure support ventilation was provided with a expiratory positive pressure (EPAP) level of 4 (2) cmH_2O to offset intrinsic PEEP. Exclusion criteria were: immediate need for intubation (coma, respiratory arrest), systolic BP < 90 mmHg, ECG evidence of arrythmia or ischaemia. Nebulized bronchodilator was delivered in-line with the ventilator (see Chapter 17) and patients encouraged to use NIPPV continuously for the first 4–6 hours.

Tolerance of NIPPV was good and physiological improvement occurred rapidly. There were no complications and no deaths. Two out of the 17 patients required intubation and conventional ventilation 35 minutes and 89 hours after starting NIPPV, respectively. Average IPAP setting was 18 (5) cmH_2O, and no patient required inspiratory pressures above 25 cmH_2O. NIPPV has also been successfully applied in children with status asthmaticus (see Chapter 15).

These data suggest that NIPPV is a feasible first line intervention in acute severe asthma. However, until a randomized study of NIPPV versus conventional ventilation is carried out, NIPPV may be considered in selected cases, but for individuals with rapid deterioration, intubation and IPPV remains the preferred option.

NIPPV IN ACUTE EXACERBATIONS OF CYSTIC FIBROSIS (CF)/BRONCHIECTASIS

As with many other non-COPD indications there has been no controlled examination of NIPPV in acute ventilatory decompensation in CF patients, although the treatment is used widely on clinical grounds. Anecdotal evidence suggests that NIPPV may be particularly helpful in acidotic, hypercapnic patients, who are tiring and having difficulty clearing secretions. In this situation physiotherapy during NIPPV may prove helpful, and an improvement in PaO_2 achieved without a concommitant increase in $PaCO_2$. Piper et al.[18] found that the use of NIPPV stabilized hypercapnic CF patients, and Hodson and colleagues[19] showed that volume preset NIPPV can be used to bridge CF patients to heart–lung transplantation by successfully avoiding intubation (see Chapter 13).

Most workers find that optimal $PaCO_2$ control may be difficult to achieve in CF patients presumably due to high V/Q mismatch as a result of extensive small airways disease. However, even small falls or stabilization in $PaCO_2$ may be beneficial and many patients derive considerable symptomatic relief. Humidification may be particularly helpful in CF patients. In addition a high proportion have additional nasal pathology such as polyps therefore a full facemask may be preferable. For those with nasal blockage who cannot tolerate a full facemask, a nasopaharyngeal airway or intranasal stents (formed using small shortened endotracheal tubes either unilaterally or bilaterally) may allow succesful application of NIPPV.[20]

Similar considerations apply in patients with bronchiectasis due to other causes. In this group, as in CF patients, NIPPV can be used logically in an attempt to avoid intubation as the outcome in patients with bronchiectasis receiving intubation and conventional IPPV is poor. By the same token, it should be noted that patients who fail acute NIPPV have a very poor prognosis

NIPPV IN ARF DUE TO NEUROMUSCULOSKELETAL DISEASE

NIPPV may offer major advantages over endotracheal intubation and ventilation in patients with neuromuscular or chest wall disease. Clearly extreme bulbar weakness is a contraindication to non-invasive techniques, but patients with milder level of bulbar compromise can use NIPPV effectively. Vianello *et al.*[21] have compared a non-invasive approach to endotracheal intubation (ETT) in patients with ARF due to Duchenne muscular dystrophy (DMD). Five out of the seven patients treated with NIPPV had a successful outcome compared to only one out of six treated conventionally. However, a minitracheostomy was used for secretion clearance in three NIPPV patients. Of importance is the fact that ICU stay was considerably reduced (12.6 days NIPPV, 31.5 days ET-IPPV). In another study[22] of NIPPV in DMD in which most patients presented acutely NIPPV was used successfully in a high dependency or ICU environment. Intensive physiotherapy during NIPPV proved a crucial part of the success of the technique and no patient in this study required minitracheostomy. Restrictive chest wall patients have been included in several open studies of weaning using NIPPV yielding success rates comparable or better than those with COPD. However, in view of the smaller numbers of these patients and heterogeneous pathology there have been no randomized controlled trials. These would almost certainly be unethical in the stable chest wall disease group or those with non-progressive or slowly progressive neuromuscular conditions such as previous poliomyelitis, in whom there is a excellent argument to try NIPPV first before resorting to endotracheal intubation. Age should not be a bar to a trial of NIPPV, as there is no evidence that elderly restrictive patients fare poorly, unless there is multiple underlying pathology. Clearly, in the neuromuscular group patient selection is of prime importance and indications, contraindications, the patient's wishes, and prognosis should carefully reviewed (see Chapters 14, 15 and 20 for a discussion of the practicalities and ethics of NIPPV in progressive neuromuscular disease).

NIPPV IN CHEST TRAUMA

CPAP has been found helpful in patients with rib fractures and hypoxaemia, and when used in conjunction with regional anaesthesia may reduce ICU and hospital stay compared with conventional mechanical ventilation. The use of bilevel pressure support to stabilize a flail chest and minimize basal atectasis has been described in two case reports,[23,24] but at present the evidence supports CPAP as first line non-invasive therapy. Chest trauma patients must be very carefully watched for the development of a pneumothorax while receiving positive pressure respiratory support.

NIPPV POST-EXTUBATION IN NON-COPD PATIENTS

In COPD patients who failed a trial of extubation Hilbert and coworkers[25] have shown in a retrospective study that NIPPV reduces the need for re-intubation (see also Chapter 7). Another French group[26] has recently examined the role of NIPPV as a systematic extubation and weaning tool in ARF. Half the patients enrolled in this randomized controlled study had COPD, but around a quarter had restrictive disorders and the remainder a mixed obstructive/restrictive pathology. According to the protocol subjects who failed a 2 hour trial of spontaneous breathing were randomized to either conventional pressure support ventilation (PSV) via endotracheal tube (ETT), or extubation and pressure support NIPPV. The level of pressure support was then gradually reduced in both groups. There was no difference in the rate of successful weaning (defined by absence of reintubation within 5 days of extubation) (ET-IPPV 75%, NIPPV 76.5%), ICU stay, hospital stay or mortality between the two groups. However, the mean period of daily ventilatory support and complications related to endotracheal intubation were significantly reduced in the NIPPV group.

Use of NIPPV in patients with acute respiratory insufficiency after early extubation has also been explored in a post-surgical population (most having undergone lung or liver transplantation).[27]

PSV with CPAP produced significant improvements in oxygenation, ventilatory variables and oxygen consumption. These acute indices did not differ in patients receiving CPAP or CPAP plus PSV for 30-minute periods. Haemodynamic variables were unchanged compared with values obtained during spontaneous breathing. After an initial CPAP versus bilevel PSV trial patients then continued to receive PSV with CPAP at least six times a day subsequently. Median duration of NIPPV was 2 days (range 1–20 days). The authors conclude that NIPPV is feasible, and early use may reduce the frequency of intubation related complications in this high risk immunosuppressed post-transplantation group.

In a further series[28] of patients with mixed obstructive/restrictive ventilatory defects who had failed a trial of extubation, NIPPV facilitated weaning and transfer from the ICU to high dependency or general ward facilities. This was an uncontrolled study, but 20/22 difficult to wean patients were successfully transferred to NIPPV and discharged home within a median of 9 days following a median stay of 31 days on ICU, indicating economic advantages to the technique by reducing ICU stay. It should be noted that this case series was exceptional in that around half the patients (mainly those with chronic chest wall or neuromuscular disease) were discharged home with nocturnal ventilatory support, whereas in the studies described above, NIPPV was discontinued before hospital discharge. This discrepancy can be explained by differences in selection, as patients with a major component of chronic disease, rather than acute major precipitant to decompensation, are more likely to require support long term.

NIPPV IN PATIENTS WITH ARF WHO REFUSE ENDOTRACHEAL INTUBATION

Many individuals with endstage or terminal pulmonary or cardiac disease wish to avoid any intervention which will protract poor quality survival and deprive them of the ability to participate in decision-making. However, they are not averse to trying therapies which may palliate symptoms or improve prognosis. These considerations are also be applicable to some patients in whom intubation and IPPV in the ICU is judged likely to be futile, but who might be helped symptomatically by NIPPV.

Meduri and team[29] have studied the use of facemask NIPPV in patients with ARF ($n = 11$) who expressly refused intubation, but agreed to a trial of NIPPV. Underlying diagnoses included COPD, congestive cardiac failure, lung cancer, lymphoma, end stage pulmonary fibrosis, and quadriplegia. Success of the intervention was judged by improvement in physiological indices and discharge from the ICU. (It is of course notable that these patients were admitted to the ICU in the first place.) Importantly, all subjects tolerated mask ventilation well and only two developed late intolerance after improvement in their condition had occurred. Gas exchange abnomalities were corrected or improved in 10/11 patients. Seven patients were discharged from the ICU and five (45%) were discharged home. As in other patient groups studied, success was predicted by a significant improvement in arterial pH after one hour of NIPPV, and in all survivors respiratory acidosis and hypoxaemia were corrected within 6 hours of initiating NIPPV. The authors remark that even though treatment was unsuccessful in some cases, facemask ventilation was still effective at relieving dyspnoea in those individuals who did not survive the admission, suggesting a potential palliative role in this population.

It should be emphasized that NIPPV can be tried in an attempt to palliate symptoms in patients with terminal disease in whom there are no major contraindications (Chapter 5), but that if this treatment becomes burdensome or is clearly ineffective after several hours, it can be relatively easily withdrawn and efforts concentrated on relieving symptoms by other means (see Chapter 14).

GENERAL APPLICABILITY OF NIPPV IN NON-COPD CAUSES OF ARF

While the value of NIPPV has been confirmed in non-COPD ARF patients by one randomized trial, it should be noted that these patients were carefully selected and the intervention was carried out in an ICU. For conditions such as acute pulmonary oedema, CPAP therapy should be considered first, while in other situations such as status asthmaticus, the role of NIPPV is not yet proven and conventional ventilation is the treatment of choice in severe cases.

In a recent survey of French ICUs[30] NIPPV was used in 42% of hypoxaemic and 46% of hypercapnic ARF patients. NIPPV was followed by intubation and conventional mechanical ventilation (CMV) in 39% of cases. Mortality was lower in patients receiving NIPPV compared with CMV but this is likely to be due to patient selection and use of NIPPV earlier in the illness. Predictive factors for failure of NIPPV were poor tolerance and illness severity.

As is the case in COPD patients, NIPPV and conventional ventilation should be regarded as complementary techniques in non-COPD causes of ARF. Introduced earlier in the course of the illness, NIPPV may reduce the need for intubation and associated complications. However, if applied inappropriately if may potentially delay intubation and worsen prognosis. As patients with hypoxaemic ARF are often unstable and the failure rate with NIPPV in non-COPD groups is higher than in COPD patients, close monitoring in a location where intubation can be swiftly carried out is indicated (e.g. in an HDU).

REFERENCES

1 Meduri GU, Conoscenti CC, Menashe P, Nair S. Noninvasive face mask ventilation in patients with acute respiratory failure. *Chest* 1989; **95**: 865–70.
2 Elliott MW, Carroll MA, Wedzicha JA, Branthwaite MA. Nasal positive pressure ventilation can be used successfully at home to control nocturnal hypoventilation in COPD. *Am Rev Respir Dis* 1990; **141**: A322–A322.
3 Pennock BE, Crawshaw L, Kaplan PD. Non-invasive nasal mask ventilation for acute respiratory failure. Institution of a new therapeutic technology for routine use. *Chest* 1994; **105**: 441–4.
4 Kramer N, Meyer TJ, Meharg J, Cece RD, Hill NS. Randomized prospective trial of noninvasive positive pressure ventilation in acute respiratory failure. *Am J Respir Crit Care Med* 1995; **151**: 1799–1806.
5 Wysocki M, Tric L, Wolff MA, Millet H, Herman B. Noninvasive pressure support ventilation in patients with acute respiratory failure. A randomized comparison with conventional therapy. *Chest* 1995; **107**: 761–8.
6 Ambrosino N, Foglio K, Rubini F, Clini E, Nava S, Vitacca M. Non-invasive mechanical ventilation in acute respiratory failure due to chronic obstructive airways disease: correlates for success. *Thorax* 1995; **50**: 755–7.
7 Antonelli M, Conti G, Rocco M, *et al.* A comparison of noninvasive positive pressure ventilation and conventional mechanical ventilation in patients with acute respiratory failure. *N Engl J Med* 1998; **339**: 429–35.
8 Confalonieri M, Potena A, Carbone G, Della Porta R, Tolley E, Meduri GU. Acute respiratory failure in patients with severe community-acquired pneumonia. A propective randomized evaluation of noninvasive ventilation. *Am J Respir Crit Care Med* 1999; **160**: 1585–91.
9 Keenan SP, Kernerman PD, Cook DJ, Martin CM, McCormack D, Sibbald WJ. The effect of noninvasive positive pressure ventilation on mortality in patients admitted with acute respiratory failure: a meta-analaysis. *Crit Care Med* 1997; **25**: 1685–92.
10 Antonelli M, Conti G, Bufi M, *et al.* Non-invasive ventilation for the treatment of acute respiratory failure in patients undergoing solid organ transplantation: a randomized trial. *JAMA* 2000; **283**: 235–41.
11 Hilbert G, Gruson D, Vargas F, *et al.* Noninvasive ventilation in immunosuppressed patients with pulmonary infiltrates, fever, and acute respiratory failure. *N Engl J Med* 2001; **344**: 481–7.
12 Hill NS. Noninvasive ventilation for immunocompromised patients. *N Engl J Med* 2001; **344**: 522–3.
13 Hoffman B, Welte T. The use of noninvasive pressure support ventilation for severe respiratory insufficiency due to pulmonary oedema. *Int Care Med* 1999; **25**: 15–20.
14 Rusterholz T, Kempf J, Berton C, Gayol S, Tournod C, Zaehringer M. Noninvasive pressure support ventilation (PIPSV) with face mask in patients with acute cardiogenic pulmonary edema (ACPE). *Int Care Med* 1999; **25**: 21–8.

15 Mehta S, Jay GD, Woolard RH, *et al.* Randomized prospective trial of bilevel versus continuous positive airway pressure in acute pulmonary edema. *Crit Care Med* 1997; **25**: 620–8.

16 Masip J, Betbese AJ, Paez J, *et al.* Non-invasive pressure support ventilation versus conventional oxygen therapy in acute cardiogenic pulmonary oedema: a randomised trial. *Lancet* 2000; **356**: 2126–32.

17 Meduri GU, Cook TR, Turner RE, Cohen M, Leeper KV. Noninvasive positive pressure ventilation in status asthmaticus. *Chest* 1996; **110**: 767–74.

18 Piper AJ, Parker S, Torzillo PJ, Sullivan CE, Bye PT. Nocturnal nasal IPPV stabilizes patients with cystic fibrosis and hypercapnic respiratory failure. *Chest* 1992; **102**: 846–50.

19 Hodson ME, Madden BP, Steven MH, Tsang VT, Yacoub MH. Non-invasive mechanical ventilation for cystic fibrosis patients – a potential bridge to transplantation. *Eur Respir J* 1991; **4**: 524–7.

20 Edenborough FP, Wildman M, Morgan DW. Mangement of respiratory failure with ventilation via intranasal stents in cystic fibrosis. *Thorax* 2000; **55**: 434–6.

21 Vianello A, Bevilacqua M, Arcano G, Ritrovato L, Gallan F, Frigo GF. Non-invasive ventilatory approach to treatment of acute respiratory failure in Duchenne's muscular dystrophy. *Eur Respir J* 1998; **12**: 129S.

22 Simonds AK, Muntoni F, Heather S, Fielding S. Impact of nasal ventilation on survival in hypercapnic Duchenne muscular dystrophy. *Thorax* 1998; **53**: 949–52.

23 Sivaloganathan M. Management of flail chest. *Hosp Med* 2000; **61**: 811.

24 Abisheganaden J, Chee CB, Wang WT. Use of bilevel positive airway pressure ventilatory support for pathological flail chest complicating multiple myeloma. *Eur Respir J* 1998; **12**: 238–9.

25 Hilbert G, Gruson D, Portel L, Gbikpi-Benissan G, Cardinaud JP. Noninvasive pressure support ventilation in COPD patients with postextubation hypercapnic respiratory insufficiency. *Eur Respir J* 1998; **11**: 1349–53.

26 Girault C, Daudenthun I, Chevron V, Tamion F, Leroy J, Bonmarchand G. Noninvasive ventilation as a systematic extubation and weaning technique in acute on chronic respiratory failure. A prospective randomized controlled study. *Am J Resp Crit Care Med* 1999; **160**: 86–92.

27 Kilger E, Briegel J, Haller M, *et al.* Effects of non-invasive positive pressure ventilatory support in non-COPD patients with acute respiratory insufficiency after early extubation. *Int Care Med* 1999; **25**: 1374–80.

28 Udwadia ZF, Santis GK, Steven MH, Simonds AK. Nasal ventilation to facilitate weaning in patients with chronic respiratory insufficiency. *Thorax* 1992; **47**: 715–18.

29 Meduri GU, Fox RC, Abou-Shala N, Leeper KV, Wunderink RG. Noninvasive mechanical ventilation via face mask in patients with acute respiratory failure who refused endotracheal intubation. *Crit Care Med* 1994; **22**: 1584–90.

30 Richard JC, Carlucci A, Wysocki M, *et al.* French multicenter survey: noninvasive versus conventional mechanical ventilation. *Am J Respir Crit Care Med* 1999; **159**: A367.

5

Starting NIPPV: practical aspects

A K SIMONDS

INTRODUCTION

The following account is a guide to starting mask ventilation. There are no absolute recipes for success, but the key to a favourable outcome lies in the selection of appropriate patients, the availability of suitable equipment, familiarity with the technique, and adequate staffing levels. A team approach with a continuing NIPPV education programme for all members is likely to improve results.

Individuals suitable for an acute trial of mask ventilation should fulfil these criteria:

- Acute respiratory failure (see Box 5.1).

Box 5.1 *Acute respiratory failure (ARF)*

The presence of any two of the following:

- Dyspnoea at rest and respiratory rate (RR) > 25 minute
- $Paco_2$ > 6.0 kPa (45 mmHg). (NIPPV can be used in normocapnic patients but success rates may be lower.)
- pH < 7.35
- Pao_2 < 8.0 kPa (60 mmHg) on air or Pao_2:Fio_2 ratio < 250 when receiving Fio_2 0.5 or more

---

- Normal or near normal bulbar function
- Ability to clear bronchial secretions
- Haemodynamic stability
- Functioning gastrointestinal tract
- Able to co-operate with treatment.

ABSOLUTE CONTRAINDICATIONS TO NIPPV

- Immediate need for intubation, e.g. respiratory arrest
- Coma
- Severe haemodynamic instability (e.g. need for vasopressors)
- More than two-system organ failure (in patient in whom ICU care is indicated)
- Severe bulbar weakness
- Extensive facial trauma or upper airway obstruction.

RELATIVE CONTRAINDICATIONS

- Highly confused or unco-operative patient
- Evolving myocardial infarction
- Unstable angina
- Moderate bulbar weakness
- Poor or absent cough reflex
- Recent oesophageal or gastric surgery
- Facial deformity.

GOALS OF NIPPV

(a) NIPPV can be used to assist ventilation at an earlier stage than endotracheal intubation (ETI) is indicated with the aim of averting the need for ETI. (b) NIPPV can be carried out as a trial with a view to ETI if NIPPV fails or (c) NIPPV can be considered a maximum level of ventilatory treatment in a patient in whom ETI and ICU care is contraindicated.

The checklist below has been used to teach the introduction of NIPPV to a number of medical and ancillary staff. It is in the nature of guidelines that the advice is didactic and some of the comments may seem obvious. The use of several types of ventilator is described. For other ventilators the same basic principles apply when establishing settings on volume preset and pressure preset equipment. A flow chart summarizing decision-making when starting NIPPV in acute exacerbations of COPD is shown in Figure 5.1.

Further information on the initiation of NIPPV in paediatric patients is given in Chapter 15.

CHECKLIST FOR NIPPV

First check patient suitability:

1 Does the patient fulfil criteria for ARF, as listed above? Measurement of arterial blood gas tensions is mandatory.
2 Have conventional medical measures been fully explored? Ensure that controlled oxygen therapy (i.e. 24% or 28% O_2 via Venturi mask) is used in hypercapnic patients, and that bronchodilator, steroid, antibiotic and/or diuretic therapy is

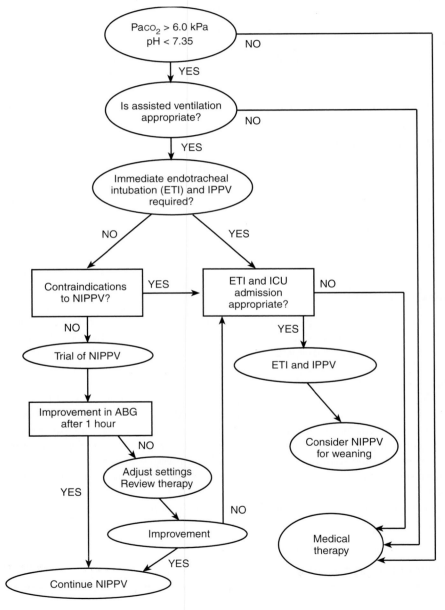

Figure 5.1 *Flow-chart for NIPPV in acute exacerbations of COPD.*

prescribed and delivered optimally. Is conventional intubation and ventilation the treatment of choice? For example, in patients with contraindications to NIPPV, or conditions such as acute severe asthma with hypercapnia, or gross sputum retention.

3 Next, remember that NIPPV is not universally successful. Consider the following: what are the reversible features in this case? Assess the patient's quality of life and prognosis. Is short- or long-term benefit likely? What are the patient's and family's views? Do the patient and family want active treatment? What are their expectations from treatment?

4 It is crucial to decide in advance what you are going to do if NIPPV fails, taking advice from senior team members where appropriate. Would it be logical to proceed to intubation and conventional ventilation? In this situation it is essential that anaesthetic/ICU staff are involved. In some cases it may be appropriate to provide NIPPV, but not to proceed to ETT and ventilation if NIPPV fails.

Assuming you wish to go ahead:

5 Where should NIPPV be carried out? This is discussed in Chapters 3, 4, 7 and 8. Patients with severe respiratory failure in whom intubation and ventilation is indicated if NIPPV fails, should be cared for in an ICU, and this is likely to be the site of management in post-extubation respiratory failure. In other patients a respiratory or general high dependency (intermediate care) unit offers a better nurse : patient ratio and usually a dedicated NIPPV team, so is the area of choice. NIPPV can be safely and effectively carried out on a general/respiratory ward area with appropriately trained staff,[1] but this is not ideal in moderately or severely acidotic patients (i.e. if pH < 7.30). Clearly the location of the patient may be influenced by bed availability, particularly in countries such as the UK where there is an ICU bed shortage and a limited number of high dependency units, but patient safety should always be the main priority.

Equipment

WHICH VENTILATOR?

6 Types of ventilator are described in Chapter 2. There are very little data to suggest that one ventilator is superior to others in ARF. In theory volume or pressure preset ventilators may be preferable in the circumstances shown in Boxes 5.2 and 5.3. These issues are discussed fully in Chapter 2. However, staff familiarity with the ventilator is an extremely important determinant of success

---

Box 5.2 *Situations in which pressure preset ventilator* may *be preferable*

Presence of pneumothorax or bullous lung disease
Persisting airleak post-surgery
Problematic symptoms of gastric distension
Positive expiratory pressure required e.g. atelectasis

Box 5.3 *Situations where volume preset ventilator* may *be preferable*

Labile airflow resistance or pulmonary compliance
Very high thoracic impedance e.g. severe chest wall disease

---

and it is generally better to use a ventilator you are familiar with than one which might be theoretically superior, but with which you have minimal experience. In some units, only one type of ventilator is available.

7   It is advisable to assemble the ventilator and circuit and check that it works, BEFORE taking it to the bedside. Ensure that the tubing connected with the exhalation valve is adjacent to the mask. With some of the bilevel pressure support systems such as the BiPAP (Respironics Inc.), it is possible to use one of a number of exhalation port options such as the whisper swivel valve, plateau valve, circuit with simple exhalation port, or mask with expiratory ports (Figure 5.2) – see Chapter 2. Ensure you have one exhalation option in place. Consult the operator manual to re-aquaint yourself with the operating characteristics of the machine. It is, of course, a remarkable fact of life that this key information often missing when it is most needed, therefore basic advice regarding the set-up of various models is given below.

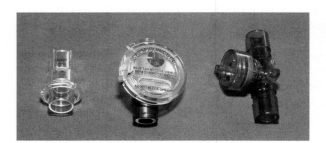

Figure 5.2 *Exhalation port options. Left to right: whisper swivel valve, plateau valve, expiratory valve.*

8   EXPLAIN what you are going to do, why you are doing it, and the sensations the patient is likely to experience. If time allows you may be able to introduce the patient to another individual using NIPPV.

9   It is helpful to start by entraining O_2 connected by tubing to a porthole in the mask or via T-piece in the circuitry (Figure 5.3) if baseline Po_2 is less than 7.0 kPa, as patients are more likely to become claustrophobic using the mask if hypoxaemia is not rapidly corrected. A flow rate of 1–2 L/min is usually sufficient, unless the patient is extremely hypoxaemic, but aim to raise Sao_2 to > 88% at least.

10 The fitting of the mask is crucial to the success of the technique. A small nasal mask is usually suitable for females, males need a medium, MS or MN. Try to match the mask to the contours and size of the patient's face. Mask fitting templates are available from some manufacturers (e.g. Respironics Inc., ResMed). If the patient uses dentures it is helpful to keep these in place. If the patient is confused, very dyspnoeic, or mouth breathing, a full facemask is

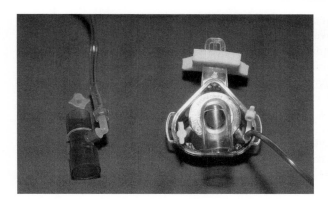

Figure 5.3 *Oxygen entrainment via porthole in mask or T-piece in circuit.*

usually a better choice, but this can make some individuals feel claustrophobic. Where possible use the mask the patient prefers. Further details on masks and other interfaces are given in Chapter 2.

11 Make sure that the patient is lying comfortably on the bed, propped by pillows in a semi-reclining position to minimize dypnoea. It is best to let him/her hold the mask firmly to the face at first. Remind them that they should breathe through their nose and keep their mouth shut, if using a nasal mask. Once the patient is happy to continue breathing through the mask, secure it in place using the headgear. Time spent fitting the mask and building the patient's confidence at this stage is well-invested.

INITIAL VENTILATOR SETTINGS

FOR THE BIPAP (RESPIRONICS INC.) VENTILATOR MODELS (FIGURE 5.4)

Add O_2 1–2 L/minute as above if PaO_2 < 7 kPa.
In adults set an inspiratory pressure (IPAP) of around 10–14 cmH_2O. Set EPAP at 4 cmH_2O.

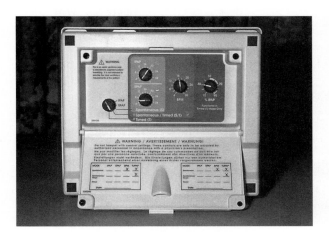

Figure 5.4 *BiPAP S/T (Respironics Inc.).*

Use the machine in spontaneous/timed (S/T) mode. S mode (assist only) may be sufficient if central drive is not depressed, but is not advisable in neuromuscular or central hypoventilation cases, or severely hypercapnic patients.

Set a back-up respiratory rate of around 10–12 breaths/minute.

Check SaO_2 and ABG after one hour as above. Increase inspiratory pressure by 2 cmH$_2$O increments to reduce PCO_2. Most individuals (apart from those with neuromuscular disease or children) will need an inspiratory pressure of > 12 cmH$_2$O.

Some patients with neuromuscular disease and COPD may benefit from a higher level of EPAP (up to 6 cmH$_2$O) – see Chapter 3. High levels of EPAP (> 7 cmH$_2$O) reduce effective pressure support and can prove counter-productive.[2]

FOR THE VPAP (RESMED) VENTILATOR (FIGURE 5.5)

Add O$_2$ at 1–2 L/minute as above if PaO$_2$ > 7 kPa.

The VPAP settings are determined using a menu indicated on a liquid crystal display (LCD) window on the front of the machine. To access the set-up menu, press the three right-hand buttons on the control panel simultaneously while turning the ventilator on. A cursor will appear on the LCD window by each setting in turn. The first to appear is MODE. Using the option buttons which scroll the screen up or down, select CPAP, S, S/T or T mode.

IPAP and EPAP levels are set in turn using the option buttons to increase and decrease the values to the desired levels. The machine is preset with default values of IPAP 10 cmH$_2$O, EPAP 8 cmH$_2$O. Try initial values of IPAP 10 cmH$_2$O, EPAP 4 cmH$_2$O in adults. In S mode only IPAP and EPAP levels require setting. In S/T mode IPAP maximum time and back-up rate (bpm) also need to be entered. For IPAP maximum time, approx 3 seconds is suggested, (but do not exceed 50% of respiratory cycle), and for breaths per minute 10–12/min is a reasonable starting level.

Other optional settings include mask alarm, delay time before maximum pressure is delivered and overheat default. In an emergency these optional variables can be safely left at the default setting and subsequently adjusted as required. Note

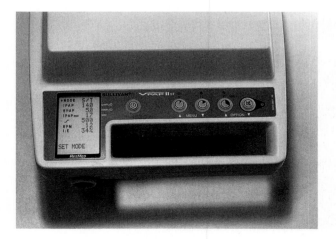

Figure 5.5   VPAP S/T (Resmed).

that in the set-up menu there is an ON/OFF option for a humidifier, if used. The settings can be locked by using the patient mode in option YES. Locking of the settings is recommended for home use, but not when initially titrating therapy.

Once you have established the settings, begin treatment by pressing the START/STOP button. You will notice that an S icon appears on the LCD when the patient triggers a breath spontaneously and a T icon appears when the machine automatically cycles from EPAP to IPAP.

Titrate IPAP and EPAP settings according to patient comfort and arterial blood gas results. Increase IPAP by 2 cmH$_2$O increments until optimal results are achieved. If synchronization is poor, check for leaks and adjust IPAP max. Further advice on problem-solving is given in Chapter 6.

FOR THE NIPPY VENTILATOR MODELS (B&D ELECTROMEDICAL)

Add O$_2$ 1–2L/minute as above if Pao$_2$ < 7 kPa.

Start at a low pressure setting e.g. C or D (10–15 cmH$_2$O) – see Figure 5.6. Set an inspiratory time of approx 1 second and an expiratory time of around 2.5 seconds. Trigger sensitivity should be low (0.5 cmH$_2$O) to reduce the work of breathing. The high pressure alarm should be set between 30 and 40 cmH$_2$O, low pressure alarm at around 8–10 cmH$_2$O (and below IPAP level). Gradually increase inspiratory pressure as the patient settles into using the machine, and titrate inspiratory and expiratory time to comfort. Most adults will need a pressure of > 12 cmH$_2$O. Adjust pressure by increasing by one alphabetical letter setting at a time e.g. E to F, and Fio$_2$ according to arterial blood gas tensions.

The NIPPY 2 differs from the standard NIPPY model in that EPAP (PEEP) can be added, there is a flow rather than pressure trigger, inspiratory pressure is set numerically rather than by alphabetical scale, and there are high and low flow alarms. The Nippaed model is a paediatric version of the NIPPY 2. The circuitry for the NIPPY and NIPPY 2 are different in that the NIPPY utilizes an exhalation valve, while the NIPPY2/Nippaed use a single tube with the requirement for an exhalation port in the mask.

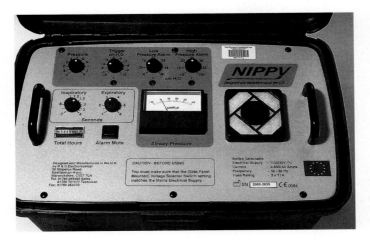

Figure 5.6 *NIPPY (B&D Electro-medical).*

FOR THE PV 401 VENTILATOR (BREAS MEDICAL LTD)

The PV 401 is set up using a multifunction button on the LCD on the front of the machine similar to that on the PV 403 (Figure 5.7). The machine is turned on by pressing the ON/OFF button for 2 seconds. Two modes are available: pressure support ventilation (PSV) or pressure controlled ventilation (PCV) – see Chapter 2 for a further description of modes. To change between the modes press the MODE button for one second. To adjust all other settings, press the function button indicated by an up and down arrow. The function button allows one to scroll through a series of parameters and alter these in turn using the + and – buttons. Where a Yes or No selection is required press + for Yes and – for No. In order of appearance on the menu, set pressure e.g. 10–14 cmH$_2$O, breaths per minute (e.g. 10–12), inspiratory time e.g. 1–2 seconds (available only in PCV mode), inspiratory trigger, plateau, and expiratory trigger (only in PCV mode). Default values of –0.5 cmH$_2$O for inspiratory trigger, setting 6 for plateau and 30% for expiratory trigger are suggested.

The alarms are fixed by pressing ALARM SET button, and then Yes by selecting the + button. The Low pressure alarm is activated if a set percentage of the pressure level is not reached within 15 seconds e.g. due to leak or disconnection of circuitry. A value of 60–70% of inspiratory pressure is suggested.

An estimated tidal volume can also be set so that the low tidal volume alarm is activated if this value is not achieved. Alarm function can be checked by switching off power to trigger power failure alarm, occluding the circuitry to trigger the high pressure alarm, and creating a leak to activate the low pressure and low volume alarms. The settings are locked by pressing and holding both the + and – buttons

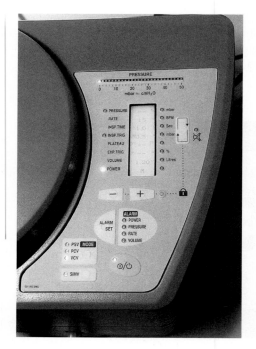

Figure 5.7 *PV403 (Breas Medical).*

for 5 seconds. To unlock, press the same buttons simultaneously for five seconds. It is only possible to adjust settings in unlocked mode. Note that the ON/OFF green light shines continuously when the machine is operated by mains supply and flashes intermittently when the machine is operated by external battery.

FOR THE PV 403 (BREAS MEDICAL LTD) (FIGURE 5.7)

This ventilator combines pressure and volume preset modes. For the pressure preset options (PCV and PSV), set up is as for the PV 401. For volume controlled mode (VCV) set tidal volume by pressing function button until Volume LED is lit. Use the + or – buttons to adjust tidal volume. A range of 300 mL to 1600 mL is available. Tidal volume requirement is greater with non-invasive ventilation than invasive ventilation because of inevitable leaks and upper airway deadspace. A tidal volume of 8–10 mL/kg is a reasonable starting point. Next set rate and inspiratory time. If the combination of rate and tidal volume selected is impossible for the machine to deliver, the preset tidal volume will be delivered but rate may be incorrect. In this eventuality the volume and rate LEDS will flash as a warning. In the VCV mode there are alarms for high and low pressure and high rate (see Box 5.4).

Box 5.4 Summary of settings for PV 401 and 403

	PCV mode	PSV mode	VCV mode
Pressure	Yes	Yes	No
Rate	Yes	Yes	Yes
Inspiration time	Yes	No	Yes
Inspiration trigger	Yes	Yes	Yes
Plateau	Yes	Yes	No
Expiration trigger	No	Yes	No
Tidal volume	No	No	Yes

FOR THE HARMONY VENTILATOR (RESPIRONICS INC.)

Set-up principles are similar to the BiPAP. However, the Harmony S/T differs from the standard BiPAP model in that device controls are on the top of the machine and IPAP, EPAP and back-up rate set by slide control knobs (Figure 5.8). IPAP rise time can be adjusted. Controls are protected by a plastic cover is opened by pressing on the recessed plastic locking tab directly below the panel cover with a pencil, ball point pen tip or screwdriver. There are power and patient disconnect alarms, and a DC battery is available.

FOR THE BROMPTONPAC (VOLUME PRESET VENTILATOR)

Start with a fairly low flow ($\dot{V}$) setting (left hand knob) – around 0.7–0.8 L/second. Very tachypnoeic patients will require a shorter TI (inspiratory time) and TE (expiratory time) than patients with reduced ventilatory effort (e.g. COPD blue bloaters). Remember that the patient will usually be triggering the ventilator, so

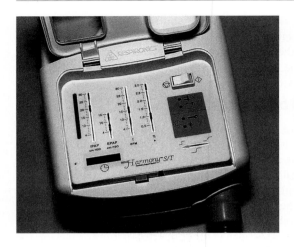

Figure 5.8 *Harmony (Respironics Inc.).*

they will normally determine the TE. An average TI setting is around 1 second, with a TE set at 2.5 seconds. However, respond to what the patient feels is comfortable. It is helpful to ask 'Are you getting a big enough breath?' and adjust the flow accordingly, and 'Does the breath feel long enough?' and adjust TI accordingly. If the patient feels that the breaths are coming too fast, TE may be too short. A more usual reason is patient anxiety which should respond to reassurance.

Alarms: expect an inflation pressure of 20–40 cmH$_2$O. The delivered pressure reflects the pressure in the upper airway, not necessarily that in the lung. With volume preset ventilators you should be able to reduce peak inflation pressure in patients at risk of pneumothorax (e.g. by reducing flow rate or increasing TI). Pressure preset machines will not exceed the inspiratory pressure setting. The upper pressure alarm should be set at around 30–40 cmH$_2$O. This may need to be reset higher in the occasional patient e.g. those with cystic fibrosis and sputum retention, or severe thoracic impedance.

The low pressure alarm should be set at around 8–12 cmH$_2$O. In the first 24 hours of NIPPV a balance should be struck between avoiding leaks and keeping the whole ward awake with the low pressure alarm. The usual reason for the alarm going off is because the pressure falls due to leaks from the mouth or around mask. The ventilator will alarm if the patient keeps talking when using a nasal mask! Some patients need a chin strap to keep the mouth shut during sleep.

HIGH DEPENDENCY UNIT VENTILATORS

The BiPAP Vision (Respironics Inc.) offers CPAP, Bilevel S/T and PAV/T modes. It also provides visual data on flow/pressure profiles and patient effort, a range of alarms and optional oxygen mixer. After switching on (rear of machine), an exhalation port check should be carried out as described by instructions which appear on the set-up screen. Press the Monitoring key and set the alarms. Using the MODE key select CPAP, S/T or PAV mode. Press the Set Up Parameters screen and adjust the CPAP or IPAP and EPAP and rate settings on the screen. Activate the new mode key.

PAV mode is an optional extra mode supplied with the Vision: the principles of proportional assist ventilation are described in Chapter 2. Since PAV is dependent on the patient's respiratory effort it should not be used in patients with significantly depressed ventilatory drive. The Vision offers a quickstart PAV menu for patients with obstructive disease, restrictive disease or normal lungs, or a custom option. Key controls are flow assist (FA) which is used to overcome resistance and volume assist (VA) used to overcome elastance. An increase in flow assist will amplify inspiratory flow rate and volume assist will increase tidal volume. The % Set control determines the amount of support provided. This should be adjusted to comfort. Bilevel (BiPAP) ventilation is available as an important back-up in case the patient become apnoeic or ventilatory drive falls. Using the quickstart option the VA and FA are preset at 30% of the allowable range. These can be adjusted using the % Set control until the patient is comfortable. Suggested EPAP level is 4 cmH$_2$O with a PAV pressure limit of 30 cmH$_2$O and PAV volume limit of 1.5 L. If comfort cannot be achieved using the quickstart mode, the custom option can be tried. It is suggested that initial setting are % Set 80%, VA 5 cmH$_2$O/L, FA 2 cmH$_2$O/L/s, EPAP 4 cmH$_2$O with back ventilation of IPAP 15 rate 8, timed inspiration 1.0 s and rise time 0.1 s. To titrate VA, gradually increase VA until the patient feels a sensation of too much air/pressure per breath, then decrease slightly to provide optimal assistance. Next increase FA gradually until the patient feels flow is too fast; turn back slightly to establish optimal flow. Note that the % Set control varies both VA and FA simultaneously.

The Vision guide should be consulted for more comprehensive instructions.

MONITORING

Monitor progress in all patients with oximetry. Aim for a Sa$_{O_2}$2 of > 88%, but judge each case individually. An Sa$_{O_2}$ of 88% may be entirely acceptable in a severe COPD patient, but an Sa$_{O_2}$ > 95% is more appropriate in a neuromuscular patient with normal lungs. If a suitable level is not achieved increase O$_2$ flow rate and/or adjust ventilation depending on Pa$_{CO_2}$. In severely ill patients ECG monitoring and an arterial line will facilitate management. The patient will need close observation and encouragement during the initial period of NIPPV, to build confidence. Relief of dyspnoea and a reduction or abolition of accessory muscle activity are encouraging signs. Those in whom NIPPV is started electively, often take longer to acclimatize as symptoms are relieved more slowly.

Be patient and wait at least 30–60 minutes before checking arterial blood gas tensions with the patient on NIPPV, unless the situation seems to be very rapidly deteriorating. DO NOT expect a major change in Pa$_{CO_2}$. The aim is adequate oxygenation and a reduction in respiratory acidosis, without an uncontrolled increase in Pa$_{CO_2}$. Nasal ventilation is relatively inefficient and so blood gases should improve gradually rather than rapidly. A rise in pH and fall in Pa$_{CO_2}$ after the first hour of NPPV are good prognostic signs. Gradually increase ventilator flow rate or inspiratory pressure to improve P$_{CO_2}$ control. An increase in inspiratory time (TI) may help improve P$_{O_2}$ if the patient can tolerate this – otherwise increase supplemental O$_2$ flow rate and/or improve overall ventilation. An increase in EPAP

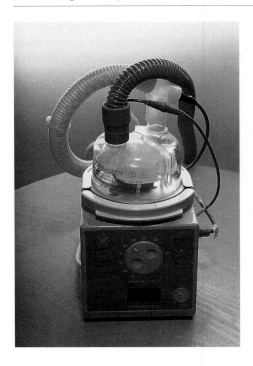

Figure 5.9 *Heated water bath humidification (Fisher & Paykel).*

may help patients with upper airway obstruction or atelectasis. The recipient is unlikely to feel much better unless PaO_2 increases to at least 7.0–8.0 kPa, or SaO_2 is > 88%. Many patients with acute exacerbations are sleep deprived and as soon as dyspnoea lessens and gases improve they fall asleep. REM sleep rebound is common, leading to reduction in postural muscle tone, potential upper airway obstruction, leaks and desynchronization. The body twitching and deep level of sleep associated with REM sleep can be confused with signs of CO_2 narcosis. Providing CO_2 is not rising markedly, a review of settings including an increase in EPAP to maintain upper airway patency, adjustment in IPAP to improve overall ventilation and switch to a full facemask may be all that is required.

Humidification

Humidification is not routinely required, but may be valuable in patients with tenacious secretions or rhinitis. A heat and moisture exchanger (e.g. Portex thermovent) can be used, or for more intensive humidification a heated water bath system (e.g. Fisher & Paykel) (Figure 5.9).

How much time should the patient spend on NIPPV?

Studies have shown a wide range in duration of use of NIPPV in acute exacerbations. In several recent randomized controlled trials in acute exacerbations of

COPD, average use was 6–8 hours in the first 24 hours and this tailed off gradually over the next few days. In most of these studies patients were initially encouraged to use NIPPV as much as possible, particularly during sleep. Primary failure of therapy requiring intubation is most likely within the first 24 hours, therefore attention should be maximally focused on compliance within this period. The successful use of sequential NIPPV has been described, i.e. several hours of NIPPV alternated with periods of spontaneous breathing. In practice this probably occurs anyway as patients discontinue NIPPV for meals and visits from relatives etc. depending on symptom control. It is notable that in the only randomized trial of NIPPV in acute COPD which did not show benefit, NIPPV was employed for just three-hour periods in the morning and afternoon. It seems logical therefore to encourage use for as long as the patient can tolerate for at least the first 24 hours and then gradually reduce support, according to clinical progress.

Tolerance of NIPPV

Initially some patients may only be able to tolerate NIPPV for short periods. It is important to explore whether this is because ventilation is inadequate, patient and ventilator are not synchronized, the mask is uncomfortable, the patient is confused, or other medical problems have developed. However, where ventilatory efficiency has been optimized as far as possible, short periods of use are often better than nothing, so encourage the patient and gradually increase use – especially at night.

If patients who have previously setlled well into NIPPV become desynchronized, in the absence of obvious problems such as mouth leak, it is vital to check arterial blood gas tensions and carry out a physical examination to exclude the development of intercurrent events such as pneumothorax, atelectasis or pulmonary oedema.

Swapping to a different ventilator

This may be required for a number of reasons (Box 5.5):

Box 5.5 *Reasons for swapping to a different ventilator*

- Patient requires higher IPAP level than provided by current machine
- Patient requires EPAP which is not available on current machine
- Patient develops gastric distension or problematic leaks on volume preset machine. Swap to pressure preset machine
- Ventilation poorly controlled on pressure preset machine. Consider swap to volume preset ventilator (see Chapter 2)
- Patient requires ventilator with additional features not available with current model; e.g. battery pack, alarms, dual 220/110 voltage
- Elective stepping down from ICU ventilator to home ventilator
- Patient preference

NIPPV failure

This is reported to occur in between 5% and 40% of patients[3-8] with an average failure rate of around 20%. Early failure occurs within the first 24–48 hours of therapy, whereas late failure can be defined as need for intubation or death after 48 hours following the initial successful application of NIPPV.[9] Technical problems and poor tolerance are probably contributory factors to the primary failure of the technique, but are not common reasons for late failure as compliance rates in those who succeed with or fail therapy after 48 hours are similar.[9] As discussed in Chapter 3, severe acidosis and failure to increase pH and reduce hypercapnia after 1 hour of NIPPV are useful predictors of a poor outcome. Moretti *et al.*[9] found a late failure rate of 23%. This was again correlated with pH on admission, but was also more likely to occur in individuals with severe functional limitation before admission, and in the presence of medical complications such as hyperglycaemia.

If NIPPV is failing and the patient is having problems tolerating the therapy, he/she should either be intubated, or if this is felt inappropriate NIPPV should be withdrawn while continuing with full symptomatic measures (Figure 5.1).

Practical problems

In one study[10] of the acute use of NIPPV the incidence of side effects was: mask discomfort 32%, dry nose 20%, air leaks 16%, eye irritation 16%, gastric distension 8%. Not surprisingly, mask symptoms and nasal bridge sores increase when NIPPV is used intensively during a phase of acute illness and are less common during long-term nocturnal domiciliary use. By and large, side effects do not cause NIPPV to be discontinued, but they do limit the efficiency of treatment. Problem-solving is discussed in Chapter 6.

STARTING NIPPV IN PATIENTS WITH A TRACHEOSTOMY OR ENDOTRACHEAL TUBE

Patients should be medically stable and fulfil minimal criteria (Box 5.6) before a switch from invasive to non-invasive ventilation can be safely achieved (see Chapter 7).

Box 5.6 *Criteria for extubation/decannulation and use of NIPPV*

- Able to breathe spontaneously for 5 minutes
- Alert and able to tolerate mask
- No evidence of moderate or severe bulbar weakness
- Intact upper airway
- Minimal bronchial secretions
- Low Fio_2 requirement (normally < 0.4)
- Normal gastrointestinal function

It is sensible to first ensure arterial blood gas tensions can be controlled in the intubated patient using the ventilator you intend to employ with the mask interface. As deadspace and leaks are minimized in intubated patients, the tidal volume or inspiratory pressure required will be lower than in a patient using a mask. Providing there is a reasonable leak around the tracheostomy tube or ETT you can allow the patient to try mask ventilation before he or she is extubated/decannulated. If a cuffed tracheostomy or ETT is in use, it is essential to deflate the cuff first and then occlude the trachestomy/ETT so that the patient breathes through the upper airway.

Bear in mind that a patient breathing through a nasal mask with an ETT or tracheostomy tube *in situ* will have an increased respiratory workload breathing around the tube, and therefore the sensation they experience will not mimic NIPPV exactly. Our usual practice is to carry out suction, then extubate/decannulate the patient on to the mask system with O_2 entrained at 1–2 L/minute. Monitor Sao_2, heart rate, blood pressure and transcutaneous $CO_2/Etco_2$ (where possible), and check arterial blood gas tensions after 40–60 minutes, depending on progress. Oxygen flow rate, and ventilator settings can then be adjusted to optimize blood gas tensions as described above.

STARTING AN NIPPV SERVICE

A survey in 1997[11] showed that only 48% of units admitting acute respiratory patients in the UK are able to provide NIPPV. Considering that these hospitals will inevitably admit patients with acute excerbations of COPD, and NIPPV in this group has been demonstrated to be effective (Chapter 3), there is a need to create or expand NIPPV facilties in a significant number of acute hospitals. The UK is not alone in this respect.[12] Plant et al.[13] have estimated that up to 20% of patients admitted with an acute exacerbation of COPD may benefit from NIPPV. In ICUs familiar with the technique NIPPV is now being used in 16% of patients with acute respiratory failure requiring mechanical ventilation. There are no statistics on the use of NIPPV for weaning, but here too use is evidence-based.[14,15] There is therefore ample justification to set up a service, and evidence that cost savings will ensue.[13] Services should always be designed to meet local needs and therefore any advice on setting up an NIPPV cannot be prescriptive. However, the following points may be of value:

- NIPPV needs to be available on a 24-hour basis. While the decision to start NIPPV should usually be made by medical staff, initiation of NIPPV should be multidisciplinary and in most successful programmes nursing staff, physiotherapists and respiratory support technicians play a key role in initiating and monitoring therapy.
- A rolling educational programme is essential to maintain skills and train new staff members. With a high medical trainee and nursing staff turnover, skills and confidence can quickly be lost even in experienced units.
- Protocols and guidelines play an important role in training and quality control, but need to need interpreted with flexibility and common sense. Some units may

find a standardized ventilator start-up protocol as described by Plant et al.[1] helpful.

- The average unit may require around three ventilators initially, but clearly this depends on case load, ICU use etc. It is sensible to stick to one or two models of ventilator (at least one of which should provide bilevel pressure support) to improve staff (and patient) familiarity, and simplify teaching.
- Do not economize on mask interfaces. A range of full facemasks, nasal masks and nasal plugs of all sizes should be available. Even the most experienced NIPPV operator will fail if the patient finds the mask is uncomfortable.
- Initiation of NIPPV in unstable patients is best carried out in an HDU. There needs to be a strong and seamless link with ICU staff to ensure that patients who require intubation are safely managed. NIPPV can be performed successfully on a general respiratory ward[1] in selected patients, but this requires an experienced team and adequate nursing levels. Management of patients with a pH of < 7.30 is not advisable on a general ward.
- In most patients with an acute episode of ventilatory failure NIPPV will be required for a few days. Over time it is inevitable that a small number of patients (often with restrictive problems) will be identified who will benefit from long-term home NIPPV. These patients should be referred to a centre with experience in domiciliary ventilation.
- Regular audit should not only help improve performance but will also alert colleagues as to the most appropriate patients to refer. Patients requiring NIPPV need inpatient care and follow-up by a respiratory physician.

REFERENCES

1   Plant PK, Owen JL, Elliott MW. Early use of noninvasive ventilation for acute exacerbations of chronic obstructive pulmonary disease on general respiratory wards: a multicentre randomised controlled trial. *Lancet* 2000; **355**: 1931–5.
2   Elliott MW, Simonds AK. Nocturnal assisted ventilation using bilevel positive airway pressure: the effect of expiratory positive airway pressure. *Eur Respir J* 1995; **8**: 436–40.
3   Bott J, Carroll MP, Conway JH, *et al*. Randomised controlled trial of nasal ventilation in acute ventilatory failure due to chronic obstructive airways disease. *Lancet* 1993; **341**: 1555–7.
4   Brochard L, Mancebo J, Wysocki M, *et al*. Noninvasive ventilation for acute exacerbations of chronic pulmonary disease. *N Engl J Med* 1995; **333**: 817–22.
5   Kramer N, Meyer TJ, Meharg J, Cece RD, Hill NS. Randomized prospective trial of noninvasive positive pressure ventilation in acute respiratory failure. *Am J Respir Crit Care Med* 1995; **151**: 1799–1806.
6   Wood KA, Lewis L, Von Harz B, Kollef MH. The use of noninvasive positive pressure ventilation in the Emergency Department. Results of a randomized clinical trial. *Chest* 1998; **113**: 1339–46.
7   Celikel T, Sungur M, Ceyhan B. Comparison of non-invasive positive ventilation with standard medical therapy in hypercapnic acute respiratory failure. *Chest* 1998; **114**: 1636–42.

8   Ambrosino N, Foglio K, Rubini F, Clini E, Nava S, Vitacca M. Non-invasive mechanical ventilation in acute respiratory failure due to chronic obstructive airways disease: correlates for success. *Thorax* 1995; **50**: 755–7.

9   Moretti M, Cilione C, Tampieri A, Fracchia C, Marchioni A, Nava S. Incidence and causes of non-invasive mechanical ventilation failure after initial success. *Thorax* 2000; **55**: 819–25.

10 Foglio C, Vitacca M, Quadri A, Scalvini S, Marangoni S, Ambrosino N. Acute exacerbations in severe COLD patients. Treatment using positive pressure ventilation by nasal mask. *Chest* 1992; **101**: 1533–8.

11 Doherty MJ, Greenstone MA. Survey of non-invasive ventilation (NIPPV) in patients with acute exacerbations of chronic obstructive pulmonary disease (COPD) in the UK. *Thorax* 1998; **53**: 863–6.

12 Nava S, Confalonieri M, Rampulla C. Intermediate respiratory intensive care units in Europe: a European perspective. *Thorax* 1999; **53**: 798–802.

13 Plant PK, Owen JL, Elliott MW. One year period prevalence study of respiratory acidosis in acute exacerbations of COPD: implications for the provision of non-invasive ventilation and oxygen provision. *Thorax* 2000; **55**: 550–4.

14 Nava S, Ambrosino N, Vitacca M, Orlando A, Prato M, Rubini F. Randomised prospective study of the use of non-invasive mechanical ventilation (NIMV) in the weaning from invasive mechanical ventilation in severe COPD patients. *Eur Respir J* 1996; **9**: 281s.

15 Girault C, Daudenthun I, Chevron V, Tamion F, Leroy J, Bonmarchand G. Noninvasive ventilation as a systematic extubation and weaning technique in acute on chronic respiratory failure. A prospective randomized controlled study. *Am J Resp Crit Care Med* 1999; **160**: 86–92.

16 Evans TW. International Consensus Conferences: Non-invasive positive pressure ventilation in acute respiratory failure. *Int Care Med* 2001; **27**: 166–78.

FURTHER READING

British Thoracic Society Guidelines: Non-invasive ventilation in acute respiratory failure. Standards of Care Committee. *Thorax* 2002; **57**: 192–211. Also available at British Thoracic Society website: *www.brit-thoracic.org.uk*

Mehta S, Hill NS. Non-invasive ventilation: state of the art. *Am J Respir Crit Care Med* 2001; **163**: 540–77.

Non-invasive positive pressure ventilation in acute respiratory failure: Report of an International Consensus Conference in Intensive Care Medicine.[16]

6

Problem solving in acute NIPPV

S HEATHER, A K SIMONDS AND S WARD

GENERAL APPROACH TO NIPPV PROBLEMS

NIPPV is not a universal panacea in patients with respiratory insufficiency. There is an established failure rate of around 5–40% depending on the application (see Chapters 3–5 and Chapter 7) and these may be primary failures (i.e. failure to initiate therapy), or late failures in patients already established on NIPPV. Success rates are improved by the appropriate selection of patients and choice of equipment. Having said that, there are number of fairly consistent problems that limit effectiveness but which can be dealt with successfully using the simple measures outlined below. A diagnostic approach to the problem is, however, vital. It should also be recognized that, by and large, correction in arterial blood gas tensions is more gradual using non-invasive ventilation than invasive techniques, as ventilation is wasted through leaks and upper airway and equipment deadspace, and support is usually intermittent rather than continuous. It is always best to identify *why* a problem has arisen, and consider whether it may be due to an underlying change in pathology rather than a simple equipment issue. This is especially the case in a patient who has previously coped well with NIPPV. In this situation if inflation pressure suddenly rises, or the patient becomes more confused, clinical re-examination is mandatory. The individual may, for example, be developing increasing bronchospasm or a pneumothorax requiring nebulized bronchodilator, a chest drain etc. A minor alteration in IPAP level is clearly not the solution here, although as a secondary issue ventilator settings may need to be adjusted. Assuming medical problems are optimally addressed, we have found the following step by step strategy useful in dealing with common NIPPV problems on the wards.

THE STEP BY STEP STRATEGY

Persistent hypercapnia

PROBLEM

$PaCO_2$ increases after initiation of NIPPV, or falls only slightly. The causes are: inspiratory pressure, tidal volume or back-up respiratory rate too low, leaks, rebreathing, asynchrony, insufficient duration of time on NIPPV, inappropriate oxygenation.

ACTION

Increase the pressure or volume setting. Pressure should be increased by around $2 cmH_2O$ at a time. A higher back-up respiratory rate may help, but bear in mind that most patients with intact ventilatory drive will be triggering the ventilator and back-up rate may only be utilized during sleep. Ensure that ventilation is not wasted due to leaks, or desynchronization between patient and ventilator (see below). Occasionally a swap to a more powerful ventilator is required (see Chapter 2).

Consider whether *rebreathing* is occurring. Mask and tubing deadspace should be minimized. A minimum EPAP of at least $4 cmH_2O$ is necessary to flush circuit deadspace when using bilevel single circuit ventilators such as BiPAP/Harmony (Respironics Inc.) and VPAP (ResMed). Exhalation in these systems is achieved using a whisper swivel exhalation valve, disposable circuit with exhalation port, mask with exhalation port, or plateau exhalation valve (Figure 5.2). Carbon dioxide clearance varies between the exhalation devices, and in small adult or paediatric patients requiring low inspiratory pressures a trial of a different exhalation system e.g. switch to a plateau valve may improve CO_2 control.[1]

Ensure the patient is not being over-oxygenated. A discussion of ideal SaO_2 level during ventilation is given in Chapter 5. It is important that during periods of spontaneous breathing off NIPPV controlled oxygen therapy is used in patients with significant hypercapnia. Uncontrolled oxygen therapy during these periods can easily offset the value of time spent using NIPPV.

Is the patient spending insufficient time on the ventilator? Encourage more sustained periods of use, particularly during sleep, and address compliance issues (see below). A NIPPV chart detailing start and stop times of NIPPV should be employed. Setting negotiated targets with individual patients is usually helpful.

Leaks

PROBLEM

Leaks from mask causing inefficient ventilation, eye irritation, noise, dry mouth and nasal symptoms.

ACTION

Take time to ensure the mask is a good fit. Leaks may be reduced by adjustment of headgear strapping, but be careful not too pull the straps too tight as this will distort the silicone cushion and lead to discomfort, pressure sores and further leaks. A full facemask will deal with persistent mouth leaks. These may also be reduced by a chin strap or cervical collar, but some patients find these additions constraining. Be prepared to try different mask types and use the fitting templates provided unless you are very experienced in mask fitting. In a minority of patients (in our opinion) an individually customized mask may be required. Simple advice to the patient to avoid mouth breathing and excessive talking during NIPPV is obviously sensible. As soon as possible train the patient to put their own mask on, as they are best placed to get the tension in the strapping and position as comfortable as possible. Ideally, keep dentures in place in edentulate patients. Accept that some minor leaks are inevitable, and that pressure preset ventilators will compensate for these.

Persistent hypoxaemia

PROBLEM

PaO_2 remains low on NIPPV.

ACTION

Ensure optimum ventilation (i.e. CO_2 control). Increase entrained O_2 flow via T-piece into circuit, ventilator oxygen mixer, or porthole in mask. An increase in Ti and EPAP may also be helpful to recruit alveoli and increase functional residual capacity (FRC). Increasing EPAP to around 6/7 cmH₂O may be particularly helpful in patients with atelactasis or pulmonary oedema (see Chapters 3 and 5 for advantages and disadvantages of EPAP).

Progressive and intractable hypoxaemia (as with progressive and uncontrolled hypercapnia or respiratory acidosis), should provoke consideration of the need for intubation and conventional ventilation.

Asynchrony between patient and ventilator

PROBLEM

Patient not triggering ventilator and interbreathing.

ACTION

Desynchrony is usually due to inappropriate ventilator settings resulting in persistent hypercapnia and hypoxaemia, leaks, or anxiety, and occur more often in patients with high ventilatory drive (e.g. in some heart failure, asthma, emphysema, intersitial lung disease and cystic fibrosis patients). Adjust inspiratory pressure/volume, respiratory rate and supplemental oxygen as described above. A very common cause of desynchrony is mouth breathing in a patient using a nasal mask or nasal plugs. By breathing through the mouth, the ventilator will not be triggered and will cycle at the back-up respiratory rate. This will be interpreted as an imposed rate by the patient, and during wakefulness is likely to be uncomfortable and confusing. It may also lead to breath stacking. If the patient cannot breath through his/her nose, swap to a full facemask. Ventilator performance may also contribute to asynchrony. If the patient's inspiratory flow demand is not met by the ventilator, or cycling to expiration does not occur effectively, poor co-ordination will result. COPD patients benefit from use of a set inspiratory time rather than a preset flow level determining the end of inspiration – this facility is available on some bilevel ventilators.[2,3] The diagnosis of complex asynchrony problems may be helped by the use of a ventilator such as the Vision (Respironics Inc.) which provides visual screen information on flow profiles.

NB: Ensure that the ventilator is functioning correctly. Exhalation valves may sometimes stick, or the ventilator may cycle inappropriately. If in doubt, substitute the ventilator with a similar model.

Hypocapnia/respiratory alkalosis

PROBLEM

$PaCO_2$ or $[H^+]$ falls too low after initiation of NIPPV.

ACTION

Minute ventilation is too high. Decrease IPAP or delivered volume.

Back-up respiratory rate may be also too high. Hypocapnia is most likely to occur in neuromuscular patients with highly compliant lungs and chest wall; it is unusual in COPD patients. Stridor and laryngospasm may occasionally be seen in patients in whom CO_2 is driven down too fast, as the glottis closes as a protective mechanism. If this occurs discontinue ventilation, reassure the patient and start again gently at a much lower inspiratory pressure/tidal volume.

Confusional state/aggressive behaviour

PROBLEM

The patient is agitated causing difficulty in initating and/or maintaining NIPPV.

ACTION

Patients suffering from severe hypercapnia and hypoxaemia are often disorientated and confused. When initiating NIPPV in such a patient it may be virtually impossible to explain your actions. This situation will not be rectified until you have improved the respiratory acidosis, hypercapnia and hypoxaemia.

Where possible, the patient should be moved to an area where constant supervision is available e.g. an HDU or ICU. Use a full facemask and correct hypoxaemia as soon as possible with entrained O_2.

Stay with the patient if you can, and ensure alterations in personnel and the environment around the patient are minimized. It may be necessary to hold the mask in place until changes in blood gas tensions occur.

NIPPV can almost always be applied without the need for sedation. In a highly confused patient who repeatedly removes the mask, sedation may be indicated. However, under these rare circumstances it is imperative that the patient is closely monitored, as if NIPPV is not then introduced successfully hypercapnic coma may ensue with disastrous consequences. The preference of our medical team is to use small doses of haloperidol (e.g. 2 mg PO, IM or IV), or diamorphine in patients with pulmonary oedema.

If these measures do not control agitation, or sedation is contraindicated, intubation and IPPV should be considered, or NIPPV discontinued and symptomatic measures used in those in whom therapy is palliative.

Unexpected high inflation pressures and/or difficulty inflating chest

PROBLEM

In patients on a volume preset ventilator, peak inflation pressures are high or the user experiences difficulty in inflating chest using any type of ventilator at previously adequate pressure levels. A sudden increase in inflation pressure may be due to bronchospasm, mucus plugging of airway, atelectasis, consolidation or pulmonary oedema reducing lung compliance. Tracheal stenosis, or more acutely, granulation tissue around a previous tracheostomy site in a recently decannulated patient will increase large airway resistance. Nasal congestion can contribute significantly. Clinical examination is required to differentiate these problems. Peak inflation pressure can be reduced in patients using volume preset ventilaton by increasing Ti and reducing tidal volume.

Nasal problems

PROBLEM

Nasal soreness, congestion or streaming, nasal bridge sore.

ACTION

The patient may experience problems with the nasal airway particularly when they are acutely unwell and using the ventilator for prolonged periods during the day as well as at night.

Nasal bridge pressure sore (Figure 6.1)
Much can be done to prevent pressure sores by ensuring that the patient is using a mask that fits them correctly. However, in patients using NIPPV intensively, the development of pressure sores is fairly common.

ActionFor treatment of pressure sores see Chapter 17.

In order to allow pressure sores to heal more rapidly, it is helpful to use an alternative interface for two to three days, for example switch to nasal plugs or a bubble mask.

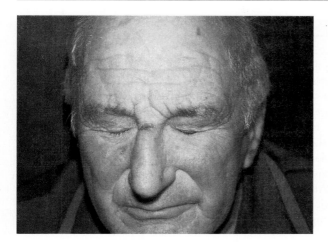

Figure 6.1 *Nasal bridge sore following a course of acute NIPPV.*

Rhinitis/nose bleeds

Some patients experience drying and crusting of the nasal muscosa, while in others profuse streaming can result.

ActionShort term use of 0.5% ephedrine nose drops help with early congestion. For longer term problems a nasal steroid preparation such as beclamethasone and fluticasone can be employed. Ipratropium bromide spray or aqueous drops may reduce nasal streaming. It should be recognized that mouth leaks cause a compensatory increase in flow through the nose and so dealing with these with a full facemask is logical, and will also offload the nasal airway. NIPPV is not routinely used in conjunction with heated humidification as the patient retains the ability to breathe through the nose or mouth. However, when NIPPV is being used intensively, time spent on the ventilator combined with the increased volumes of air passing through the airways can lead to cooling and drying of the mucous membranes which if severe is best addressed by humidification using either heat and moisture exchangers or a heated water bath system (Figures 2.9, 5.9).

Gastric distension

PROBLEM

Abdominal pain, distention and flatulence during and after NIPPV use.

ACTION

This is common in patients with neuromuscular disease, and paradoxically those with high thoracic impedance. In both groups, inspired air inflates the stomach more easily than the lungs. Repositioning in bed may help, as does the avoidance of carbonated drinks. Decrease the pressure or tidal volume, or if this fails try swapping from a volume to pressure limited model. It is not advisable to use NIPPV in patients with an ileus, therefore check for bowel sounds before initiating non-invasive therapy in post-operative patients.

Rapid eye movement (REM) sleep rebound

PROBLEM

Strictly speaking this is not a problem, and occurs as patients with acute on chronic ventilatory failure may be severely sleep deprived. Once effective NIPPV has been initiated, a natural response is to 'catch up' on missed REM sleep (REM rebound). Consequently, the patient may experience almost immediate and prolonged periods of REM sleep and during these may become deeply unresponsive with loss of intercostal and accessory muscle tone, and frequent twitching. In this state, the individual will be much more ventilator dependent, and as upper airway tone and neck muscle tone is reduced IPAP or tidal volume may need to be increased. Restlessness and REM sleep related twitching of arms and legs may be mistaken for hypercapnic coma and can be distinguished by careful blood gas monitoring.

ACTION

The patient should be in an area where close supervision is possible. Wherever possible, oxygen saturation and transcutaneous or end tidal carbon dioxide monitoring should be used to ensure ventilation is effective. A soft cervical collar can be used to help maintain neck position to reduce upper airway obstruction, an increase in EPAP will also help. REM rebound is beneficial to the patient's recovery and should not be unnecessarily interrupted. It is usually accomplished within the first 24 hours of therapy.

Troublesome cough

PROBLEM

Sometimes patients beginning treatment with NIPPV experience intense and productive coughing due to an airway cooling and drying effect, and mobilization of secretions. This is, of course, more common in patients with airway inflammation due to cystic fibrosis/bronchiectasis, asthma and COPD.

ACTION

Heated humidification is usually the answer, combined with physiotherapy to clear secretions (see Chapter 17). Ensure that airflow obstruction is adequately treated with bronchodilator, steroids, antibiotics, etc.

Claustrophobia

PROBLEM

Claustrophobia is not uncommon in dyspnoeic patients and may be made worse by the use of a mask.

ACTION

Use a small interface such as nasal plugs, the Monarch system or Simplicity mask (Respironics Inc.) where possible. Ensure optimal correction of hypoxaemia. Allow the patient to hold the mask in place and keep in control of the situation, if able. In an extreme case of claustrophobia in patients requiring long-term NIPPV, a programme of desensitization using a psychotherapeutic approach was successful.

Ventilator over-dependence

PROBLEM

The opposite of poor tolerance in that the patient feels unable to discontinue ventilation for long periods.

ACTION

True physiological dependence needs to be excluded by monitoring respiratory pattern, and arterial blood gas tensions during periods of spontaneous breathing, non-invasive monitoring using an oximeter and transcutaneous or end tidal CO_2 monitor is helpful. Measurement of lung function and respiratory muscle strength is needed to assess ventilatory capacity. We find it helpful to correct arterial $PaCO_2$ and base excess as completely as possible before discontinuing ventilatory support as this will optimize the patient's own ventilatory drive (and possibly muscle function) and make it easier for them to assume spontaneous breathing. It is sometimes felt that as the patient is acclimatized to a chronic level of hypercapnia, it is best to aim for a $PaCO_2$ level of 7 or 8 kPa. In our experience this makes weaning more difficult for some patients. For patients in whom dependence has become psychological, a gradual approach using increasing periods off the ventilator during periods of distraction e.g. at visiting time, when watching videos etc., combined with a pulmonary rehabilitation programme and breathing control advice is often successful.

REFERENCES

1   Ferguson GT, Gilmartin M. CO_2 rebreathing during BiPAP ventilatory assistance. *Am J Respir Crit Care Med* 1995; **151**: 1126–35.
2   Kacmarek RM. New ventilator options for long-term mechanical ventilation in the home. In: Hill NS (ed.) *Long-term mechanical ventilation*, 1st edn. New York: Marcel Dekker, 2001: 375–409.
3   Calderini E, Confalonieri M, Puccio PG. Patient–ventilator asynchrony during non-invasive ventilation: the role of the expiratory trigger. *Int Care Med* 1999; **25**: 662–7.

7

Non-invasive mechanical ventilation in the Intensive Care Unit and High Dependency Unit

MARCO CONFALONIERI AND STEFANO NAVA

INTRODUCTION

Until 15 years ago, mechanical ventilation (MV) was limited to the Intensive Care Unit (ICU) because patients needed to be immobile and sedated. Over the last decade the great interest in non-invasive mechanical ventilation in the form of nasal intermittent positive pressure ventilation (NIPPV) has opened new horizons in the field of MV and ways in which to apply it. Indeed, as the consequence of various clinical and physiological evidence,[1] NIPPV has become a first-line intervention in the management of severe exacerbations of chronic obstructive pulmonary disease (COPD). Moreover, it has been shown that NIPPV can be applied at an earlier stage in the evolution of ventilatory failure than would be usual when a patient is intubated and that the NIPPV can be administered even outside the ICU. Mechanical ventilation without the need of an ICU admission is an attractive option given the high costs of ICU care, but caution should be exercised as NIPPV does have limitations and should be used only in selected patients: most controlled studies of NIPPV in acute respiratory failure (ARF) have been performed on

Table 7.1 *Prospective randomized controlled studies on NIPPV in patients with ARF according to the location*

	Number of studies	References	Study population
ICU	5	1, 2, 3, 4, 5	COPD (2 studies) Non-COPD (1) Hypoxaemic ARF (2)
HDU or RICU	3	10, 11, 12	COPD (weaning) CAP, COPD
Ward	3	7, 8, 9	COPD (3)
Emergency Room	1	6	Hypercapnic or hypoxaemic ARF

patients cared for in an ICU setting (Table 7.1). To date there have been 12 prospective randomized controlled studies on NIPPV in acute respiratory failure (ARF): five were performed in general ICUs,[1–5] one in an emergency room,[6] three in pneumology wards[7–9] and three in respiratory intermediate ICUs.[10–12] Five of the randomized studies on NIPPV in ARF involved selected patients with exacerbation of COPD,[1,4,7,9,12] and the others involved the following types of patients: acute severe hypoxaemic,[3] post-transplant,[5] severe pneumonia,[11] weaning from invasive mechanical ventilation (IMV) for COPD exacerbation,[10] patients admitted to an emergency room for ARF of different causes,[6] and non-COPD patients admitted to an ICU.[2]

This chapter will summarize the evidence on where and how NIPPV should be performed, highlighting ICU and High Dependency Unit (HDU) applications.

WHO SHOULD BE ADMITTED TO AN ICU OR HDU FOR NIPPV?

Acute hypercapnic respiratory failure

The literature on NIPPV in ARF is abundant, but conclusive results have been obtined only in ARF due to an exacerbation of COPD. A meta-analysis by Keenan and co-workers[13] showed that NIPPV can reduce the need for endotracheal intubation with survival benefits in this population and indeed this conclusion would have been further strengthened had the results of more recent studies been included in the meta-analysis.[9,11,12] Unfortunately, a meta-analysis cannot focus on what is the ideal setting in which to apply NIPPV or the best population to receive it. Most studies on NIPPV were performed in ICUs and Respiratory High Dependency Units (RHDUs), but a number of COPD patients with ARF were treated in general wards. Nonetheless, it should be emphasized that the positive results reported with NIPPV were observed only in selected COPD patients with the majority excluded. Patients with COPD needing immediate intubation have regularly been excluded from all studies published to date. This means that wherever NIPPV is performed, facilities for prompt endotracheal intubation should be readily available (Table 7.2).

Table 7.2 *Failure of NIPPV and need for endotracheal intubation (in ICU or RHDU)*

- Respiratory arrest or apnoea with loss of consciousness or airways protection reflexes absent
- Severe haemodynamic instability (systolic blood pressure < 70 mmHg, uncontrolled severe arrhythmia)
- Respiratory rate > 35 breaths per minute (and increasing with regard to baseline)
- Pao_2/Fio_2 < 150 (and decreasing with regard to baseline)
- Increasing $Paco_2$ > 20% and/or decreasing pH with regard to baseline
- Multiple organ failure (MOFS)
- Bronchial hypersecretion and need to airway clearance
- Agitation and/or need of heavy sedation

Indeed, a major problem regarding the use of NIPPV out of an ICU is the possible need for rapid intubation and conventional ventilation.

No authors have compared outcomes of patients treated in different settings, but this would in any case be difficult because the severity of respiratory impairment of the patients in the studies differed greatly. In fact, all the studies performed in a general ward concerned patients with a mean pH > 7.29, whilst patients admitted to ICU or RHDU had a more severe respiratory acidosis (pH < 7.29). This pH value can reasonably be considered as a cut-off point for deciding whether a patient should be admitted to an ICU/RHDU for NIPPV or whether he can stay in a general ward. This has been recently demonstrated in a large number of patients in the Yorkshire (YONIV) study.[9] The severity of illness and the presence of co-morbid conditions must also be taken in account when deciding the optimal location for treatment. These two factors have been reported to be correlated with failure of NIPPV in ARF.[14] Yet other factors must be considered before admitting

Table 7.3 *Where should NIPPV be used in COPDs?*

Medical Ward
- To prevent 'overt' ARF (pH from 7.30 to 7.35)

Respiratory High Dependency Unit
- To treat severe ARF (pH ≤ 7.30)but only if:
    Haemodynamic stability
    Pao_2/Fio_2 ≥ 1.5
    No sepsis
    Minimal spontaneous capacity
    Normal sensorium
    NO multiple organ failure

ICU
- To treat severe ARF (pH < 7.30) and in presence of one of the following contraindications for RHDU:
    Pao_2/Fio_2 < 1.5
    No spontaneous activity
    > 1 organ failure

In all the other conditions: Intubation

a patient to an ICU, e.g. prior quality of life, functional status and central nervous system impairment. Table 7.3 is a schematic recommendation of where COPD patients should be treated in the case of an episode of acute hypercapnic respiratory failure.

Acute hypoxaemic respiratory failure (see also Chapter 4)

While many studies support the use of NIPPV in patients with acute hypercapnic respiratory failure, some controversy exists with respect to its efficacy in hypoxaemic patients. Almost all the randomized controlled trials concerning hypoxaemic patients were performed in ICUs,[2,3,5] but one was carried out in a RHDU.[11] The success rate of NIPPV was overall not significantly higher than that of standard medical treatment, but was much lower in a single study on non-COPD patients.[2] However, recent studies comparing NIPPV with invasive mechanical ventilation in hypoxaemic patients found a significant shortening in the time spent in the ICU and duration of MV in the group non-invasively ventilated.[3] Nevertheless, once again it should be remembered that the clearest positive results in hypoxaemic ARF were found only in randomized studies performed in a single, highly skilled ICU.

Use of NIPPV for weaning

The process of discontinuing MV constitutes a major clinical challenge, especially in patients with chronic obstructive pulmonary disease, in whom weaning is particularly difficult. The rate of weaning failure can exceed 60% in COPD patients, representing a major cause of prolonged use of ICU resources. NIPPV can be used in the weaning process of COPD patients with ARF at various stages. A recent multicentre, randomized trial in patients with an exacerbation of COPD showed that NIPPV was more successful in weaning than a conventional approach.[10] In this study, patients with hypercapnic respiratory failure who failed a T-piece trial 48 hours after intubation were randomly assigned to receive either NIPPV after immediate extubation or invasive pressure support ventilation and further weaning according to conventional criteria. Patients who received NIPPV during weaning had a shorter weaning time, spent less time in the ICU, had a lower incidence of nosocomial pneumonia, and improved 60-day survival rates. The application of NIPPV prevented the development of nosocomial pneumonia, a common complication of endotracheal intubation which is known to contribute to mortality. Another study applying NIPPV a few days after intubation in patients affected by hypercapnic respiratory failure due either to COPD or restrictive thoracic disease, showed similar results, even though the incidence of infectious complications did not achieve statistical significance.[15] One recent study reported the use of NIPPV for weaning patients without pre-existing COPD, most of them following transplant procedures.[16] This study, too, showed that nosocomial pneumonia can be reduced using non-invasive pressure support ventilation, and that the duration of MV, the length of admission, and need for reintubation were also reduced. These studies were performed in an ICU and an RHDU, and suggest that NIPPV may allow patients to be extubated earlier than usual, and that this approach might not

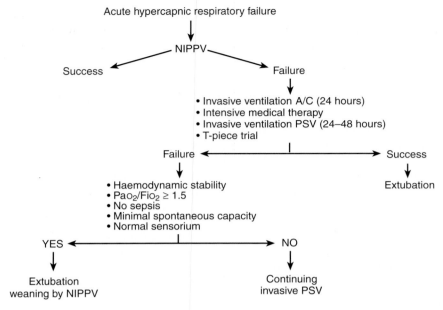

Figure 7.1 *Proposed flow-chart of the management of patients affected by acute hypercapnic respiratory failure.*

only be more rapid but also more successful than conventional weaning procedures. Nevertheless, it must be acknowledged that careful selection of patients and the skills and experience of the team involved in respiratory care are crucial to the success of NIPPV. Further clinical investigations are needed to be able to extend results from small clinical trials to routine clinical practice and to establish NIPPV definitively as a first-line option in weaning procedures. A proposed flow-chart of the management of patients affected by acute hypercapnic respiratory failure is shown in Figure 7.1.

Perioperative care

Post-operative respiratory failure is a well known complication of thoracic and upper abdominal surgery characterized by reductions in functional residual capacity, forced vital capacity, and PaO_2. NIPPV and continuous positive airway pressure (CPAP) via a nasal or facial mask are often used to treat post-operative respiratory failure. An RHDU or surgical ICU seems to be the ideal location to treat these patients non-invasively. Randomized studies are not always available for patients with post-operative ARF, nonetheless, a number of uncontrolled series of patients showed that mask CPAP and NIPPV have beneficial effects in avoiding reintubation. Patients treated with NIPPV for post-operative ARF were usually haemodynamically stable and without multiorgan failure. Pinilla *et al.*[17] and Jousela *et al.*[18] reported that the use of CPAP after weaning in patients undergoing aorto-coronary bypass surgery improved pulmonary gas exchange but failed to modify the prevalence of post-surgical atelectasis. Both CPAP and bilevel positive airway pressure (BiPAP) decreased the extravascular lung water content after extubation,[19] and lung mechanics and arterial oxygenation improved,[20] following similar surgical procedures. A recent paper demonstrated that CPAP may also be effective to improve oxygenation in less than one hour in post-operative patients with severe non-hypercapnic failure, avoiding at the same time endotracheal intubation.[21] With regard to 'general' surgery patients, bilevel ventilation has been shown to increase the efficiency of gas exchange, without any adverse effect (i.e. pleural leaks) in patients undergoing lung resectional surgery,[22] while CPAP promoted a more very rapid recovery of pulmonary function after upper abdominal surgery.[23] In another study performed in obese patients after gastroplasty, bilevel ventilation improved lung mechanics and arterial PaO_2 post-operatively on day 1, and these physiological benefits were maintained on long-term basis.[24]

Another 'perioperative' use of mask MV may be the application of NIPPV as a bridge to lung transplantation for particular categories of patients (those with cystic fibrosis, COPD), although no controlled studies have been published on this issue. Also, there are no controlled data on the use of NIPPV before surgery in chronically ill respiratory patients at risk of surgical complications.

MONITORING, STAFFING AND VENTILATORS FOR NIPPV (see also Chapters 3 and 5)

The optimal monitoring and staffing levels for NIPPV in patients with ARF have not yet been established. Most monitoring and staffing considerations presented in literature reviews and editorials are experienced-based rather than evidence-based.

Staff to assist during NIPPV

There is, however, one controlled study giving evidence-based results on staffing needs during NIPPV. Nava and co-workers[25] showed that NIPPV requires the same level of assistance as invasive MV during the first 48 hours but after this period significantly less human resources are needed by patients receiving non-invasive ventilation compared with those undergoing invasive ventilation. This study was performed in a RHDU caring for patients more severely ill than those usually admitted to a general ward. Although severity of illness is a key point in deciding which levels of assistance and monitoring are more appropriate, nursing assistance cannot fall below a minimum level. The optimal nurse-to-patient ratio for NIPPV is 1 : 2–1 : 3, but during the first hours of application NIPPV can be very time-consuming and indeed can require the maximum of assistance (nurse-to-patient ratio 1 : 1). In North America the direct care and management of ventilators and ventilated patients is carried out by respiratory therapists. In Europe this role is often taken by physiotherapists.[26] The optimal therapist-to-patient ratio is 1 : 6, but only during the day since in most countries work shifts do not cover the whole 24 hours. Finally it should be emphasized that to ensure the best results of NIPPV it is important that the team undergoes adequate training and a continuous education programme.

Monitoring during NIPPV

Although some studies on NIPPV do not discuss scheduled criteria for the monitoring of patients non-invasively ventilated it should be stressed that accurate monitoring is essential for the success of NIPPV. In fact, monitoring is imperative in patients with acute and post-critical respiratory disease, as such patients have a high risk of sudden and unexpected deterioration. Patient–ventilator interaction and the patient's response to NIPPV needs to be supervised carefully, especially during the first 48 hours, for optimal application of NIPPV. Patients cannot be monitored accurately during NIPPV if the nurse-to-patient ratio is inadequate (e.g. less than 1 : 5). The bedside presence of a nurse trained and familiar with NIPPV or a respiratory therapist is important for adjusting the mask and eliminating excessive air leaks. Despite recent technological advances, there is still no substitute for direct clinical examination of patients to identify early indicators of muscle fatigue, neurological deterioration, or the development of other complications. Moreover, during the first 30–60 minutes of NIPPV, a physician or a respiratory therapist must evaluate the response of the patient, as determined by arterial blood gas concentration, adequacy of exhaled tidal volume (V_{Texp} should be at least 5 mL/kg), the presence of respiratory distress, and then adjust ventilator settings if necessary. The severity of neurological dysfunction can be best assessed using the Kelly score (Table 7.4),

Table 7.4 *Kelly and Matthay Neurologic Status Score (modified from Ref. 27)*

Grade no.	Description
1	Alert, follows complex 3-step command
2	Alert, follows simple commands
3	Lethargic, but arousable and follows simple commands
4	Stuporous, only intermittently follows simple commands
5	Comatose, brainstem intact
6	Comatose with brainstem dysfunction

specifically designed for critically ill respiratory patients.[27] Severity of illness scores may be a guide to predicting failure of NIPPV, as reported by several authors.[28–30] Invasive monitoring should be limited to more severely ill patients admitted to the ICU. Most patients treated with NIPPV can be adequately monitored using non-invasive methods, particularly in an HDU or RHDU. Basic physiological non-invasive parameters include heart rate and rhythm, blood pressure, continuous oximetry with alarms, end tidal CO_2, respiratory rate and breathing pattern, neuro-muscular drive ($P_{0.1}$), maximal inspiratory pressure, tidal volume/dynamic lung volumes, and flow and pressure waveforms. This information should be available before starting NIPPV, but that does not necessarily imply that all these parameters must be measured in all patients. More sophisticated and expensive monitoring may be used in specialist centres. This includes measurement of transdiaphragmatic pressure (Pdi), electrical or magnetic phrenic nerve stimulation, indirect calorimetry, colour-Doppler echocardiography, respiratory inductive plethysmography, and electromyography of the respiratory muscles.

Use of ICU rather than custom built NIPPV ventilators for NIPPV

The majority of the randomized clinical trials used ICU ventilators via a facemask, but a number of workers have reported good results with custom built NIPPV ventilators. It has been shown that the so-called 'home ventilators' performed *in vitro* as well or even better than the traditional ICU ventilators. Nevertheless, some failures of NIPPV with portable home devices may be attributable to limitations in the ability of these devices to generate pressure support rather than to the existence of a condition refractory to NIPPV.[31] Another major problem encountered with home devices using a single tube circuit is CO_2 rebreathing,[32] but this can be prevented by applying a higher level of PEEP. The principal limitation to the use of home ventilators during ARF is the scarce monitoring facilities provided by these devices. In fact, most custom built NIPPV ventilators do not allow direct 'on line' monitoring of pressure, volume or flow. Furthermore, the evaluation of patient–ventilator asynchrony is very difficult if not impossible without visualization of flow and pressure waveforms (Figure 7.2). These are important features, especially during the first period of ventilation when it is important to assess the patient–ventilator interaction, respiratory mechanics, and expired V_T.[33,34] Indeed, most portable ventilators do not have a gas blender so the operator does not know exactly what concentration of oxygen the patient is receiving. In addition, a bench study has recently demonstrated the inaccuracy of tidal volume delivered by some home mechanical ventilators when the pressure imposed on the ventilator is

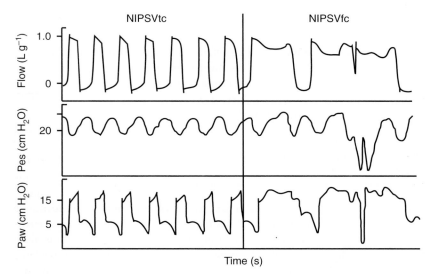

Figure 7.2 *Airway pressure (Paw), flow, and oesophageal pressure (Pes) in a patient non-invasively ventilated for acute respiratory failure with a time-cycling (right) and a flow-cycling (left) pressure support mode. The tracings clearly show that patient–ventilator asynchrony is evident during conventional flow-cycling non-invasive pressure support (NIPSV) and not during time-cycling NIPSV (modified from Ref. 33).*

increased to simulate high airway resistance.[35] In other words, some of the commercially available devices fail to provide the desired V_T reliably during volume ventilation. This represents an evident limitation to the use of these devices when the respiratory load is increased, as it is during ARF.

Regarding the use of masks, the optimal interface and ventilator design have not been determined, and this may vary between patients. The commercially available masks currently consist of five types: (1) full facemask; (2) nasal masks; (3) nasal pillows or plugs; (4) mouthpieces; (5) custom-fabricated nasal masks. The major clinical advantages for the full facemask compared with the nasal mask are: the ability to reach higher airway pressure, use of mouth respiration, fewer air-leaks, a requirement for less co-operation. By contrast, the main disadvantages are: less comfort, the inability to speak, eat and drink during ventilation, and the increased risk of aspiration if vomiting occurs.

Nasal pillows seem to be useful to substitute both face and nasal masks in the event of troublesome nose skin abrasion. There is only one study, performed however in stable patients, that systematically assessed the impact of different types of interfaces on gas exchange and patient's tolerance.[36] The main findings of the study were that facemask and nasal pillow produced a greater fall in $PaCO_2$ than nasal masks but that the use of nasal mask resulted in a better acceptance of ventilation than the other two interfaces. It was also suggested that nasal pillows can be as effective as facemasks in reducing $PaCO_2$ and increasing pH, but the presence of expiratory leaks made adequate monitoring of V_T difficult. Taking this information into account, the pillows may be used to alternate with the facial mask, to alter the site of pressure, if nose skin abrasions occur. This approach may prove a way to enhance tolerance of NIPPV and therefore allow duration of ventilation per day to be increased. NIPPV was however tolerated significantly better when administered via a nasal mask, using a compliance scale ranging from 'very poor' to 'excellent', suggesting that in its use during chronic ventilation nasal masks are preferable. Bearing in mind that this was a physiologic study, designed only to assess short-term effects, any extrapolation to long-term situations should be made with caution, but it may suggest that in patients with chronic hypercapnic respiratory failure, irrespective of the underlying pathology, NIPPV outcome can be affected by the type of interface.

ROLE OF INTERMEDIATE CARE UNITS AND DIFFERENCES IN USE IN EUROPE

It is well demonstrated that general ICUs are expensive and there are ethical and economic concerns when chronically ill patients are admitted, because these patients may require a long stay in the ICU not only for the severe disease underlying ARF but also for ICU-related complications. The possibility of treating patients with acute-on-chronic respiratory disease in settings which entail less cost while offering an optimal level of assistance is an attractive alternative to the use of the traditional general ICU. The principal differences between an ICU and a HDU or RHDU and between a HDU and the general ward are the level of nursing assistance and monitoring. The HDU offers an intermediate care level between the ICU and the general ward, that can be general or specialized (e.g. RHDU, Coronary

Care Unit). HDU care is cheaper than ICU care because of lower staffing costs. Another key feature of HDUs is the preferential use of non-invasive monitoring and non-invasive mechanical ventilation. The introduction of NIPPV into clinical practice has been a powerful stimulus for the development of specialized respiratory care units with a concentration of staff expertise.[37] The RHDU is an ideal place for initiating NIPPV in patients who are not clinically stable. The potential advantages of RHDUs are not only their lower costs compared with those of an ICU, but also greater comfort and quality of care for the patient. Increasing RHDU beds will not automatically alleviate ICU bed crises but can increase flexibility. Appropriate care should reduce or prevent ICU-type complications, and hence improve outcome and reduce overall length of stay.

The number of RHDUs opened has been increasing in the last 15 years, initially in the USA but recently in Europe too. Many RHDUs and HDUs are set up within a general ward with staff rotating through both areas, but several units have dedicated and specialized staff. A flexible approach to staffing could help to cater for the needs of chronic respiratory patients requiring NIPPV while ensuring that the rest of the ward is not understaffed. The RHDU was defined by the Italian Association of Hospital Pneumologists[38] as:

> An area for the monitoring and treatment of patients with acute respiratory failure due to a primary respiratory cause and of patients with acute-on-chronic respiratory failure. Non-invasive monitoring techniques and non-invasive mechanical ventilation should be principally employed as first line of treatment: however, when mandatory, invasive monitoring techniques must be used. Similarly, when non-invasive mechanical ventilation fails, conventional mechanical ventilation by endotracheal intubation or tracheostomy must be provided. Tracheostomy may be provided *in situ* or in the ICU.

Although the idea of a single-organ intermediate intensive care unit has spread in several European countries, its practical impact has to be assessed in a variety of ways. Some units act essentially as specialized ICUs, whereas others are merely non-invasive monitoring units. According to a recent unpublished survey, Italy has the largest number of respiratory units. In France these units are numerous and widely spread geographically, but the organization and division by level (according to the monitoring system available) is the most advanced. In other countries, such as the United Kingdom, the lack of a sufficient number of specialist units may have contributed to an insufficient availability of NIPPV for ARF in general hospitals.[39] It has been suggested that the ideal number of RHDU beds per head of population would be 1/100,000, but in Europe only France seems to have a ratio close to this ideal. The European Respiratory Society has instituted a task force to examine RHDU practices across Europe, highlighting the importance of this area to respiratory and intensive care physicians.

REFERENCES

1   Brochard L, Mancebo J, Wysocki M, *et al*. Noninvasive ventilation for acute exacerbation of chronic obstructive pulmonary disease. *N Engl J Med* 1995; **333**: 817–22.

2   Wysocki M, Tric L, Wolff MA, Millet H, Herman B. Noninvasive pressure support ventilation in patients with acute respiratory failure: a randomized comparison with conventional therapy. *Chest* 1995; **107**: 761–8.

3   Antonelli M, Conti G, Rocco M, *et al*. A comparison of noninvasive positive-pressure ventilation and conventional mechanical ventilation in patients with acute respiratory failure. *N Engl J Med* 1998; **339**: 429–35.

4   Kramer N, Meyer TJ, Meharg J, Cece RD, Hill NS. Randomized, prospective trial of noninvasive positive pressure ventilation in acute respiratory failure. *Am J Repair Crit Care Med* 1995; **151**: 1799–1806.

5   Antonelli M, Conti G, Bufi M, *et al*. Noninvasive ventilation for treatment of acute respiratory failure in patients undergoing solid organ transplantation. *JAMA* 2000; **283**: 235–41.

6   Wood KA, Lewis L, Von Harz B, Kollef MH. The use of noninvasive positive pressure ventilation in the emergency department: results of a randomized clinical trial. *Chest* 1998; **113**: 1339–46.

7   Bott J, Carroll MP, Conway JH, *et al*. Randomized controlled trial of nasal ventilation in acute ventilatory failure due to chronic obstructive airways disease. *Lancet* 1993; **341**: 1555–7.

8   Barbé F, Togores B, Rubì M, Pons S, Maimò A, Agustì AG. Noninvasive ventilatory support does not facilitate recovery from acute respiratory failure in chronic obstructive pulmonary disease. *Eur Respir J* 1996; **9**: 1240–5.

9   Plant PK, Owen JL, Elliott MW. Early use of non-invasive ventilation for acute exacerbations of chronic obstructive pulmonary disease on general respiratory wards: a multicentre randomised controlled trial. *Lancet* 2000; **355**: 1931–5.

10 Nava S, Ambrosino N, Clini E, *et al*. Noninvasive mechanical ventilation in the weaning of patients with respiratory failure due to chronic obstructive pulmonary disease. A randomized controlled trial. *Ann Intern Med* 1998; **128**: 721–8.

11 Confalonieri M, Potena A, Carbone G, Della Porta R, Tolley E, Meduri GU. Acute respiratory failure in patients with severe community acquired pneumonia. A prospective randomised evaluation of non-invasive ventilation. *Am J Respir Crit Care Med* 1999; **160**: 1585–91.

12 Celikel T, Sungur M, Ceyhan B, Karakurt S. Comparison of noninvasive positive ventilation with standard medical therapy in hypercapnic acute respiratory failure. *Chest* 1998; **114**: 1636–42.

13 Keenan SP, Kernerman PD, Cook DJ, Martin CM, McCormack D, Wibbald WJ. The effect of noninvasive positive pressure ventilation on mortality in patients admitted with acute respiratory failure: a meta-analysis. *Crit Care Med* 1997; **25**: 1685–92.

14 Moretti M, Cilione C, Tampieri A, Fracchia C, Marchioni A, Nava S. Incidence and causes of non-invasive mechanical ventilation failure after an initial (< 48 hrs) successful attempt. *Thorax* 2000; **55**: 819–25.

15 Girault C, Daudenthum I, Chevron V, *et al*. Noninvasive ventilation a systematic extubation and weaning technique in acute-on-chronic respiratory failure: a prospective, randomized controlled study. *Am J Respir Crit Care Med* 1999; **160**: 86–92.

16 Kilger E, Briegel J, Haller M, *et al*. Effects of noninvasive positive pressure ventilatory support in non-COPD patients with acute respiratory insufficiency after early intubation. *Intensive Care Med* 1999; **25**: 1374–9.

17 Pinilla JC, Oleniuk FH, Tan L, *et al.* Use of a nasal continuous positive airway pressure mask in the treatment of postoperative atelectase atelectasis in aortocoronary bypass surgery. *Crit Care Med* 1990; **18**: 836–40.

18 Jousela I, Rasanen J, Verkkala K, Lamminen A, Makelainen A, Nikki P. Continuous positive airway pressure by mask in patients after coronary surgery. *Acta Anaesthesiol Scand* 1994; **38**: 311–16.

19 Gust R, Gottschalk A, Schmidt H, Bottiger BW, Bohrer, Martin E. Effects of continuous (CPAP) and bi-level positive airway pressure (BiPAP) on extravascular lung water after extubation of the trachea in patients following coronary artery bypass grafting. *Intensive Care Med* 1996; **22**: 1345–50.

20 Matte P, Jacquet L, Van Dyck M, Goenen M. Effects of conventional physiotherapy, continuous positive airway pressure and non-invasive ventilatory support with bilevel positive airway pressure after coronary artery bypass grafting. *Acta Anaesthesiol Scand* 2000; **44**: 75–81.

21 Kindgen-Milles D, Buhl R, Gabriel A, Bohner H, Muller E. Nasal continuous positive airway pressure. A method to avoid endotracheal reintubation in postoperative high-risk patients with severe nonhypercapnic oxygenation failure. *Chest* 2000; **117**: 1106–11.

22 Aguilo R, Togores B, Pons S, Rubi M, Barbe F, Agusti AGN. Noninvasive ventilatory support after lung resectional surgery. *Chest* 1997; **112**: 117–21.

23 Stock MC, Downs JB, Gauer PK, Alster JM, Imrey PB. Prevention of postoperative pulmonary complications with CPAP, incentive spirometry, and conservative therapy. *Chest* 1985; **87**: 151–7.

24 Joris JL, Sottiaux TM, Chiche JD, Desaive CJ, Lamy ML. Effect of bi-level positive airway pressure (BiPAP) nasal ventilation on the postoperative restrictive syndrome in obese patients undergoing gastroplasty. *Chest* 1997; **111**: 665–70.

25 Nava S, Evangelisti I, Rampulla C, Compagnoni ML, Fracchia C, Rubini F. Human and financial costs of noninvasive mechanical ventilation in patients affected by COPD and acute respiratory failure. *Chest* 1997; **111**: 1631–8.

26 Norrenberg M, Vincent JL. A profile of European intensive care unit physiotherapists. *Intensive Care Med* 2000; **26**: 988–94.

27 Kelly BJ, Matthay MA. Prevalence and severity of neurological dysfunction in critically ill patients. Influence on need for continued mechanical ventilation. *Chest* 1993; **104**: 1818–24.

28 Ambrosino N, Foglio K, Rubini F, Clini E, Nava S, Vitacca M. Non-invasive mechanical ventilation in acute respiratory failure due to chronic obstructive pulmonary disease: correlates for success. *Thorax* 1995; **50**: 755–7.

29 Confalonieri M, Aiolfi S, Gandola L, Scartabellati A, Della Porta R, Parigi P. Severe exacerbations of chronic obstructive pulmonary disease treated with BiPAP by nasal mask. *Respiration* 1994; **61**: 310–16.

30 Soo Hoo GW, Santiago S, Williams AJ. Nasal mechanical ventilation for hypercapnic respiratory failure in chronic obstructive pulmonary disease: determinants of success and failure. *Crit Care Med* 1994; **22**: 1253–61.

31 Lofaso F, Brochard L, Hang T, Lorino H, Harf A, Isabey D. Home versus intensive care pressure support devices. *Am J Respir Crit Care Med* 1996; **153**: 1591–9.

32 Gary T, Ferguson GT, Gilmartin M. CO_2 rebreathing during BiPAP ventilatory assistance. *Am J Resp Crit Care Med* 1995; **151**: 1126–35.

33 Calderini E, Confalonieri M, Puccio PG, Francavilla N, Stella L, Gregoretti C. Patient–ventilator asynchrony during noninvasive ventilation: the role of expiratory trigger. *Intensive Care Med* 1999; **25**: 662–7.
34 Kacmarek RM. NIPPV: patient–ventilator synchrony, the difference between success and failure? *Intensive Care Med* 1999; **25**: 645–7.
35 Lofaso F, Fodil R, Lorini H, *et al*. Inaccuracy of tidal volume delivered by home mechanical ventilators. *Eur Respir J* 2000; **15**: 338–41.
36 Navalesi P, Fanfulla F, Frigerio P, Gregoretti C, Nava S. Physiologic evaluation of noninvasive mechanical ventilation delivered with three types of masks in patients with chronic hypercapnic respiratory failure. *Crit Care Med* 2000; **28**: 1785–91.
37 Nava S, Confalonieri M, Rampulla C. Intermediate respiratory intensive care units in Europe: a European perspective. *Thorax* 1998; **53**: 798–802.
38 Corrado A, Ambrosino N, Rossi A, Donner CF. Unità di Terapia Intensiva Respiratoria. *Rasseg Patol Apparat Respir* 1994; **9**: 125–38.
39 Doherty MJ, Greenstone MA. Survey of non-invasive ventilation (NIPPV) in patients with acute exacerbations of chronic obstructive pulmonary disease (COPD) in the UK. *Thorax* 1998; **53**: 863–6.

8

NIPPV in the Emergency Room and for transferring patients

A K SIMONDS

As most patients are admitted to hospital via an Emergency Room (ER) or Casualty Department, and the early use of NIPPV may reduce the need for intubation, mortality and hospital stay in patients with ARF, it is not surprising that there has been increasing interest in applying NIPPV in the ER environment. Results so far show variable efficacy.

FEASIBILITY OF NIPPV IN THE ER

The practicalities of using NIPPV as first-line therapy in severe non-traumatic ARF were explored prospectively in a case series[1] of 50 patients, who were stable haemo-dynamically and not in need of immediate intubation, on entry to an Arizona teaching hospital ER. The causes of ARF were congestive heart failure (CHF) $n = 16$, pneumonia $n = 10$, acute exacerbation of COPD $n = 9$, status asthmaticus $n = 6$ and miscellaneous conditions, including overdose and CVA. Bilevel pressure support ventilation was adjusted according to patient tolerance from a starting point of 5 cmH$_2$O, and applied via a nasal or facemask. NIPPV was successful in 43 (86%) of patients as judged by (a) improvement in arterial blood gas tensions;

(b) reduction in respiratory distress; and (c) avoidance of endotracheal intubation and IPPV. Success was distributed equally across diagnostic groups with no cause of ARF having a more or less favourable outcome. The authors report, not surprisingly, that all patients required inpatient care. However, over 50% of those who would have normally required an ICU bed were admitted to a lower level of care with consequent financial savings. Of the treatment failures, two did not tolerate NIPPV, three patients required intubation, and two failed the technique, but were not intubated because of advance directives to the contrary. These results demonstrate that NIPPV is fully feasible in the ER.

CAN SUCCESSFUL USE OF NIPPV IN THE ER BE PREDICTED?

Clearly it would be helpful to predict which patients are most likely to respond well to non-invasive respiratory support in the ER, and identify those in whom failure is likely. Poponick and colleagues[2] carried out a retrospective survey of NIPPV outcome in a large urban ER, in Cleveland, USA. A trial of bilevel pressure support was carried out in 58 patients aged 25 to 88 years with ARF. The majority of recruits had either congestive cardiac failure or an acute exacerbation of COPD. Overall, 74% of the trials of NIPPV were successful. Of the 15 unsuccessful cases, 13 required intubation and two did not respond to NIPPV but had advance directives specifying non-intubation. There was no difference between treatment failure and success groups in age, gender, Glasgow coma score or Acute Physiology and Chronic Health Evaluation II (APACHE II) score on admission. Pre-NIPPV arterial blood gas tensions were also similar but values obtained after 30 minutes of NIPPV were helpful in predicting successful avoidance of intubation (pH 7.34 v 7.27, $PaCO_2$ 8.2 v 9.7 kPa). As might be expected, NIPPV successes had a shorter duration of ventilation, and shorter ICU and hospital stay compared to NIPPV failures. The authors concluded that it is not possible to anticipate the outcome of NIPPV in the ER from diagnosis or baseline arterial blood gases, but a 30-minute trial of NIPPV allows patient success to be predicted. By extension they argue that if improvement is not seen within 30 minutes of NIPPV, intubation and mechanical ventilation is indicated. This information is in close agreement with work in acute COPD, showing that the best prognostic factors are change in pH and $PaCO_2$ after one hour of NIPPV, and pH and $PaCO_2$ on admission.[3]

In the light of these results, a randomized study of NIPPV versus conventional therapy was the obvious next step.

RANDOMIZED CONTROLLED STUDY OF NIPPV IN THE ER

Wood et al.[4] randomized 27 ER admissions with ARF to bilevel NIPPV or standard therapy in a prospective controlled trial. All patients had evidence of respiratory distress with one of the following: pH < 7.35, $PaCO_2$ > 6.0 kPa (45 mmHg), PaO_2 < 7.3 kPa (55 mmHg)/SaO_2 < 90% on room air, or alveolar-arterial gradient > 13.3 kPa (100 mmHg) with supplemental oxygen. Patients with acute asthma, pneumothorax or acute chest wall trauma were excluded, as were those with an immediate need for intubation, cardiac instability, upper airway obstruction, or who were unable co-operate with mask ventilation. As in previous ER studies the primary outcome measure was the need for intubation and IPPV; secondary endpoints were hospital mortality, length of hospital stay, complications, and demands on staff time. The average age of the patients was 59 years and the commonest diagnoses were cardiogenic pulmonary oedema, COPD, and pneumonia.

Forty-three per cent of patients receiving NIPPV required intubation and conventional ventilation compared with 45.5% in the standard therapy group ($p = $ NS). There was no difference in length of hospital stay, duration of ventilation or complications between the groups. However, the authors found that the period-time from arrival in the ER to endotracheal intubation was longer in those receiving NIPPV compared with standard therapy (26.0 v 4.8 hours, $p = 0.055$). Moreover, there was also a trend to greater hospital mortality in the NIPPV group (25% NIPPV v 0% standard therapy) although this did not reach significance ($p = 0.123$).

These results paint a different outcome picture to the prospective, uncontrolled case series, and suggest that NIPPV may lead to an adverse outcome in some patients by delaying endotracheal intubation. How can we reconcile these findings, and do they mean that NIPPV is unsuitable to apply in the ER?

OVERVIEW OF NIPPV IN THE ER

There are several important factors to be considered when analysing these results. Firstly, the randomized trial of NIPPV in the ER contained a relatively small number of patients (16 NIPPV, 11 control) despite the fact that recruitment took place over a six-month period. Trial numbers were based on the calculation that 30 patients would allow the study to detect a difference between an expected intubation rate of 70% in the conventionally treated group and 30% in the NIPPV group, with a probability of 95% and power of 80%. The fact that only 27 patients took part increases the possibility of Type I and Type II statistical errors as acknowledged by the authors. Secondly, the diagnoses of ARF were not equally distributed within the two limbs of the study. For example, there were more than double the number of cases of pneumonia, an excess of patients with cardiogenic pulmonary oedema and fewer COPD patients in the NIPPV group, compared with those receiving standard therapy, which may have biased outcome.

It is also necessary to examine protocols for instituting NIPPV in each institution. The NIPPV protocol employed by Wood et al.[4] used bilevel pressure support machines (BiPAP, Respironics Inc.) with an initial IPAP setting of 8 cmH$_2$O and EPAP of 2–4 cmH$_2$O. This low IPAP setting may well be insufficient for a number if patients and lead to poor tolerance. In addition, nasal masks were used, accompanied by chin straps in patients who were mouth breathers. Many acutely breathless patients tolerate full facemasks better. Mask ventilation was initiated by respiratory care practitioners in the ER and continued on a medical ward or ICU.

ER SPECIAL CONSIDERATIONS

There are special difficulties in managing patients in the ER. Initially, the diagnosis may be unclear and previous medical history unobtainable. Plant et al.[5] have shown that a proportion of patients with COPD may arrive with a raised $Paco_2$ and acidosis due to the inappropriate administration of high flow oxygen during transfer to hospital. Admissions to the ER will also include very severely ill patients who may die before transfer to the ICU or surgery, thereby affecting the mortality of this group. However, such patients on arrival were excluded from the NIPPV studies in ER.

An important consideration is the composition of the team applying respiratory support, Respiratory therapists and physiotherapist do not routinely work in the ER, and the number of cases recruited in the study by Wood et al.[4] would suggest that it is difficult for ER staff to obtain and maintain expertise in non-invasive ventilatory techniques. One practical option would be for patients in whom such treatment were indicated to be transferred directly to respiratory intermediate care units/HDUs or ICU where the technique could be implemented, in the same way that patients with myocardial infarction are admitted directly to coronary care units. As a complementary approach non-invasive respiratory support teams could be responsible for the initiation of NIPPV at all relevant sites in the hospital including the ER.

TRANSFER OF PATIENTS DEPENDENT ON NIPPV

Patients who require transfer while receiving NIPPV can be safely managed with the use of sensible planning. Non-invasive ventilators can be powered by an internal or external battery (Figure 8.1), electical supply from car battery via converter (e.g. Handy Mains) (Figure 8.2), or by oxygen cylinders. Small portable battery powered ventilator are becoming available e.g. the Hippy (B&D Electromedical), but these are often unsophisticated and may not meet the patient's full ventilatory needs. A list of these options is given in Box 8.1.

As with other battery systems, the battery life will depend on the electrical consumption of the ventilator which will depend to some extent on the settings. In general fully charged batteries will last from around 4–8 hours. Internal batteries

---

Box 8.1 *Examples of ventilatory equipment for transfer of patients receiving NIPPV*

Ventilator	Manufacturer	Power source
PV 401/403	Breas Ltd	External battery
BiPAP Harmony	Respironics Inc.	External battery
PLV 100, 101	Lifecare	Internal battery
Hippy	B&D Electromedical	External battery
Any ventilator via Handy Mains		Car battery
BromptonPAC	PneuPAC	Oxygen cylinder
(TransPAC)		

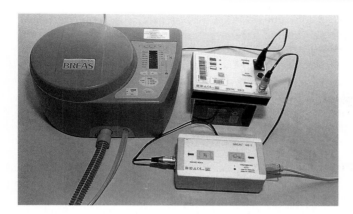

Figure 8.1 *Breas PV 401 ventilator with battery pack and charger.*

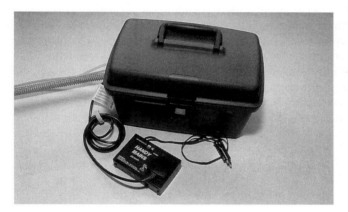

Figure 8.2 *Nippy ventilator used with Handy Mains which attaches to car battery via cigarette lighter.*

tend to have a shorter life, e.g. a few hours. We encourage our patients to test their ventilator with the battery in controlled home circumstances to get an idea of the battery life at their own ventilator settings. Guidelines[6] for the transfer of intubated and ventilated patients are relevant to non-invasively ventilated patients. It is clearly critically important to avoid the transfer of unstable patients with deteriorating conscious level, or who have become acutely 24-hour ventilator dependent. For this group efforts should be directed at stabilization and then transfer with intubation with full ventilatory support, so that safe extubation on to NIPPV can be considered after arrival.

INVESTIGATIVE PROCEDURES IN NIPPV-DEPENDENT PATIENTS

Computerized tomography and MRI scanning

These procedures need to be carried out with the patient lying supine, so that even in patients who are not 24-hour ventilator-dependent NIPPV may be required –

particularly in those with diaphragm weakness, orthopnoea or extreme breathlessness. Episodes of respiratory arrest have been reported anecdotally in NIPPV patients in whom NIPPV was temporarily discontinued while scanning took place. There is usually no problem with the mask as it does not contain metal parts. It is helpful to extend the ventilator tubing, by adding another full length, to enable to ventilator to be placed outside scanning range and accessible to medical staff. An attendant familiar with ventilator use should always attend the Radiology Department with the patient.

Colonoscopy, sigmoidoscopy

The routine use of sedation during these procedures and the fact that a lateral supine position is required means that nocturnal NIPPV recipients should be advised to use NIPPV throughout the procedure and recovery period. It is critical that the team responsible for the respiratory care of the patient liaises fully with the gastroenterologists/surgeons and anaesthetic team to insure that the non-invasive ventilator is available in theatre and the recovery suite. Extreme care is required in the use of sedation or pre-medication in this patient group, as airway control and adequate spontaneous ventilation may be compromised. Clearly such patients cannot be managed as straightforward day cases. If a significant degree of sedation is required or the procedure is likely to be protracted, then consideration should be given to carrying it out under general anaesthesia with full airway protection. The patient can then be extubated back on to NIPPV in controlled circumstances. Where possible reversible sedative agents should be used. These comments also apply to obstructive sleep apnoea patients using nasal CPAP therapy, who should be advised to use CPAP during sedation and the recovery period.

Upper gastrointestinal endoscopy/insertion of percutaneous gastrostomy (PEG)

Upper GI endoscopy can be performed in NIPPV users. The endoscope can be introduced through a T-piece connected to the mask. We have used PEG insertion in a number of 24-hour NIPPV-dependent patients with Duchenne muscular dystrophy or motor neurone disease without complications. The procedure should be carried out by an experienced operator in a well monitored area such as HDU or anaesthetic room, and careful observation maintained for the next 24 hours. The main risk in this period seems to be sputum retention; gastric distension or free peritoneal air have not been a problem.

Bronchoscopy

Fibreoptic bronchoscopy (FOB) +/- bronchoalveolar lavage (BAL) is often required to establish the cause of pulmonary infiltrates and fever in immunosuppressed patients with acute respiratory failure. In a cohort of immuncompromised patients with PaO_2/FiO_2 ratio < 100 and pH > 7.35, Antonelli et al.[7] have performed FOB

+/- BAL with the support of NIPPV via facemask. Having demonstrated satisfactory oxygenation following the application of NIPPV the bronchoscope was inserted into the nose via a T-piece seal attached to a full facemask. Pressure support of 17 cmH$_2$O with EPAP of 4 cmH$_2$O was applied, and FiO$_2$ electively increased to 1.0 during the procedure. PaO$_2$/FiO$_2$ ratio improved during NIPPV, patients tolerated the procedure well and no FOB-related complications were seen. This approach can also be considered in long-term NIPPV patients with chronic ventilatory failure who require investigation for suspected bronchial carcinoma, haemoptysis etc.

CATARACT SURGERY UNDER LOCAL ANAESTHETIC IN NIPPV PATIENTS

Comments regarding sedation during procedures are relevant in the patient undergoing cataract surgery under local anaesthetic. Following surgery, leaks from around the upper part of the nasal or facemask affecting the eyes may cause problems, and therefore consideration should be given to temporarily substituting a nasal plug system with which leaks are less likely to affect the eyes.

DENTAL SURGERY IN NIPPV PATIENTS

In patients receiving nocturnal NIPPV, sedation for tooth extraction and other dental procedures should be carried out with extreme caution. Local anaesthetic should be safe. It is prudent to carry out anything other than minor procedures under local anaesthetic in a hospital dental department with a full range of anaesthetic facilities and general anaesthetic available. The patient should of course take their ventilator with them to use in the post-operative period.

Contrary to expectation it is possible to carry out some form of minor dental surgery and scaling in patients who are 24-hour mask ventilation dependent. Nasal plug interfaces combined with pressure preset ventilaton should allow sufficient access to the mouth with a degree of compensation for a substantial and inevitable mouth leak. An alternative solution in this situation is to use negative pressure ventilation, for example with a pneumosuit or Hayek Oscillator. Patients should be familiarized with this equipment in advance of the procedure.

CONCLUSION

Further work is required to clarify the role of NIPPV in the ER, but it is clearly feasible and should be applied by a team familiar with the technique. As transfer, investigative and surgical procedures are virtually inevitable in NIPPV patients at some point, it is helpful to provide the long term NIPPV patient with written advice outlining potential problems, and the need for ventilatory support during procedures and subsequently. Many home ventilator patients (and sometimes their medical attendants) wrongly believe that they are 'unfit' to undergo any surgical procedures. While this may be the case in certain circumstances, with careful planning and support most can be managed safely and should not be denied this aspect of their care. If there is any doubt about the ability to control ventilation with NIPPV during transfer or operative procedures, the patient should be intubated, and extubated back on to NIPPV on recovery. NIPPV should be supervised by an experienced team member, and facilities available for intubation if required.

REFERENCES

1   Pollack C, Torres MT, Alexander L. Feasibility study of the use of bilevel positive airway pressure for respiratory support in the emergency department. *Ann Emerg Med* 1996; **27**: 189–92.

2   Poponick JM, Renston JP, Bennett RP, Emerman CL. Use of a ventilatory support system (BiPAP) for acute respiratory failure in the emergency department. *Chest* 1999; **116**: 166–71.

3   Ambrosino N, Foglio K, Rubini F, Clini E, Nava S, Vitacca M. Non-invasive mechanical ventilation in acute respiratory failure due to chronic obstructive airways disease: correlates for success. *Thorax* 1995; **50**: 755–7.

4   Wood KA, Lewis L, Von Harz B, Kollef MH. The use on noninvasive positive pressure ventilation in the Emergency Department. Results of a randomized clinical trial. *Chest* 1998; **113**: 1339–46.

5   Plant PK, Owen JL, Elliott MW. One year period prevalence study of respiratory acidosis in acute exacerbations of COPD: implications for the provision of non-invasive ventilation and oxygen provision. *Thorax* 2000; **55**: 550–4.

6   Intensive Care Society. *Guidelines for the transport of the critically ill adult*. London: ICS, 1997.

7   Antonelli M, Conti G, Riccioni L, Meduri GU. Noninvasive positive-pressure ventilation via face mask during bronchoscopy with BAL in high-risk hypoxaemic patients. *Chest* 1996; **110**: 724–8.

9

Negative pressure ventilation in acute respiratory failure

N AMBROSINO

Box 9.1 *Overview*

Although the first negative pressure ventilation (NPV) devices were described in the 19th century, they came into widespread clinical use during poliomyelitis epidemics of the second part of the 20th century. All negative pressure devices have two major components: an applicator, in which the sub-atmospheric pressure is generated at the surface of the body during inspiration, and a pump, which effects these pressure changes. Applicators range from chambers that cover only the anterior surface of the thorax and upper abdomen (e.g. cuirass) to chambers that cover all extra-cranial portions of the body (e.g. iron lung, some body suits).

Physiological studies suggest that NPV is able to improve breathing pattern and arterial blood gases, and to unload the respiratory muscles, thus fulfilling the aims of mechanical ventilation. Clinical studies show that NPV (by iron lung) is able to reduce the need of endo-tracheal intubation and related complications even in patients with severe respiratory acidosis.

It remains to be seen whether NPV is an alternative to invasive IPPV, and superior or inferior to mask NIPPV.

With negative-pressure ventilators the chest wall is exposed to sub-atmospheric pressure during inspiration, which results in air being drawn into the lungs through the mouth and nose. When the pressure around the chest wall returns to atmospheric, expiration occurs passively owing to the elastic recoil of the lungs and chest wall.[1-4]

HISTORICAL NOTES

Early negative pressure ventilation (NPV) devices were described in the 19th century. Alexander Graham Bell devised a negative pressure vacuum jacket for the resuscitation of infants shortly after the death of his son in 1881.[5] Drinker first developed the 'iron lung' or 'tank ventilator' in 1928.[6] In the 1950s Plum and Wolff[7] described the life-saving effect of NPV in severely ill patients with rapidly progressive acute respiratory failure (ARF) due to poliomyelitis. An anecdotal description of successful resuscitation and long-term survival of an emphysematous patient with decompensated hypercapnic ARF treated with the iron lung has been reported.[8] Conversely during the poliomyelitis epidemic, mortality decreased from 87% to 40% when NPV was replaced by positive-pressure ventilation (PPV).[9] This observation caused a marked reduction in the clinical use of NPV. Nevertheless a few investigators have continued to apply NPV to treat acute and acute on chronic respiratory failure.

NEGATIVE PRESSURE VENTILATORS

All negative pressure devices have two major components: an applicator where a negative (sub-atmospheric) pressure is generated at the surface of the body during inspiration and a pump which effects pressure changes.[1,10]

The *cuirass* (or shell) covers the anterior surface of the chest and upper abdomen. It is connected to the negative pressure pump through a tube and hose inlet on the centre. Standard sizes are available with commercial devices, whereas it is possible to tailor custom-made shells to patients with thoracic deformities such as kyphoscoliosis.[11]

All body suits like the *pneumowrap* or the *ponchowrap* applicators are fitted over a rigid grid including patient's rib cage and upper abdomen. The grid is anchored posteriorly with a backplate. The pneumowrap is attached to the negative pressure pump in a way similar to the cuirass. Different types of body suit are available[1] (Figure 9.1).

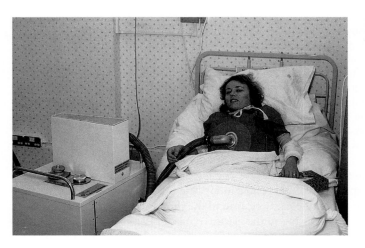

Figure 9.1 *A body suit ventilator.*

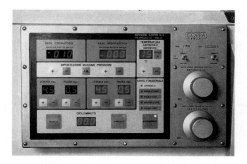

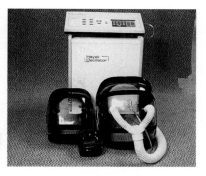

Figure 9.2 *Ventilatory variables during NPV in a contemporary iron lung (courtesy Coppa Biella).*

Figure 9.3 *High frequency external negative pressure ventilator and cuirass shells (Hayek Oscillator)*

The modern *iron lung* or *tank ventilator* is made of aluminium and plastic. All the patient's body rests on a thin mattress except his/her head, which protrudes through a porthole at one end of the ventilator. The head and the neck are supported to ensure comfort and to prevent upper airway collapse. Most tank ventilators have windows allowing patient observation and portholes through which catheters and monitor leads can be passed and which allow access to the patient for procedures. In some models the patient's head can be raised so that aspiration may be prevented. Negative pressure is generated by bellows pumps incorporated into the structure of the ventilator or by separate rotary pumps (see Figure 2.11).

Most of the pumps used are pressure cycled; that is the ventilator will continue to develop a sub-atmospheric pressure until a set level is reached. With this modality the set pressure is the independent variable, whereas the tidal volume (V_T) depends on the mechanic characteristics of the patient (besides the amount of leaks). With most tank ventilators the caregiver can set the pressure to be delivered during inspiration and expiration independently, and also inspiratory and expiratory times (Figure 9.2).[1] Volume cycled pumps have also been used, nevertheless these devices cannot compensate for variable air leaks from the applicator and their use is limited.

At the present time there are three modes for delivering NPV: intermittent negative pressure ventilation (INPV), negative/positive pressure, and continuous negative external pressure (CNEP).[1] Recently external high frequency negative pressure ventilators have been developed[12] (Figure 9.3).

INPV is the most commonly used mode. When operating in this mode the respirator generates a set negative pressure around the body to initiate (or assist) inspiration. Expiration is passive and expiratory pressure at the anterior thoracic surface is atmospheric.

During CNEP sub-atmospheric pressure surrounds the patient throughout the respiratory cycle, the patient can breathe spontaneously or the respirator can be set to superimpose cycles of increased negative pressure. The clinical importance of CNEP is somewhat similar to PEEP, but its cardiovascular effects differ.[13,14]

All negative pressure ventilators provide control mode; additionally some devices provide a 'trigger' whereby patient-generated negative pressure at the nares or tracheotomy stoma initiates a machine breath.[10] Other devices use a thermistor at the nares to trigger a breath. Nevertheless, at present these modalities are still experimental. Comprehensive reviews of negative pressure devices have been published.[2-4]

PHYSIOLOGICAL EFFECTS

The aims of mechanical ventilation in ARF are considered to be: (i) to buy time for the cause of ARF to subside; (ii) to improve pulmonary gas exchange; (iii) to increase ventilation and lung volume; and (iv) to unload the ventilatory muscles.[15,16]

Most physiological studies have been performed in stable patients with hypercapnic chronic respiratory insufficiency, their results are summarized below:

Breathing pattern and gas exchange

Tank ventilators are able to maintain normal arterial blood gases in stable patients with chronic obstructive pulmonary disease (COPD) and even in patients with little or no spontaneous respiratory effort.[17,18] Tidal volume, V_T, is linearly related to the peak negative pressure within the chamber both of tank and cuirass ventilators.[19,20]

Respiratory muscles

In stable COPD patients INPV (by iron lung or body suits) was able to reduce electrical and mechanical activity of the inspiratory muscles allowing them to rest, although the extent of respiratory muscle unloading is less than with non-invasive PPV (NIPPV).[21-23] A short period of patient training is necessary to allow optimal respiratory muscle rest.[24] The effects of INPV on electrical or mechanical activity of respiratory muscles have not been specifically investigated during ARF. Indirect evidence of the effects of INPV on respiratory muscles of COPD in ARF comes from two studies.[25,26] In these studies, INPV carried out intermittently for 7 days with an iron lung[25] or continuously by ponchowrap[26] was able to improve respiratory muscle strength and reduce Pa_{CO_2}.

Haemodynamics

Negative pressure applied to the chest wall increases venous return and can improve the performance of a right ventricle overloaded by an acute rise in pulmonary artery pressure due to hypoxic pulmonary vasoconstriction, together with the effects of hyperinflation and intrinsic PEEP. However, relative to atmospheric pressure, left ventricular pressures are decreased by NPV which means that a greater pressure output is required from the left ventricle to maintain constant systemic blood pressure, in other words, left ventricular ejection is impeded.[27] An increase in right ventricular size as a consequence of enhanced venous return may also decrease left ventricular diastolic compliance by displacing the interventricular septum. In contrast, PPV tends to reduce venous return and may increase left ventricular ejection. Independent of these changes, an increase in lung volume may reduce ventricular filling and alter pulmonary vascular resistance and capacitance.[27] As a result of these complex interactions, the effects of NPV and PPV will differ significantly according to the underlying cardiopulmonary status of the patient. Predictably, the few studies that have examined the haemodynamic effects of PPV and NPV have indicated no major advantage to either, and it should be remembered that these circulatory effects are at their most profound at the initiation of ventilatory support and during weaning. Indeed INPV with an 'iron lung' was found to show a linear relationship between the increase in venous pressure and the mean pressure applied to ventilate normal humans.[28] On the other hand no significant change in cardiac output and haemodynamics was found during INPV by cuirass ventilators in stable COPD patients,[29] whereas a reduction in CO and oxygen delivery has been observed with NIPPV (in Pressure Support modality) with and without PEEP, although this was of negligible clinical significance.[30]

High frequency INPV with a cuirass improved cardiac output in children after total cavo-pulmonary connection and tetralogy of Fallot repair.[31] In a comparative animal study iron lung ventilation with negative end-expiratory pressure was found to be haemodynamically equivalent to intermittent PPV with positive end-expiratory pressure (PEEP), whereas poncho wrap negative end-expiratory pressure ventilation had less adverse haemodynamic effects.[13] On the other hand in a study of patients with acute lung injury, CNEP was as effective as PEEP in improving lung volume and gas exchange at comparable transpulmonary pressure.[32] Cardiac index was higher with CNEP than with PEEP, and this was associated with increased transmural cardiac pressures and intra-thoracic blood volumes.[32]

Other effects

It has been reported that the application of INPV during sleep both in normal subjects and in patients with chronic respiratory insufficiency may result in obstructive sleep apnoeas or hypopnoeas.[33] However, most events were associated with only mild oxygen desaturation. Such apnoeas seem related to upper airway collapsibility at the glottic or supraglottic level,[34] but the underlying mechanism is unclear. Sleep related reduction in coordination of upper airway muscles might enhance the effect of the sub-atmospheric pressure developed in the upper airway during INPV.[34] Lower oesophageal sphincter dysfunction both in normal subjects and in COPD patients has been reported.[35] This dysfunction, at least theoretically, might induce regurgitation and eventually aspiration, but can be prevented by premedication with metoclopramide.[35]

CLINICAL STUDIES

Chronic respiratory insufficiency

The effects of INPV in chronic respiratory insufficiency resulting from neuromuscular, chest wall diseases and COPD are outside the remit of this chapter. Briefly however, chronic hypercapnic respiratory insufficiency due to *neuromuscular* and *skeletal disorders* is the main indication for long-term INPV.[18] Tank and jacket ventilators are effective but in most cases their inconvenience outweighs any advantage, and a cuirass is preferable for long-term use. Arterial blood gases improved both during the day and at night,[20] and the prognosis once treatment is instituted is usually good unless the underlying disease is progressive.[36]

Physiological and short-term clinical studies have been promising in COPD patients.[17,21] Nonetheless a double blind randomized controlled study of 184 stable COPD patients performed by Shapiro *et al.*[23] produced negative results. After an in-hospital training phase patients performed 12 weeks of either INPV by a poncho-wrap or sham treatment. Neither active nor sham treatment showed statistically significant improvements in exercise tolerance, dyspnoea, quality of life, arterial blood gases or respiratory muscle function.[23] Although most of the patients of this study[23] were not hypercapnic, the negative result has brought into question the concept of 'chronic respiratory muscle fatigue'. Almost certainly the discouraging outcome has reduced the enthusiasm for further research in this field.

Acute respiratory failure

NEUROMUSCULAR DISEASES

INPV has been used to avoid the need for endotracheal intubation during episodes of ARF in neuromuscular and skeletal disorders.[37] During poliomyelitis epidemics in the 1930s, several investigators showed that INPV reduced mortality by approximately 50%, the technique being more effective in spinal rather than in bulbar polio.[38,39] In the last case impaired airway clearance and upper airway collapsibility limited the INPV effectiveness. Furthermore during the poliomyelitis epidemic, mortality decreased substantially when INPV was replaced by PPV.[9] Indeed nowadays, if mechanical ventilation is indicated during ARF episodes, patients with neuromuscular disorders are usually treated by means of invasive or (less commonly) NIPPV. More recently only few uncontrolled or anecdotal reports are available on the effect of INPV in patients with ARF due to neuromuscular diseases. Using an iron lung, Libby *et al.* and Garay *et al.*[40,41] avoided endotracheal intubation in patients with ARF due to kyphoscoliosis. INPV by a pneumowrap was successful in patients with amyotrophic lateral sclerosis and Duchenne muscular dystrophy.[42] In a retrospective study[37] of a series of 15 patients with ARF due to different neuromuscular diseases treated by the iron lung, Corrado *et al.* reported an 80% success rate in avoiding endotracheal intubation and death.[37]

Although these reports suggest that INPV by iron lung can be effective in the treatment of ARF, many important questions remain unanswered. Prospective controlled studies should confirm the preliminary results of uncontrolled or anecdotal reports and clearly determine the effect of this technique on short- and long-term survival and length of hospital stay. The limitations of INPV must also be considered. Lack of protection of the airway and the risk of upper airway collapse with resulting obstructive apnoeas are potential risks with INPV in patients with neuromuscular diseases.

ACUTE ON CHRONIC RESPIRATORY FAILURE DUE TO EXACERBATIONS OF COPD

The role of INPV in acute exacerbations of COPD is still controversial. Early anecdotal reports[8,43–45] indicated a positive effect of INPV in this condition. Nevertheless, from the 1960s COPD patients have been routinely treated with PPV through an endotracheal tube. More recently, attempts to avoid the complications of invasive mechanical ventilation have led to innovations in mask NIPPV and a renewed interest in INPV.[46] Iron lung, cuirass and ponchowrap ventilators have been used successfully in exacerbations of COPD.[25,26,38,47–49] Montserrat et al.[26] evaluated the acute effects of INPV using a ponchowrap in 20 consecutive patients with COPD and ARF. In patients treated by INPV but not in those treated with conventional medical therapy, $PaCO_2$ and maximal inspiratory pressures improved after six hours of INPV whereas PaO_2 remained unchanged. However, six out of 20 patients were not compliant with INPV. Sauret et al.[49] treated by ponchowrap 17 COPD patients with acute on chronic respiratory failure, reporting better oxygenation and a reduction in hypercapnia and dyspnoea. These authors concluded that INPV facilitates increased oxygen supplementation and prevents the need for more aggressive ventilatory support.[49]

INPV used as first-line treatment in severe COPD patients with ARF has been found to be associated with good short- and long-term prognosis.[48] A total of 105 patients were retrospectively evaluated. All patients were treated by iron lung due to their severe respiratory acidosis. Sixty-two out of 105 (59%) were in coma on admission, and the other 43 showed neurological signs of deteriorating sensorium. Twelve patients died during hospitalization, but 93 (88.5%) were successfully weaned and followed up to 5 years. All relapses during the follow-up were treated by INPV. The survival rates after 1 and 5 years were 82 and 37% respectively, a survival better than that reported in COPD patients with ARF who received invasive PPV.[50] In a subsequent study the same authors, who have contributed greatly to the renaissance of INPV, confirmed this encouraging long-term survival.[51]

In a retrospective and uncontrolled study Corrado et al.[52] have reported a series of 150 consecutive patients (79% COPD) with hypoxic hypercapnic coma admitted to their respiratory ICU. The level of acidosis (mean level: 7.13) and the Glasgow coma scores (ranging from three to eight) were severe, and the mean Acute Physiology and Chronic Health Evaluation (APACHE) II score was 31.6. All patients underwent INPV with the iron lung. There was a 30% treatment failure rate and a 24% mortality. Six per cent of patients required endotracheal intubation because of lack of airway control. The median duration of ventilation was 27 hours (range 2–274). All successfully treated cases were discharged after a mean of 12.1 days. It should be noted that whereas all the patients in the study by Corrado et al.[52] suffered from a severe encephalopathy (Glasgow coma score < 8), alteration in sensorium was less severe and unconsciousness was an indication for intubation in all controlled studies of NIPPV in acute on chronic respiratory failure of COPD,[46] suggesting that NPV may be superior to NIPPV in some circumstances.

The Florence group has also performed a case–control study[53] designed to evaluate the effectiveness of INPV versus conventional mechanical ventilation in the treatment of acute on chronic respiratory failure in sequential patients admitted to their respiratory intermediate intensive care unit (RIICU) and four general ICUs. Twenty-six patients admitted to the RIICU and treated with INPV were matched on admission to 26 patients admitted to the ICUs and treated by IPPV via endotracheal intubation, controlling for age, sex, causes of ARF, APACHE II score (mean: 25 in both groups), pH (7.24 v 7.23 in cases (NPV) and controls (IPPV) respectively) and $PaCO_2$ (13 v 12 kPa). Mortality did not differ (23% and 27% for cases and controls respectively). Five NPV cases needed endotracheal intubation, four of whom subsequently died. The duration of ventilation in survivors was significantly lower in cases than in controls (median 16 hours v 96 hours), whereas the length of hospital stay was similar in the two groups (12 days for both). No complications were observed in cases, whereas three intubated controls developed infectious complications. The authors concluded that INPV is as efficacious and results in a similar length of hospital stay as conventional invasive PPV for the treatment of acute on chronic respiratory failure, but it is associated with a shorter duration of ventilation.[53]

It is noteworthy that patients in this study undergoing INPV were very severely ill (pH:7.24, APACHE II 25). It has been reported that NIPPV is more successful if applied early and in less severely acidotic patients.[54] The results of this study seem to indicate that INPV may be effective in a later stage of disease, with similar results to those obtained using endotracheal intubation. As suggested by Simonds[55] a possible explanation for the favourable effects of NPV in this study may be that it has a more beneficial effect on cardiopulmonary haemodynamics than NIPPV. However, direct comparisons of INPV vs NIPPV have not been performed.

One of the most interesting results of this study[53] was that INPV was performed successfully in a RIICU, which can be considered a reasonable alternative to the ICU for patients with less severe ARF. Indeed this study suggests that even though there was a difference between RIICU and ICU in the level of nursing care (nurse : patient ratio: RICCU = 1 : 3, ICU = 1 : 1) the outcome if these severe ARF patients was similar. Therefore, although no formal evaluation available, this study[53] suggests that using INPV in ARF may result in cost savings.

What do we learn from these studies?

- Prospective, randomized controlled studies of INPV v standard medical therapy and of INPV v conventional invasive mechanical ventilation are required.
- The most recent 'positive' reports come from a single Italian centre, and these results may well be influenced by the specialist medical experience of that team.
- Physiological studies suggest that INPV is able to improve breathing pattern[19–21] and arterial blood gases,[17,18] and to unload the respiratory muscles,[21–23] thus fulfilling the aims of mechanical ventilation.[15,16]
- Both uncontrolled retrospective and controlled non-randomized clinical studies show that INPV (by iron lung) is able to reduce the need for endotracheal intubation and related complications in patients with severe respiratory acidosis.
- Although recent reports are encouraging on the role of INPV in some cases of acute on chronic respiratory failure, there are many difficulties to overcome in introducing this mode to the vast majority of ICUs or RIICUs, where NIPPV is seen as the non-invasive mode of choice.[56] The reason for this preference may

be related to the fact that iron lungs are expensive and cumbersome, rather than due to the side effects reported with the devices.

OTHER APPLICATIONS

INPV and high frequency NPV are used largely in children and neonatology.[31,57] The use of CNEP in adult respiratory distress syndrome (ARDS) and in persistent flail chest deformity has been described.[58] Sawicka et al.[59] treated the cardiorespiratory complications developed during pregnancy in four patients with kyphoscoliosis. CNEP has been used in the treatment of ARF in infectious complications of lung transplantation.[60] Using INPV, Simonds et al.[61] reported successful weaning from IPPV in eight out of 10 patients with severe pulmonary disease after the failure of conventional weaning. Vitacca et al.[62] have found that INPV by a ponchowrap may be useful in reducing apnoeas during laser therapy under general anaesthesia, thus reducing hypercapnia, related acidosis and need for oxygen supplementation (and related hazard of combustion). In a subsequent study,[63] INPV compared with spontaneous assisted ventilation in paralysed patients undergoing interventional rigid bronchoscopy reduced the administration of opioids, shortened recovery time, prevented respiratory acidosis, excluded the need for manually assisted ventilation, reduced oxygen need, and afforded optimal surgical conditions.[63]

ADVANTAGES, CONTRAINDICATIONS AND SIDE EFFECTS

Advantages and contraindications of INPV are shown in Table 9.1. As with other modalities of non-invasive mechanical ventilation, the major advantage of INPV is the avoidance of endotracheal intubation and its related complications, while preserving physiological functions such as speech, cough, swallowing and feeding. As with NIPPV, bronchoscopic manoeuvres can be performed during INPV.[62,63] Nonetheless, when treating patients with INPV several limitations should be considered:

• Lack of upper airway protection, especially in unconscious and/or neurological patients may result in aspiration, given the reported effect of INPV on the lower

Table 9.1 *Advantages of INPV and contraindications to negative pressure ventilation*

Advantages	Contraindications
Avoidance or reduced need for endotracheal intubation	Gastrointestinal bleeding
Intermittent delivery of ventilation	Rib fractures
Airway suction during ventilation	Recent abdominal surgery
Physiological cough	Unco-operative patient
Bronchoscopic procedures allowed	Sleep apnoea syndrome
Normal swallowing, feeding, speech	Neurological disorders with bulbar dysfunction

Table 9.2 *Side effects reported with INPV*

Tiredness
Depression
Musculo-skeletal pain or tightness
Oesophagitis
Rib fractures and pneumothorax
Impaired sleep quality
Upper airway obstruction

oesophageal sphincter,[35] an effect to be prevented by pre-medication with metoclopramide.[35]

- Upper airway obstruction may occur[33] or be enhanced in unconscious patients, or in patients with neurological disorders associated with bulbar dysfunction and/or in those with sleep apnoea syndrome.

However, it has been reported[38] that in unconscious patients with normal bulbar function, the placement of a naso-gastric tube and the positioning of an oro-pharyngeal airway can minimize the risk of aspiration and/or airway collapsibility.

Most of the reports on side effects of INPV come from stable chronically ventilated patients (Table 9.2). In these studies the most common side effects were poor compliance, upper airway obstruction and musculoskeletal pain. All negative pressure ventilators restrict motion and back pain is a common problem. INPV has also been associated with rib fractures and pneumothorax.[64] In the study by Corrado *et al.*[53] two out of 26 (8%) subjects reported discomfort and back pain and two others suffered from vomiting during INPV. These percentages are similar to those reported for NIPPV.[46]

CONCLUSION

Despite the promising results shown by several studies in acute on chronic respiratory failure (most of them uncontrolled and/or retrospective, from one centre) 'the effectiveness, efficiency and utility of any intervention such as INPV requires the translation of trial results into general clinical practice. With limited INPV facilities and expertise in most countries, it seems NIPPV will remain the most widely applied non-invasive ventilatory method, with INPV continuing as a viable option in some centres'.[55]

REFERENCES

1   Levine S, Henson D. Negative pressure ventilation. In: Tobin MJ. *Principles and practice of mechanical ventilation*. NY: McGraw-Hill, 1994: 393–411.

2   Hill N. Clinical applications of body ventilators. *Chest* 1986; **90**: 897–905.

3   Ambrosino N, Rampulla C. Negative pressure ventilation in COPD patients. *Eur Respir Rev* 1992; **2**: 353–6.

4   Ambrosino N, Simonds AK. Mechanical ventilation. *Eur Respir Monog* 2000.
5   Woollam CHM. The development of apparaturs for intermittent negative pressure respiration 1832–1918. *Anaesthesia* 1976; **31**: 537–47.
6   Drinker P, Shaw LA. An apparatus for the prolonged administration of artificial respiration. I. A design for adults and children. *J Clin Invest* 1929; **7**: 229–47.
7   Plum F, Wolff HG. Observations on acute poliomyielitis with respiratory insufficiency. *JAMA* 1951; **146**: 442–6.
8   Bourteline-Young HG, Whittemberger JL. The use of artificial respiration in pulmonary emphysema accompanied by high carbon dioxide levels. *J Clin Invest* 1951; **30**: 838–46.
9   Lassen HCA. A preliminary report on the 1952 epidemic of poliomyelitis in Copenhagen with special references to treatment of acute respiratory insufficiency. *Lancet* 1953: **1**: 37–41.
10 Smith IE, King MA, Shneerson JM. Choosing a negative pressure ventilation pump: are there any important differences? *Eur Respir J* 1995; **8**: 1792–5.
11 Newman JH, Wilkins JK. Fabrication of a customized cuirass for patients with severe thoracic asymmetry. *Am Rev Respir Dis* 1988; **137**: 202–3.
12 Al-Saady NM, Fernando SSD, Petros AJ, Cummin AR. Sidhu VS. Bennett ED. External high frequency oscillation in normal subjects and in patients with acute respiratory failure. *Anaesthesia* 1995; **50**: 1031–5.
13 Skaburskis M, Helal R, Zidulka A. Hemodynamic effects of external continuous negative pressure ventilation compared with those of continuous positive pressure ventilation in dogs with acute lung injury. *Am Rev Respir Dis* 1987; **136**: 886–91.
14 Lockhat D, Langleben D, Zidulka A. Hemodynamic differences between continual positive and two types of negative pressure ventilation. *Am Rev Respir Dis* 1992; **146**: 677–80.
15 Slutsky AS. Mechanical ventilation. *Chest* 1993; **104**: 1833–59.
16 Tobin MJ. Mechanical ventilation. *N Eng J Med* 1994; **330**: 1056–61.
17 Ambrosino N, Montagna T, Nava S, *et al*. Short term effect of intermittent negative pressure ventilation in COPD patients with respiratory failure. *Eur Respir J* 1990; **3**: 502–8.
18 Shneerson JM. Non-invasive and domiciliary ventilation: negative pressure techniques. *Thorax* 1991; **46**: 131–5.
19 Whittemberger JL, Ferris BG Jr. Alterations of respiratory function in poliomyelitis. *Am J Phys Med* 1952; **31**: 226–37.
20 Kinnear W, Petch M, Taylor G, Shneerson JM. Artificial ventilation using cuirass respirators. *Eur Respir J* 1988; **1**: 198–203.
21 Nava S, Ambrosino N, Zocchi L, Rampulla C. Diaphragmatic rest during negative pressure ventilation by pneumowrap. Assessment in normal and COPD patients. *Chest* 1990; **98**: 857–65.
22 Belman MJ, Soo Hoo GW, Kuei JH, Shadmer R. Efficacy of positive vs negative pressure ventilation in unloading the respiratory muscles. *Chest* 1990; **98**: 850–6.
23 Shapiro SH, Ernst P, Gray-Donald K, *et al*. Effect of negative pressure ventilation in severe chronic obstructive pulmonary disease. *Lancet* 1992; **340**: 1425–9.
24 Rodenstein DO, Stanescu DC, Cuttitta G, Liistro G, Veriter C. Ventilatory and diaphragmatic EMG responses to negative-pressure ventilation in airflow obstruction. *J Appl Physiol* 1988; **65**: 1621–6.

25 Corrado A, Bruscoli G, De Paola E, Ciardi-Duprè GF, Baccini A, Taddei M. Respiratory muscle insufficiency in acute respiratory failure of subjects with severe COPD: treatment with intermittent negative pressure ventilation. *Eur Respir J* 1990; **3**: 644–8.

26 Montserrat JM, Martos JA, Alarcon A, Celis R, Plaza V, Picado C. Effect of negative pressure ventilation on arterial blood gas pressures and inspiratory muscles strength during an exacerbation of chronic obstructive lung disease. *Thorax* 1991; **46**: 6–8.

27 Pinsky MR. Cardiopulmonary interaction – the effects of negative and positive pleural pressure changes on cardiac output. In: Dantzker DR (ed.) *Cardiopulmonary critical care*. Orlando: Grune and Stratton, 1986: 89–121.

28 Beck GJ, Seanor HE, Barach AL, Gats D. Effects of pressure breathing on venous pressure: a comparative study of positive pressure breathing applied to the upper respiratory passageway and negative pressure to the body of normal individuals. *Am J Med Sci* 1952; **224**: 169–73.

29 Ambrosino N, Cobelli F, Torbicki A, *et al.* Hemodynamic effects of negative-pressure ventilation in patients with COPD. *Chest* 1990; **97**: 850–6.

30 Ambrosino N, Nava S, Torbicki A, *et al.* Hemodynamic effects of pressure support ventilation and PEEP by nasal route in patients with chronic hypercapnic respiratory insufficiency. *Thorax* 1993; **48**: 523–8.

31 Shekerdemian LS, Shore DF, Lincoln C, Bush A, Redington AN. Negative-pressure ventilation improves cardiac output after right heart surgery. *Circulation* 1996; **94** (Suppl II): II.49–II.55.

32 Borelli M, Benini A, Denkewitz T, Acciaro C, Foti G, Pesenti A. Effects of continuous negative extrathoracic pressure versus positive end-expiratory pressure in acute lung injury patients. *Crit Care Med* 1998; **26**: 1025–31.

33 Levy RD, Cosio MG, Gibbons L, Macklem PT, Martin JG. Induction of sleep apnoea with negative pressure ventilation in patients with chronic obstructive lung disease. *Thorax* 1992; **47**: 612–5.

34 Sanna A, Veriter C, Stanescu D. Upper airway obstruction induced by negative-pressure ventilation in awake healthy subjects. *J Appl Physiol* 1993; **75**: 546–52.

35 Marino WD, Pitchumoni CS. Reversal of negative pressure ventilation-induced lower esophageal sphincter dysfunction with metoclopramide. *Am J Gastroenterol* 1992; **87**: 190–4.

36 Baydur A, Layne E, Aral H, *et al.* Long term non-invasive ventilation in the community for patients with musculoskeletal disorders: 46 year experience and review. *Thorax* 2000; **55**: 4–11.

37 Corrado A, Gorini M, De Paola E. Alternative techniques for managing acute neuromuscular respiratory failure. *Sem Neurol* 1995; **15**: 84–9.

38 Corrado A, Gorini M, Villella G, De Paola E. Negative pressure ventilation in the treatment of acute respiratory failure: an old non invasive technique reconsidered. *Eur Respir J* 1996; **9**: 1531–44.

39 Crone NL. The treatment of acute poliomyelitis with the respirator. *N Engl J Med* 1934; **210**: 621–3.

40 Libby BM, Briscoe WA, Boyce B, Smith JP. Acute respiratory failure in scoliosis or kyphosis. *Am J Med* 1982; **73**: 532–8.

41 Garay SM, Turino GM, Goldring RM. Sustained reversal of chronic hypercapnia in patients with alveolar hypoventilation syndromes: long-term maintenance with noninvasive nocturnal mechanical ventilation. *Am J Med* 1981; **70**: 269–74.

42 Braun SR, Sufit RL, Giovannoni R, O'Connor M, Peters H. Intermittent negative
    pressure ventilation in the treatment of respiratory failure in progressive
    neuromuscular disease. *Neurology* 1987; **37**: 1874–5.
43 Stone DJ, Schwartz R, Neuman W, Feltman JA, Lovelock FJ. Precipitation by
    pulmonary infection of acute anoxia, cardiac failure, and respiratory acidosis in
    chronic pulmonary disease. *Am J Med* 1953; **14**: 14–21.
44 Lovejoy FW, Yu PNG, Nye RE, Joos HA, Simpson JH. Pulmonary hypertension. III.
    Physiologic studies in three cases of carbon dioxide narcosis treated by artificial
    respiration. *Am J Med* 1954; **16**: 4–11.
45 Marks A, Bocles J, Morganti L. A new ventilatory assister for patients with respiratory
    acidosis. *N Engl J Med* 1963; **268**: 61–7.
46 Ambrosino N. Noninvasive mechanical ventilation in acute respiratory failure. *Eur
    Respir J* 1996; **9**: 795–807.
47 Gunella G. Traitement de l'insuffisance respiratoire aiguè des pulmonaires chroniques
    avec le poumon d'acier: resultat dans une serie de 560 cas. *Ann Med Physique* 1980;
    2: 317–27.
48 Corrado A, Bruscoli G, Messori A, *et al.* Iron lung treatment of subjects with COPD in
    acute respiratory failure. Evaluation of short- and long-term prognosis. *Chest* 1992;
    101: 692–6.
49 Sauret JM, Guitart AC, Rodriguez-Frojan G, Cornudella R. Intermittent short-term
    negative pressure ventilation and increased oxygenation in COPD patients with severe
    hypercapnic respiratory failure. *Chest* 1991; **100**: 455–9.
50 Menzies R, Gibbons W, Goldberg P. Determinants of weaning and survival among
    patients with COPD who require mechanical ventilation for acute respiratory failure.
    Chest 1989; **95**: 398–405.
51 Corrado A, De Paola E, Messori A, Bruscoli G, Nutini S. The effect of intermittent
    negative pressure ventilation and long-term oxygen therapy for patients with COPD: a
    4 year study. *Chest* 1994; **105**: 95–9.
52 Corrado A, De Paola E, Gorini M, *et al.* Intermittent negative pressure ventilation in
    the treatment of hypoxic hypercapnic coma in chronic respiratory insufficiency.
    Thorax 1996; **51**: 1077–82.
53 Corrado A, Gorini M, Ginanni R, *et al.* Negative pressure ventilation versus
    conventional mechanical ventilation in the treatment of acute respiratory failure in
    COPD patients. *Eur Respir J* 1998; **12**: 519–25.
54 Ambrosino N, Foglio K, Rubini F, Clini E, Nava S, Vitacca M. Non-invasive mechanical
    ventilation in acute respiratory failure due to chronic obstructive pulmonary disease.
    Correlates for success. *Thorax* 1995; **50**: 755–7.
55 Simonds AK. (Editorial). Negative pressure ventilation in acute hypercapnic chronic
    obstructive pulmonary disease. *Thorax* 1996; **51**: 1069–70.
56 Nava S, Confalonieri M, Rampulla C. Intermediate respiratory intensive care units in
    Europe: a European perspective. *Thorax* 1998; **53**: 798–802.
57 Shekerdemian LS, Bush A, Shore DF, Lincoln C, Redington AN. Cardiorespiratory
    responses to negative pressure ventilation after tetralogy of Fallot repair: a
    hemodynamic tool for patients with a low-output state. *J Am Coll Cardiol* 1999; **33**:
    549–55.
58 Morris AH, Elliott GC. Adult respiratory distress syndrome: successful support with
    continuous negative extrathoracic pressure. *Crit Care Med* 1985; **13**: 989–90.

59 Sawika EH, Spencer GT, Branthwaite MA. Management of respiratory failure complicating pregnancy in severe kyphoscoliosis: a new use for an old technique? *Br J Dis Chest* 1986; **80**: 191–6.
60 Ambrosino N, Rubini F, Callegari G, Nava S, Fracchia C. Non invasive mechanical ventilation in the treatment of infectious complications of lung transplantation. *Monaldi Arch Chest Dis* 1994; **49**: 311–4.
61 Simonds AK, Sawicka EH, Carrol N, Branthwaite MA. Use of negative pressure ventilation to facilitate the return of spontaneous ventilation. *Anaesthesia* 1988; **43**: 216–9.
62 Vitacca M, Natalini G, Cavaliere S, *et al.* Breathing pattern and arterial blood gases during Nd-YAG laser photoresection of endobronchial lesions under general anesthesia: use of negative pressure ventilation. A preliminary study. *Chest* 1997; **111**: 1466–73.
63 Natalini G, Cavaliere S, Vitacca M, Amicucci G, Ambrosino N, Candiani A. Negative pressure ventilation vs spontaneous assisted ventilation during rigid bronchoscopy. A controlled randomized trial. *Acta Anesthesiol Scand* 1998; **42**: 1063–9.
64 Zibrak JD, Hill NS, Federman EC, Kwa SL, O'Donnell C. Evaluation of intermittent long-term negative pressure ventilation in patients with severe chronic obstructive pulmonary disease. *Am Rev Respir Dis* 1988; **138**: 1515–8.

10

Selection of patients for home ventilation

A K SIMONDS

INTRODUCTION

Not only have the numbers of individuals receiving home ventilation increased over the last decade, but there has also been a widening of indications for these techniques. In some areas this expansion is evidence-based, in others NIPPV is being applied where evidence to support its use is limited. The suitability of patients for home ventilation is explored below.

Assisted ventilation may be required long-term, or for a short period during an exacerbation of chronic respiratory failure. In general, ventilatory *dependency* can be classified into four categories:

- Grade 1: Assisted ventilation required for a short period during an acute illness or following an operation.
- Grade 2: Assisted ventilation required regularly during sleep.
- Grade 3: Assisted ventilation required during sleep and part of the day.
- Grade 4: Assisted ventilation required continuously 24 hours a day.

The majority of patients using non-invasive ventilation at home in Europe and the USA fall into grades 2 and 3. A small proportion require ventilation contin-

Table 10.1 *Indications for home ventilation*

Condition	Level of recommendation	Comment
(a) Chest wall disorders		
Scoliosis	C	Unlikely to be
Thoracoplasty/previous TB procedures	C	randomized controlled
Fibrothorax	C	trials as outcome without
Obesity hypoventilation syndrome		ventilatory support is death
(b) Neuromuscular disorders		
Congenital		
Myopathies	C	Unlikely to be randomized
Duchenne muscular dystrophy	C	controlled trials for reasons
Other muscular dystrophies	C	given above
Spinal muscular atrophy	C	
Hereditary sensory neuropathies e.g. Charcot–Marie–Tooth	C	
Acquired		
Old poliomyelitis	C	
Polymyositis	C	
ALS/motor neurone disease	B	Detailed studies on quality
Cervical spinal cord lesion	C	of life in progressive conditions required
(c) Neurological disorders		
Congenital central hypoventilation syndrome	C	
Brainstem CVA	C	
(d) Obstructive lung disease		
COPD	B	COPD: mixed results
Idiopathic bronchiectasis	C	cross-over trials. RCT v
Cystic fibrosis	C	LTOT required

RCT = randomized controlled trial; LTOT = long term oxygen therapy.
Guide to grading of recommendations:
A: Supported by at least one randomized controlled trials.
B: Supported by well conducted clinical studies.
C: Consensus evidence.

uously and most of these Grade 4 patients are treated with tracheostomy-IPPV, although an increasing number use 24-hour non-invasive ventilation. The number of patients in grade 1 who receive treatment for an acute respiratory failure is unknown – the indications for and outcome of this intervention are discussed in Chapters 3 and 4. Continued growth of acute non-invasive ventilation will inevitably lead to an increase in those who cannot be weaned following the acute episode and who therefore need to be considered for long-term respiratory support.

Conditions in which benefit from home ventilation has been demonstrated are listed in Table 10.1. With increasing experience in different patient groups over the last decade, indications have been extended to include more progressive disorders and paediatric neuromuscular disease, for example. Information on the outcome of home ventilation in these groups is given in Chapters 11–15. Here the indications for initiating elective domiciliary non-invasive ventilation are discussed.

ELECTIVE INDICATIONS

Starting home ventilation is a major undertaking for the individual and his/her family which has major social and financial implications. The appropriate timing of this intervention is therefore crucial. The elective introduction of any treatment presupposes that high risk patients can be identified, the natural history of the underlying respiratory disorder is known, and that the overall impact of treatment is beneficial. Assessment of the natural history of the disorder entails appropriate monitoring of the patient to detect trends in pulmonary function. Clearly, it is essential that all standard non-ventilatory therapeutic options have been fully explored before embarking on respiratory support. Each of these aspects will be considered in turn.

Identification of patients at high risk of ventilatory failure

Several longitudinal studies[1-3] have confirmed the excess morbidity and premature mortality associated with severe unfused idiopathic scoliosis. Cor pulmonale was the primary cause of death in 30% of 102 patients with untreated idiopathic scoliosis followed for 50 years.[2]

Branthwaite[3] has shown that patients with unfused idiopathic scoliosis and a vital capacity of less than 50% predicted at presentation may develop a disproportionate loss of lung volume with age. By contrast, patients with a vital capacity of more than 50% predicted were unlikely to develop respiratory problems (Figure 10.1). The age of onset of scoliosis is important with those acquiring the curvature at less than 5 years of age being at most risk of cardiorespiratory decompensation. Here, the early onset of the deformity may restrict alveolar duplication, the maturation of pulmonary vasculature, and chest wall growth. In addition, congenital scoliosis may be associated with other disorders, including congenital heart defects.[4,5] In a separate study of mortality, over 90% of individuals who experienced cardiorespiratory failure which could be attributed to the scoliosis, developed their thoracic deformity at less than 5 years of age.[3] A high thoracic curve seems to have a more adverse prognosis than a low thoracic defect probably because it places the respiratory muscles, accessory muscles and rib cage at a greater mechanical disadvantage.

In confirmation of some of these findings, Pehrsson[6] has reported results from a 20-year follow-up of lung function in adult idiopathic scoliosis. Respiratory failure occurred in 25% of patients. All those who developed respiratory decompensation had a vital capacity of less than 45% predicted, and a thoracic spinal curvature of more than 110 degrees. Wheeze was more common in those who developed ventilatory problems, although most patients did not smoke. It seems that the presence of additional respiratory pathology, such as asthma, may be sufficient to precipitate respiratory failure in those with borderline lung function.

The peak incidence of respiratory failure in the UK series[3] was during the fifth decade, although in this study and the Swedish series the age at decompensation ranged widely from 30 to 70 years.

Considering the evolution of respiratory failure in other conditions, an analysis[7] of 180 patients requiring NIPPV at the Royal Brompton Hospital has shown that

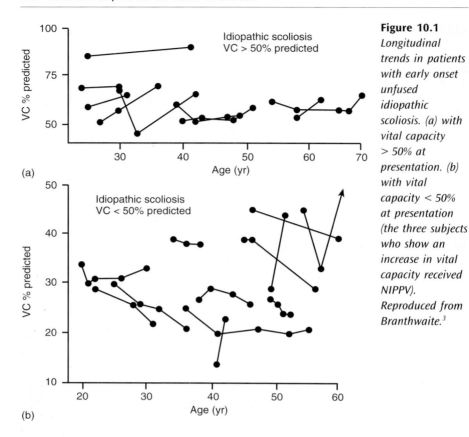

Figure 10.1
Longitudinal trends in patients with early onset unfused idiopathic scoliosis. (a) with vital capacity > 50% at presentation. (b) with vital capacity < 50% at presentation (the three subjects who show an increase in vital capacity received NIPPV). Reproduced from Branthwaite.[3]

the mean (range) age at which NIPPV was initiated for patients with previous poliomyelitis was 51.2 (25–76) years, sequelae of pulmonary tuberculosis 61.8 (45–75) years, COPD 58.2 (42–72) years and bronchiectasis 39.8 (19–61) years. In this cohort the mean age of patients with early onset idiopathic scoliosis when starting NIPPV was 49 years (range 17–74 years).

Pulmonary function tests demonstrated a mean (SD) vital capacity of 0.82 (0.37) litres in the early onset scoliosis patients, 1.1 (0.4) litres in poliomyelitis patients, and 1.2 (0.6) litres in those with previous tuberculosis. In the group with obstructive lung disease, mean (SD) FEV_1 was 0.58 (0.3) litres in COPD patients and 0.48 (0.16) litres in those with bronchiectasis.

Respiration during sleep has been compared in patients with scolioses of varying aetiology.[8] Nocturnal arterial oxygen saturation was lowest in patients with a paralytic scoliosis associated with a severe reduction in vital capacity, and in older patients with non-paralytic scoliosis. The degree of scoliosis did not correlate well with the extent of nocturnal desaturation. In patients with neuromuscular disease,[9] minimum arterial oxygen saturation during sleep was correlated with vital capacity, and the percentage fall in vital capacity on changing from the erect to supine position. There was a relationship between daytime arterial blood gas tensions and nocturnal desaturation, but the wide scatter in results makes it difficult to predict the degree of nocturnal desaturation on the basis of diurnal values alone. Maximum inspiratory mouth pressures are not closely correlated with nocturnal saturation.

Braun et al.[10] have demonstrated that in patients with neuromuscular disorders, a vital capacity of less than 55% predicted and mouth pressures of less than 30% strongly predict the development of daytime hypercapnia. In Duchenne muscular dystrophy patients the presence of a daytime $PaCO_2$ of > 6 kPa and base excess of > 4 mmol/L is strongly predictive of significant nocturnal desaturation[11] (see Chapter 15).

Regarding high risk COPD patients, there is a clear relationship between the degree of airflow obstruction and the risk of cardiorespiratory failure. However, the predictive value of FEV_1 for nocturnal desaturation is not high, and the best predictor of oxygenation during sleep is wake arterial oxygen saturation. The presence of obstructive sleep apnoea complicating COPD to can produce profound nocturnal desaturation. The coexistence of these disorders is relatively common, and often characterized by symptoms of obstructive apnoea, disproportionate hypoxaemia to the degree of airflow obstruction, and polycythaemia. COPD patients who develop chronic hypercapnia will almost inevitably have a history of previous acute ventilatory decompensation at the time of an infective exacerbation.

MONITORING

Having identified high risk patients, the purpose of follow-up is to detect a progressive fall in lung function and the development of nocturnal hypoventilation, before progression to frank diurnal respiratory failure and cor pulmonale occurs. Early diagnosis and intervention is important as results suggest that the outcome of nocturnal ventilation is less good in those with longstanding cor pulmonale and pulmonary hypertension.[7] As a routine, standard treatment measures should be optimized and advice given regarding general health, and the maintenance of ideal body weight. Weight gain with age is an important hazard in patients with limited respiratory reserve. Hormone replacement therapy is probably advisable in postmenopausal female scoliotic patients to prevent the development of osteoporosis and progression of the curvature. In most patients the presence of a morning headache, fatigue and poor sleep quality correlates well with the degree of nocturnal hypoventilation. A headache on waking may be wrongly ascribed to musculoskeletal pain resulting from a cervical scoliosis. It is important to have a high index of suspicion for nocturnal hypoventilation in patients with severe restrictive chest wall disorders. We have been referred several hypercapnic, scoliotic patients who had undergone extensive investigation of morning headaches with temporal artery biopsy and CT scan of the brain, before arterial blood gas measurement was considered.

Some individuals may present with nocturnal confusion and overt psychiatric features, although this is uncommon.[12] A recent patient referred with severe respiratory muscle weakness due to motor neurone disease presented with temper tantrums and confusion on waking associated with profound hypercapnic respiratory failure.

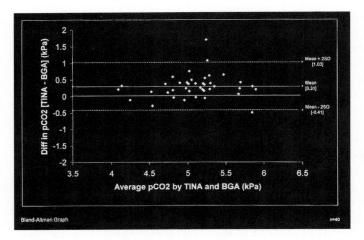

Figure 10.2 *Bland–Altman plot of relationship between transcutaneous and arterial P_{CO_2} using Radiometer TINA (transcutaneous CO_2) electrode. Courtesy of Derek Cramer, Royal Brompton Hospital. BGA: arterial blood gas analysis.*

In addition to a careful review of symptoms, routine assessment should include pulmonary function tests, measurement of arterial blood gas tensions and the monitoring of respiration during sleep. A progressive fall in lung volumes (notably vital capacity and total lung capacity) is usually seen in restrictive disorders. As indicated above, individuals with mild to moderate nocturnal hypoventilation will usually develop a raised venous base excess prior to the development of overt diurnal respiratory failure. This finding should prompt overnight investigation. Nocturnal monitoring in this situation should include oximetry and either transcutanous or end-tidal CO_2. End-tidal CO_2 measurements are relatively reliable in patients with restrictive disorders, but do not accurately represent alveolar P_{CO_2} in subjects with severe airflow obstruction. Transcutaneous CO_2 measurement has been found to follow changes in arterial P_{CO_2} reliably,[13] although some investigators dispute this.[14] The response time of the electrode is inevitably slower than oximetry so that a maximum reading represents the peak level achieved during an episode of hypoventilation rather than an accurate representation of CO_2 fluctuations during individual hypopnoeas. Meticulous skin preparation before the CO_2 electrode is applied and regular calibration is essential. We use a Radiometer electrode heated to 41 degrees which can be left safely in place for 8 hours. A Bland–Altman plot of the relationship between arterial and transcutaneous CO_2 values using this system is shown in Figure 10.2. Additional monitoring of chest wall movement and oronasal airflow is helpful to characterize apnoea and hypopnoeas, especially in conditions such as Duchenne muscular dystrophy and motor neurone disease where bulbar weakness predisposes the individual to upper airway obstruction, as well as hypoventilation. Full polysomnograhy is not essential, but it is important that at least some REM sleep is observed, as early nocturnal hypoven-

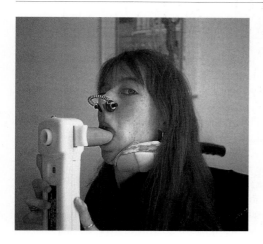

Figure 10.3 *Mouth pressure meter for measuring Pi_{max} and Pe_{max} (Precision Medical Ltd.).*

tilation will always be manifest in this sleep stage.[15] Clinical experience suggests that the development of diurnal respiratory failure in the presence of preserved inspiratory muscle strength ($> 70\,cmH_2O$) is highly indicative of a significant component of upper airway obstruction during sleep.[15]

Global respiratory muscle strength is best measured using a mouth pressure meter (e.g. Precision Medical Ltd., Pickering, Yorkshire) (Figure 10.3). Using this device, expiratory muscle strength (Pe_{max}) is measured at the mouth as the patient makes a maximum expiratory effort against a closed airway from total lung capacity. Likewise, inspiratory muscle strength (Pi_{max}) can be gauged from the pressure obtained at the mouth during a maximum inspiratory effort from residual volume or functional residual capacity. The meter includes a small leak to prevent erroneously high pressures being generated by the buccal muscles. Accurate measurement depends on full patient co-operation, and preserved bulbar function. Reference normal ranges depend partly on the type of mouthpiece used, but a Pi_{max} and Pe_{max} above $80\,cmH_2O$ excludes significant weakness of the inspiratory and expiratory muscles.[16]

Transdiaphragmatic pressure generation is a more specific assessment of diaphragm muscle function and can be measured by passage of oesophageal and gastric balloons linked to a pressure transducer. In the presence of a low transdiaphragmatic pressure, phrenic nerve stimulation in the neck will clarify the functional integrity of the phrenic nerves. Measurement of mouth pressures and transdiaphragmatic pressure during a maximal voluntary effort are dependent on patient co-operation. Cervical root excitation using a magnetic stimulator over C_{3-5}, and transcutaneous phrenic nerve stimulation in the supraclavicular fossa both circumvent the volitional element and may be useful to confirm true weakness, when poor effort is suspected.

During regular follow-up the views and motivation of the patient, together with social/psychological factors can be explored so that the individual and family are well-prepared for the introduction of home ventilation. Patients often find it helpful to meet other individuals who are already using home ventilation.

CAN VENTILATORY FAILURE BE PREVENTED OR DELAYED?

The hypothesis that prophylactic use of NIPPV might prevent the development of ventilation failure in normocapnic Duchenne muscular dystrophy patients with a vital capacity of 20–50% predicted has been tested by Raphael and coworkers in a randomized controlled study.[17] They found no evidence that this prophylactic application delayed or prevented the development of daytime hypercapnia; indeed the strategy was poorly tolerated and associated with a number of disadvantages (see Chapter 15).

There are some data to support the use of intermittent positive pressure hyper-inflation of the lungs using positive pressure devices to reverse a fall in lung volumes in restrictive chest wall conditions.[18] Barois and Estournet-Mathiaud recommend intermittent positive pressure hyperinflation in children with congenital conditions such as spinal muscular atrophy to promote alveolar expansion, improve chest wall compliance and mobilize secretions,[19] but this use has not been subject to controlled studies.

TREATMENT OPTIONS FOR VENTILATORY INSUFFICIENCY

There are a number of treatment options which are worth exploring in patients with stable hypercapnia and mild to moderate nocturnal hypoventilation. These may allow the use of home ventilation to be delayed for up to several years.

Drug therapy

The tricyclic drug protriptyline can control moderate nocturnal hypoventilation[20,21] and is usually more successful in restrictive disorders than COPD. It appears to work by reducing REM sleep-related hypoventilation, although an independent effect on upper airway tone may play a part.[22] Low doses (5–10 mg at night) are sufficient. Higher doses (as used to treat depression) are associated with significant anticholinergic side effects including dry mouth, constipation, urinary hesitancy and impotence. Protriptyline should be given with caution in individuals with a history of prostatism, and all users should be warned of the risk of photosensitivity. It is not possible to predict which individuals will respond to protriptyline. In some patients improvement in nocturnal and diurnal arterial blood gas tensions is maintained over years,[23] in others the effect is transient,[24] or side effects preclude long-term use.[21] Unfortunately the manufacture of protriptyline is likely to be suspended in 2001 (although supplies may last a further few years) as the drug has been superceded for use in depression, its original indication. Fluoxetine has similar REM suppressant properties, but fewer side effects than protriptyline. It has been shown to reduce REM-related sleep-disordered breathing in obstructive sleep apnoea,[25] however it is not yet clear whether fluoxetine also has an independent effect on upper airway muscle tone like protriptyline, or is as effective as protriptyline at controlling nocturnal hypoventilation. The use of other REM suppressants for sleep-disordered breathing is currently being explored.

Almitrine has been shown to produce a sustained increase in nocturnal and diurnal oxygenation in COPD patients. The precise mechanism of action is unclear, but almitrine has been shown to have a stimulant effect on carotid and aortic body chemoreceptors,[26] and improves ventilation–perfusion matching by a direct effect on the pulmonary vascular bed.[27] In many countries, however, the drug is not freely available.

Medroxyprogesterone stimulates hypercapnic ventilatory drive during wakefulness and sleep, and can produce a small fall in $PaCO_2$ in some patents with chronic respiratory failure.[28] However, side effects including fluid retention and impotence in males limit its application.

Acetazolamide increases urinary bicarbonate ion excretion and shifts the ventilatory response to hypercapnia to the left. Occasional short term benefit has been seen in patients with hypercapnic COPD,[29] although care should be taken to avoid worsening the level of acidosis in patients with acute on chronic ventilatory decompensation. Acetazolamide may have a minor role in central sleep apnoea,[30] but as with other respiratory stimulants, side effects are troublesome.

Long-term oxygen therapy (LTOT)

LTOT is unequivocally the treatment of choice in COPD patients who fulfil the criteria listed in Table 10.2. Until the results of trials comparing nocturnal nasal ventilation and LTOT in COPD are available, LTOT should be first-line treatment and nasal ventilation considered only in hypercapnic COPD patients who tolerate oxygen therapy poorly (see Chapter 12). LTOT is usually inadvisable in severe restrictive disorders because of the risk of provoking uncontrolled hypercapnia. However, Strom and colleagues[31] have recently examined the role of domiciliary oxygen therapy in patients with severe thoracic spine deformities. In the group studied, almost 40% had additional pathology contributing to hypoxaemia (e.g. COPD, previous pulmonary tuberculosis). It seems that a proportion of patients with a significant component of ventilation–perfusion mismatch due a combination of chest wall disease and parenchymal lung disease may benefit initially from oxygen therapy, although survival in patients over the age of 65 years was poor and a growing number of patients required home ventilation with time. These findings underline the importance of close monitoring of any hypercapnic patient receiving oxygen therapy. Overnight assessment of oximetry and transcutaneous CO_2 is strongly recommended.

Table 10.2 *Criteria for prescribing long-term oxygen therapy (LTOT)*

Proven benefit
Patients with COPD with steady state values of:
- FEV_1 less than 1.5 litres
- FVC less than 2.0 litres
- PaO_2 on air of less than 7.3 kPa (55 mmHg)

Potential benefit
- Patients with other chronic irreversible lung disease e.g. interstitial lung disease or bronchiectasis with PaO_2 of less than 7.3 kPa
- Patients with symptomatic pre-terminal respiratory failure due to any aetiology e.g. bronchial carcinoma

Continuous positive airway pressure (CPAP) in respiratory failure

The use of CPAP in obstructive sleep apnoea in considered in Chapter 16. CPAP has been shown to reduce the work of breathing in COPD patients during exercise. It may also be of value in patients with respiratory decompensation due to a combination of obstructive sleep apnoea and COPD (overlap syndrome), and in those in whom bulbar weakness outstrips general respiratory muscle weakness. However, in most patients with ventilatory failure due to chest wall disease, neuromuscular conditions or COPD, CPAP is unable to offload respiratory muscles to the same extent as assisted ventilation, and does not control severe nocturnal hypoventilation.

Intermittent courses of non-invasive ventilation

A final strategy that may be employed before the introduction of home ventilation is intermittent courses of in-hospital non-invasive ventilation. Clearly this is of value in patients who develop an acute hypercapnic exacerbation of chronic lung disease, but occasionally patients who experience a gradual decline in ventilatory function may derive sustained improvement in arterial blood gas tensions and a reduction in symptoms after a short course of intensive nocturnal and diurnal NIPPV lasting approximately seven to ten days. Some of these patients may be maintained in good health by two or three courses of NIPPV a year. Similar improvements in arterial blood gas tensions have been seen after two weeks of negative pressure ventilation. The mechanism of action of this short period of treatment is under investigation, but it may work via a reduction in ventilatory load and 'resetting' of hypercapnic drive. Alternatively (or additionally) an improvement in respiratory muscle function and/or mechanics may occur. Most patients initially maintained on intermittent courses of NIPPV will ultimately require domiciliary ventilation, although in-hospital courses of treatment may be helpful in individuals who cannot cope with ventilatory equipment in the home for social or practical reasons. Further studies are required to examine the long-term outcome and cost-effectiveness of this approach, which should currently be regarded as experimental. Short course NIPPV should be distinguished from the practice of giving non-invasive ventilation on a regular weekly outpatient basis. This approach is controversial,[32] and we have not found it helpful.

CRITERIA FOR STARTING DOMICILIARY VENTILATION

There are no hard and fast rules, but assuming all standard treatment has failed and the patient is motivated to try non-invasive ventilation, most authorities proceed to treatment in the presence of symptomatic diurnal respiratory failure when mean overnight SaO_2 is less than 90% and PCO_2 exceeds 7 kPa. In severely hypercapnic patients with marked symptoms and stable underlying disease, the decision to start treatment is relatively easy. Recurrent admissions for acute hypercapnic exacerbations are also an important influencing factor. In those with milder, more intermittent symptoms a controlled trial to determine the optimum time for initiating therapy is probably indicated. As indicated above, at present there is NO indication for NIPPV to be used prophylactically (i.e. before CO_2 retention has developed) in neuromuscular disease or any other disorder.

CONSENSUS RECOMMENDATIONS

The proceedings from a consensus conference on the clinical indications for NIPPV in chronic respiratory disease have recently been published.[33] For patients with neuromusculoskeletal disease the following suggestions are made:

1 Disease documentation
   - Before considering a restrictive thoracic patient for NIPPV a physician with skills in NIPPV must establish and document an appropriate diagnosis on the basis of history, physical examination, and diagnostic tests, and asssure optimal treatment of other underlying disorders (such as performing a multi-channel sleep study to detect associated apnoea if clinically indicated).
   - The most common disorders would include a sequelae of polio, spinal cord injury, neuropathies, myopathies and dystrophies, amyotrophic lateral sclerosis (ALS), chest wall deformities and kyphoscoliosis.
2 Indications for usage
   - Symptoms (such as fatigue, dyspnoea, morning headache) and one of the following:
     (a) $Pa_{CO_2} > 6.0$ kPa.
     (b) Nocturnal oximetry demonstrating oxygen saturation $< 88\%$ for 5 consecutive minutes.
     (c) For progessive neuromuscular disease, maximal inspiratory pressures < 60 cmH$_2$O or FVC $< 50\%$ predicted.

For COPD patients the following recommendations were made:

1 Disease documentation
   - Before considering a COPD patient for NIPPV, a physician with skills and experience in NIPPV must establish and document an appropriate diagnosis on the basis of history, physical examination, and the results of diagnostic tests and assure optimal management of COPD with such treatments as bronchodilators, oxygen when indicated, and optimal management of underlying disorders (such as performing a multichannel sleep study to exclude sleep apnoea if clinically indicated).
   - The most common obstructive lung diseases would included chronic bronchitis, emphysema, bronchiectasis, and cystic fibrosis.
2 Indications for use
   - Symptoms (such as fatigue, dyspnoea, morning headache) and
   - Physiologic criteria (one of the following):
     (a) $Pa_{CO_2} > 7.3$ kPa (55 mmHg)
     (b) Pa_{CO_2} 6.7–7.2 kPa (50–54 mmHg) and nocturnal desaturation (oxygen saturation $< 88\%$ for 5 continuous minutes while receiving oxygen therapy at 2 L/minute.

(c) Pa_{CO_2} 6.7–7.2 kPa and hospitalization related to recurrent (two or more admissions in a 12-month period) episodes of hypercapnic respiratory failure.

Comment on consensus guidelines

Although it is important in diagnostic terms to establish the presence of other or related conditions such as obstructive sleep apnoea (OSA), it should be noted that OSA, for example, is likely to exacerbate nocturnal hypoventilation in restrictive and obstructive lung disease patients and therefore *add* to the indications for nocturnal ventilatory support. The indications for domiciliary NIPPV in COPD are undoubtedly still controversial, as discussed in Chapter 12. It is perhaps most likely that a subgroup of COPD patients may benefit, but further randomized controlled trials of NIPPV plus LTOT versus LTOT alone are required to settle the issue, and examine the cost-effectiveness of the intervention. Guidelines are being prepared by a task force from European Respiratory Society, but these are unlikely to differ greatly from those above.

INITIATION OF NON-INVASIVE VENTILATION AND COMPLIANCE

Familiarization with the technique during a brief hospital admission is advisable to address any initial teething problems, educate the patient and family, ensure the correct ventilatory settings, and instill confidence in all concerned. Advice on the choice of equipment, practical aspects of starting NIPPV and organization of home care is given in Chapters 2, 5 and 18, respectively. Evidence suggests that long-term compliance with NIPPV is less good if treatment is started on an outpatient basis.[34]

Criner et al.[35] found that 65% (26/40) of patients were continuing to use domiciliary NIPPV at 6-month follow-up, and a further 7.5% had progressed to tracheostomy ventilation. This compliance rate seems disappointingly low, as a UK-based study found that only 5/180 (3%) discontinued NIPPV due to poor tolerance.[7] All patients voluntarily discontinuing NIPPV in this study had COPD. Leger et al.[36] showed that 85% of scoliotic patients continued NIPPV long-term in a French multicentre series, whereas this figure was lower at 56% in COPD patients. These results are partly explained by higher morbidity and mortality rates in COPD patients, as individuals discontinue NIPPV due to illness as well as poor tolerance. However, as 50% of the patients in the report by Criner et al.[35] had COPD, it is evident that long-term compliance rates are worse in patients with obstructive disease – perhaps reflecting the lesser degree of physiological improvement derived from NIPPV in obstructive versus restrictive disorders. Although not all studies included an accurate measurement of the duration of time spent at the prescribed mask pressure level (and can therefore be contested), overall compliance rates with NIPPV are almost certainly superior to comparable figures for CPAP use in obstructive sleep apnoea patients.

REFERENCES

1   Nachemson A. A long term follow up study of non-treated kyphoscoliosis. *Acta Orthop Scand* 1968; **39**: 466–76.

2   Freyschuss V, Nilsonne U, Lundgren KD. Idiopathic scoliosis in old age. 1. Respiratory function. *Arch Med Scand* 1968; **184**: 365.

3   Branthwaite MA. Cardiorespiratory consequences of unfused idiopathic scoliosis. *Br J Dis Chest* 1986; **80**: 360–9.

4   Reckles LN, Peterson HA, Bianco AJ, Weidman WH. The association of scoliosis and congenital heart disease. *J Bone Joint Surg* 1975; **57**: 449–55.

5   Simonds AK, Carroll N, Branthwaite MA. Kyphoscoliosis as a cause of cardiorespiratory failure – pitfalls of diagnosis. *Respir Med* 1989; **83**: 149–50.

6   Pehrsson K, Bake B, Larsson S, Nachemson A. Lung function in adult idiopathic scoliosis: a 20 year follow up. *Thorax* 1991; **46**: 474–8.

7   Simonds AK, Elliott MW. Outcome of domiciliary nasal intermittent positive pressure ventilation in restrictive and obstructive disorders. *Thorax* 1995; **50**: 604–9.

8   Sawicka EH, Branthwaite MA. Respiration during sleep in kyphoscoliosis. *Thorax* 1987; **42**: 801–8.

9   Bye PT, Ellis ER, Issa FG, Donnelly PM, Sullivan CE. Respiratory failure and sleep in neuromuscular disease. *Thorax* 1990; **45**: 241–7.

10 Braun NMT, Arora NS, Rochester DF. Respiratory muscle and pulmonary function in polymyositis and other proximal myopathies. *Thorax* 1983; **38**: 616–23.

11 Hukins CA, Hillman DR. Daytime predictors of sleep hypoventilation in Duchenne muscular dystrophy. *Am J Respir Crit Care Med* 2000; **161**: 166–70.

12 Elliott MW, Branthwaite MA. Occult respiratory failure as a cause of neuropsychiatric symptoms in patients with chest wall deformity and neuromuscular disease. *Respir Med* 1991; **85**: 431–3.

13 McLellan PA, Goldstein RS, Ramacharan V, Rebuck AS. Transcutaneous carbon dioxide monitoring. *Am Rev Respir Dis* 1981; **124**: 199–201.

14 Sanders MH, Kern NB, Costantino JP, *et al.* Accuracy of end-tidal transcutaneous P_{CO_2} monitoring during sleep. *Chest* 1994; **106**: 472–83.

15 Piper AJ, Sullivan CE. Breathing and neuromuscular disease. In: Saunders NA, Sullivan CE (eds). *Sleep and Breathing*, 2nd edn. New York: Marcel Dekker, 1994: 777.

16 Green M, Moxham J. Respiratory muscles in health and disease. In: Barnes PJ (ed.) *Respiratory medicine: recent advances*. Oxford: Butterworth-Heinemann, 1993: 252–75.

17 Raphael J-C, Chevret S, Chastang C, Bouvet F. Randomised trial of preventive nasal ventilation in Duchenne muscular dystrophy. *Lancet* 1994; **343**: 1600–4.

18 Simonds AK, Parker RA, Branthwaite MA. The effect of intermittent positive-pressure hyperinflation in restrictive chest wall disease. *Respiration* 1989; **55**: 136–43.

19 Barois A, Estournet-Mathiaud B. Spinal muscular atrophy: respiratory management as a function of clinical aspects. In: Robert D, Make BJ, Leger P *et al.* (eds). *Home mechanical ventilation*, 1st edn. Paris: Arnette Blackwell, 1995: 261–75.

20 Simonds AK, Parker RA, Sawicka EH, Branthwaite MA. Protriptyline for nocturnal hypoventilation in restrictive chest wall disease. *Thorax* 1986; **41**: 586–90.

21 Carroll N, Parker RA, Branthwaite MA. The use of protriptyline for respiratory failure in patients with chronic airflow limitation. *Eur Respir J* 1990; **3**: 746–51.

22 Bonora M, St John WM, Bledsoe TA. Differential elevation by protriptyline and depression by diazepam of upper airway respiratory motor activity. *Am Rev Respir Dis* 1985; **131**: 41–5.

23 Simonds AK, Carroll N, Shiner R, James R, Idzikowski C, Branthwaite MA. Long term suppression of REM sleep in the treatment of sleep disordered breathing. *Thorax* 1988; **43**: 851P.

24 Series F, Cormier MY, La Forge J. Long term effects of protriptyline in patients with chronic obstructive pulmonary disease. *Am Rev Respir Dis* 1993; **147**: 1487–90.

25 Kopelman PG, Elliott MW, Simonds AS, Cramer D, Ward S, Wedzicha JA. Short term use of fluoxetine in asymptomatic obese subjects with sleep related hypoventilation. *Int J Obes* 1992; **16**: 825–30.

26 Laubie M, Schmitt H. Long lasting hyperventilation induced by almitrine: evidence for a specific effect on carotid and thoracic chemoreceptors. *Eur J Pharmacol* 1980; **61**: 123–36.

27 Melot C, Naerije R, Rothschild T, Mertens P, Mols P, Hallemans R. Improvement in ventilation perfusion matching by almitrine. *Chest* 1983; **83**: 528–33.

28 Skatrud JB, Dempsey JA, Iber C, Berssenbrugge A. Correction of CO_2 retention during sleep in patients with chronic obstructive pulmonary disease. *Am Rev Respir Dis* 1981; **124**: 260–8.

29 Skatrud JB, Dempsey JA. Relative effectiveness of acetazolamide versus medroxyprogesterone acetate in correction of carbon dioxide retention. *Am Rev Respir Dis* 1983; **127**: 405–12.

30 White DP, Zwillich CW, Pickett CK, Douglas NJ, Findley LS, Weil JV. Central sleep apnea. Improvement with acetazolamide therapy. *Arch Int Med* 1982; **142**: 1816–19.

31 Strom K, Pehrsson K, Boe J, Nachemson A. Survival of patients with severe thoracic spine deformities receiving domiciliary oxygen therapy. *Chest* 1992; **102**: 164–8.

32 Gutierrez M, Beroiza T, Contreras G, *et al*. Weekly cuirass ventilation improves blood gases and inspiratory muscle strength in patients with chronic airflow limitation and hypercarbia. *Am Rev Respir Dis* 1988; **138**: 617–23.

33 Consensus Conference. Clinical Indications for noninvasive positive pressure ventilation in chronic respiratory failure due to restrictive lung disease, COPD, and nocturnal hypoventilation – a Consensus conference report. *Chest* 1999; **116**: 521–34.

34 Elliott MW, Simonds AK, Carroll MP, Wedzicha JA, Branthwaite MA. Domiciliary nocturnal nasal intermittent positive pressure ventilation in hypercapnic respiratory failure due to chronic obstructive lung disease: effects on sleep and quality of life. *Thorax* 1992; **47**: 342–8.

35 Criner GJ, Brennan K, Travaline JM, Kreimer D. Efficacy and compliance with non-invasive positive pressure ventilation in patients with chronic respiratory failure. *Chest* 1999; **116**: 667–75.

36 Leger P, Bedicam JM, Cornette A, *et al*. Nasal intermittent positive pressure ventilation. Long term follow-up in patients with severe chronic respiratory insufficiency. *Chest* 1994; **105**: 100–105.

11

Domiciliary non-invasive ventilation in restrictive disorders and stable neuromuscular disease

A K SIMONDS

INTRODUCTION

In this chapter the outcome of domiciliary non-invasive ventilation in restrictive disorders is discussed. Use of NIPPV in specific situations such as during pregnancy and pulmonary rehabilitation is also considered. In all these areas case series data (sometimes extensive) are now available, but there have been few randomized controlled studies in patients with chest wall or neuromuscular disease. As patients with ventilatory failure due to restrictive ventilatory disorders were originally treated with negative pressure ventilation and tracheostomy-IPPV (T-IPPV), use of these techniques and NIPPV will be compared and contrasted. It is important to note that these findings should be interpreted bearing in mind that ventilatory modes have evolved over the last few decades; there has been a gradual change in the indications and patient selection for ventilatory support, and a growing public debate on the ethics of life-saving therapies and the quality of life which results.

NEGATIVE PRESSURE VENTILATION (NPV) IN RESTRICTIVE DISORDERS

As described in Chapter 1, negative pressure ventilation (NPV) achieved prominence in the 1950s as a tool to deal with respiratory insufficiency due to poliomyelitis. It is an interesting phenomenon that many individuals who required temporary support with NPV following poliomyelitis in their youth, have subsequently required NIPPV in later life due to ventilatory decompensation. A renaissance of interest in physiological mechanisms of action of NPV followed in the 1970s and 1980s.

Twenty years' experience with NPV in 40 patients with neuromuscular disease has been described by Splaingard et al.[1] Most recipients were aged between 6 and 40 years and had muscular dystrophy. The majority used tank ventilation in the home; a few were ventilated using a cuirass or pneumosuit. Only three received supplemental oxygen therapy. Survival for the group ranged from 6 months to 19 years with 5 and 10-year survival rates of 76% and 61% respectively. This is despite the fact that 35% of patients had Duchenne muscular dystrophy (DMD). The authors also helpfully consider nine patients in whom NPV was unsuccessful. Six of these were under 3 years of age and developed problems with upper airway obstruction and/or recurrent aspiration. One patient died of electrical power failure. In the older age group NPV failed in individuals with a severe thoraco-cervical scoliosis which limited the efficacy of the neck seal of the tank ventilator. Most of these NPV failures were successfully treated with tracheostomy ventilation. The patients in this series were recruited through the period 1962 to 1982 and it is likely that NIPPV would now be the treatment of choice in at least some of the patients with NPV-induced upper airway obstruction or neck seal problems.

An account of an even longer experience (46 years) with domiciliary NPV has recently been published.[2] It describes the use of NPV, mouth ventilation and NIPPV in 560 patients with neuromuscular disease treated at the Rancho Los Amigos Medical Center, California, USA from 1949 to 1995. The vast majority (500) had acute poliomyeltis and were recruited at the beginning of the series. Most of these (76%) were weaned off NPV within two years. The report recounts the subsequent course in the polio patients who were still ventilator dependent after two years, and a further group who had other forms of neuromuscular and chest wall disease (e.g. 15 DMD, four myopathy, two spinal muscular atrophy, two amyotrophic lateral sclerosis (ALS), five scoliosis). In total, long-term follow-up data were available on 79 patients. It is notable that 14/25 post-polio patients and all non-DMD and myopathy patients treated with NPV ultimately required transfer to tracheostomy ventilation, largely because hypercapnia could not be adequately controlled. Nine out of ten deaths occurred in the patients using NPV, although not all these could be attributed to respiratory causes. Interestingly 67% of patients receiving positive pressure non-invasive ventilation reported favourable outcomes (improved sense of independence and well-being) compared with only 29% receiving NPV. Problems such as machine discomfort and self-discontinuation of ventilation occurred more than twice as often in negative pressure users, compared with those receiving NIPPV or mouth ventilation and crucially, hospital admission rates *increased* a surprising 8-fold after initiation of NPV, but *decreased* by 36% in those started on NIPPV/MIPPV.

Although striking, these results should be interpreted with caution as the study has a number of limitations. As the authors admit, over the long period of recruitment, equipment evolved, medical teams changed, patient population shifted from being almost entirely comprised of post-polio cases to a heterogeneous mix with small numbers in each category, and patient groups were not matched. These major limitations notwithstanding, the results suggest that NPV is less efficient than positive pressure non-invasive ventilation. In addition, the findings imply that a deterioration in lung function and the number of hospital admissions may be reduced in those with non-progressive pathologies receiving NIPPV.

The long-term effectiveness of cuirass ventilation in chest wall disease has been explored by Jackson et al.[3] Pre-treatment vital capacity for the group was 30% predicted with a mean $PaCO_2$ of 8.2 kPa. Five-year survival was 60% (15/25); three patients swapped to positive pressure ventilation. $PaCO_2$ in suvivors decreased to 6.1 kPa after one year of cuirass ventilation and was 6.8 kPa after 5 years. Interestingly, survival was not correlated with age, lung volumes or arterial blood gas tensions at presentation.

Sawicka and colleagues[4] analysed the outcome in 51 patients with restrictive disorders using a variety of negative pressure devices including cuirass, pneumosuit and tank ventilator. Five patients had progressive neuromuscular disorders and, of the remainder, around half had stable neuromuscular conditions and half chest wall disease. A reduction in breathlessness and improvement in exercise tolerance and arterial blood gas tensions was seen in all patients. The efficiency of NPV was limited by upper airway obstruction in approximately 20% of patients. This was treated with either a tracheostomy or protriptyline.

In another study of patients group with stable ventilatory failure due to restrictive disorders, 6 months of domiciliary therapy with a pneumosuit resulted in significant improvements in arterial blood gas tensions and inspiratory muscle strength. Three out of 31 of these patients developed upper airway obstruction during sleep. An even higher incidence of upper airway obstruction during NPV was found by Bach et al.[5] They demonstrated that 26/37 patients with chronic paralytic/restrictive disorders developed multiple desaturation episodes during sleep using NPV and these were attributable to upper airway obstruction. As described in Chapter 15 obstructive apnoeas complicating NPV are also a feature in Duchenne muscular dystrophy.[6] Sleep disordered breathing was recorded in 11/12 DMD patients using negative pressure body ventilators. Almost certainly the increased incidence of obstructive sleep apnoea in patients using NPV is due to the dissociation between lower respiratory muscle activity and the activation of the muscles maintaining upper airway patency, and this problem will be worsened in patients with bulbar weakness. Several groups[5,6] have advocated the addition of CPAP to NPV to overcome upper airway obstruction, but this complicates management considerably, and the problem is now more easily addressed using NIPPV.

NPV VERSUS NIPPV

There has never been a prospective comparison of domiciliary NPV with NIPPV in restrictive chest wall disease. The efficacy of NIPPV versus NPV via pneumosuit has been examined in short-term physiological studies[7] using the ability to offload the respiratory muscles as the main endpoint. In awake normal subjects and patients with obstructive lung disease diaphragm electromyographic activity, trans-diaphragmatic pressure, pressure time integral coefficient of variation of tidal volume and PCO_2 were all lower during NIPPV compared with NPV, indicating that NIPPV is the more efficient technique. This impression is borne out by the results of a crossover study[8] where restrictive patients ($n = 15$) receiving chronic noctur-nal NPV were swapped to NIPPV. Arterial blood gas values improved from PaO_2 7.5 (1.2), $PaCO_2$ 7.1 (1.2) using NPV to PaO_2 9.6 kPa, $PaCO_2$ 6.3 (0.7) kPa ($p < 0.005$) on NIPPV, and no patient opted to return to NPV.

Paediatric NPV

A role for NPV is likely to remain in the paediatric population. This ranges from the application in children with phrenic nerve injury following cardiac surgery in whom recovery of phrenic nerve function is anticipated,[9] to use in children central hypoventilation syndromes[10] and neuromuscular or chest wall disease. Successful outcomes in these situations have been well demonstrated, but in many cases NIPPV is now an option and the use of NPV is waning. In a recent UK survey[11] of domiciliary ventilation in children, only 7% were receiving NPV.

NIPPV

Following its introduction in the early 1980s, NIPPV entered mainstream clinical practice in 1986–87, therefore long-term experience is inevitably more limited than with NPV. However the total database of patients receiving NIPPV is expanding rapidly and now far exceeds the number of patients using domiciliary negative pressure techniques. As with NPV, domiciliary NIPPV was first applied in patients with restrictive ventilatory pathology. In a large French multicentre series[12] the 3-year probability of continuing domiciliary NIPPV was between 75% and 80% for patients with scoliosis and post-tuberculous restrictive disease. Similar results are seen in a single centre UK cohort[8] which showed a 5-year actuarial probablity of continuing domiciliary NIPPV of 79% (95% CI 66–92) for scoliotic patients, 100% in post-polio patients, 94% (95% CI 83–100) in patients with post-tuberculous lung disease, and 81% (95% CI 61–100) in those with neuromuscular disorders exclud-ing poliomyelitis (Figure 11.1). This compares with five-year figures of 43% in COPD patients and less than 20% in bronchiectaisis. In this study the probability of continuing NIPPV equates almost completely with survival as the main reason for discontinuing NIPPV was death. In the French cohort, 7% of scoliotic patients discontinued NIPPV voluntarily, and 3% progressed to tracheostomy ventilation. Almost a third of DMD patients transferred to T-IPPV. Both the UK and French series demonstrated that arterial blood gas tensions during NIPPV were well maintained long-term. Importantly, the French data show that the probability of survival for 5 years for scoliosis patients using NIPPV is significantly better than survival rate using long-term oxygen therapy alone (73% NIPPV v 60% oxygen

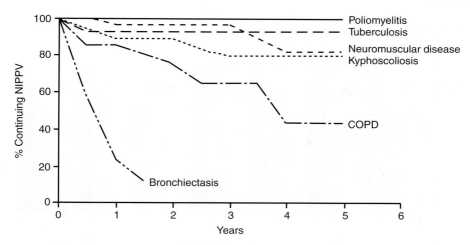

Figure 11.1 *Survival using long-term NIPPV (redrawn from Ref. 8). NB: Probability of continuing NIPPV is equivalent to survival as main reason for discontinuation was death.*

therapy). As expected a survival advantage was also seen in post-tuberculous lung disease patients (60% v 53%).

Effects of NIPPV on morbidity and quality of life

Improvements in morbidity are also consistently seen in NIPPV users. Leger *et al.*[12] report significant reductions in inpatient days for at least 2 years after the initiation of NIPPV in patients with scoliosis, post-tuberculous lung disease and DMD, implying that worthwhile economic savings can be made.

A UK subgroup who received the SF 36 health status questionnaire gave comparable results to other groups with chronic disorders such as diabetes mellitus and ischaemic heart disease. Although physical function was reduced in contrast to age-matched population norms, mental health and energy/vitality were similar (Figure 11.2). Sleep quality is a significant contributor to quality of life scores and contrary to popular belief, patients using nocturnal NIPPV rated their sleep quality as average (67%) or very good (27%), with only 5% describing sleep quality as poor.

Most recipients found that the main limiting factors of NIPPV were inconvenience (19%), nasal symptoms/mask problems (9%), gastric distension (3%) and noise (3%).[8] It can be seen that nasal side effects and mask problems are less prevalent during chronic NIPPV than acute NIPPV, as use is less intensive and a greater period of time is available to optimize mask fit and mimimize side effects.

Paediatric NIPPV

This topic is discussed in Chapter 15. However, currently the main indication for paediatric NIPPV is congenital neuromusculoskeletal disease. Fauroux *et al.*[13] report

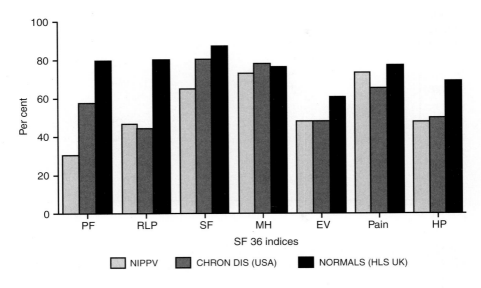

Figure 11.2 *Health status (quality of life) measured using the SF 36 in patients using domiciliary NIPPV, in a US group with chronic diseases and in UK age-matched normal subjects. PF: Physical function; RLP: role limitation related to physical function; SF: social function; MH: mental health; EV: energy and vitality; Pain: total pain; HP: health perception. 0 = minimum score; 100 = maximum score (redrawn from Ref. 7).*

from the ANTADIR central data collection agency that of 287 children developing chronic respiratory failure in the period 1992–93, 176 had restrictive disorders and 158 children received home ventilation.

Mechanisms of action

Several mechanisms have been proposed to explain the physiological effects of long-term ventilatory support, particularly the fact that nocturnal application of treatment is translated into improvements in daytime blood gas tensions. These are:

- Relief of chronic respiratory muscle fatigue
- Improvement in central respiratory drive
- Improvement in chest wall/lung mechanics
- Improvement in sleep efficiency and quality
- Alteration in cardiopulmonary/renal haemodynamics.

As indicated in Chapter 12 it may be that the relative importance of these mechanisms differs in restrictive chest wall disorders and obstructive lung disease, and of course the explanations are not mutually exclusive. It has often been assumed that respiratory muscle fatigue is an important factor in the development of ventilatory failure. However, the presence of fatigue is difficult to confirm in practice. In addition, although some uncontrolled studies have demonstrated small improvements in respiratory muscle strength after NIPPV,[14,15] others have not;[16,17] and it may be that these increases in respiratory muscle strength are due to an improvement in general well-being and/or a learning effect.

Hill[18] examined the efficacy of NIPPV by withdrawing it from restrictive patients who had acclimatized to the technique for at least 2 months. All had demonstrated improvements in symptoms and arterial blood gas tensions following initiation. A week after withdrawal patients experienced an increase in breathlessness, morning headaches, and somnolence *in the absence* of any change in daytime blood gas tensions, pulmonary function or respiratory muscle strength. Moreover, nocturnal monitoring without NIPPV showed greater desaturation, a larger rise in $PaCO_2$, and an increase in tachypnoea and tachycardia compared with results when receiving NIPPV – suggesting that one of the prime mechanisms of action is via control of nocturnal hypoventilation.

The effects of withdrawal of NIPPV after successful implementation have also been observed by Piper *et al.*[14] In 14 scoliotic and neuromuscular patients treated with nocturnal NIPPV for at least 6 months, mean (SD) arterial blood gas tensions measured while breathing spontaneously during the day improved from PaO_2 7.5 (1.2) kPa, $PaCO_2$ 8.2 (1.6) kPa to PaO_2 10.2 (1.3) kPa, $PaCO_2$ 6.4 (0.7) kPa, and maximum inspiratory mouth pressure rose from 41 to 65 mmHg ($p < 0.003$). During full polysomnography without ventilatory support breathing during sleep was improved compared with a pre-NIPPV study, but was still abnormal. The REM sleep-related fall in SaO_2 and rise in transcutaneous CO_2 tension were 20% and 1.5 kPa respectively, compared with values of 41% and 2.8 kPa in the baseline study before NIPPV. There was no difference in effects between patients with scoliosis and those with primary neuromuscular disease and in both patient groups there was no correlation between the increase in respiratory muscle strength and improvement in nocturnal gas exchange. As a result the authors argue that the improvement in nocturnal gas exchange following NIPPV be due to a reduction in hypoxic and hypercapnic induced arousals with consequent beneficial effects on sleep quality. Sleep fragmentation and deprivation caused by arousal are known to have a negative effect on ventilatory drive and therefore it is postulated that central drive is increased by the enhanced sleep quality.

In support of this theory, Annane *et al.*[17] have shown that the reduction in $PaCO_2$ that occurs after initiation of NIPPV in patients with neuromuscular disease and scoliosis is correlated with an increase in the slope of the ventilatory response to CO_2 ($r = -0.68$, $p = 0.008$). This study too showed no improvement in respiratory muscle strength or lung mechanics. An additional mechanism contributing to increased chemosensititvty to CO_2 may be the washout of CO_2 stores following correction of overnight hypercapnia.

However, Schonhofer *et al.*[19] have challenged the belief that correction of nocturnal hypoventilation is of key importance, in a study using ventilatory support solely during the day in patients who remained awake. There was no significant difference in improvement in arterial blood gas tensions in patients using daytime and night-time ventilator support, although clearly support during sleep is more convenient for patients.

COMPLIANCE WITH NIPPV

In general, compliance with long-term NIPPV is usually higher in restrictive patients compared with those with COPD. In a series reported by Criner et al.,[20] 15% of restrictive patients discontinued NIPPV at six months, whereas 20% of these with COPD did not continue therapy.

PREGNANCY AND SCOLIOSIS/NEUROMUSCULAR DISEASE

Normal pregnancy is associated with major physiological changes including an increase in minute ventilation by 40%, reduction in functional residual capacity, and rise in cardiac output by about 2.5 L/minute. Despite these challenges, the outlook for the majority of females with mild adolescent onset idiopathic scoliosis during pregnancy is good. Breathlessness and back pain are usually no more common than in the normal population,[21] and providing the scoliosis is stable at the start of the pregnancy, progression of the curve is unlikely. Genetic counselling is strongly advisable, particularly in those with early onset scoliosis, as the curvature may be the consequence of genetic disorders such as neurofibromatosis or Marfan syndrome. Genetic counselling is also important in patients with neuromuscular disease. It is becoming increasingly obvious that some scolioses, previously labelled as 'idiopathic' may be the presenting feature of mild variants of congenital muscular dystrophy or myopathies.

Patients with scoliosis who are most at risk of cardiorespiratory complications during pregnancy are those with a vital capacity of less than one litre (or < approximately 40% predicted). Pulmonary hypertension is an absolute contraindication to pregnancy. Pre-pregnancy counselling clinics have now been established at some centres so that the risks to the mother and fetus can be carefully assessed. These include:

- Genetic risk to infant
- Risk of cardiorespiratory complications in mother
- Risk of progression of scoliosis during pregnancy
- Obstetric complications e.g. pelvic deformity
- Anaesthetic problems e.g. difficult intubation, problems with siting epidural block, poor tolerance of anaesthetic agents in patients with NMD, post-operative ventilatory failure/weaning problems.

At the Royal Brompton/Queen Charlotte's Hospital Scoliosis Pre-pregnancy Clinic, investigations include full pulmonary function tests, arterial blood gas measurement, ECG, echocardiogram, and sleep study if nocturnal hypoventilation is suspected. We have found sleep studies particularly helpful in predicting which patients are unlikely to cope with added ventilatory load. Figure 11.3 shows overnight monitoring of arterial oxygen saturation and transcutaneous CO_2 in (a) a patient with a Pott's kyphoscoliosis who underwent an uneventful pregnancy but required NIPPV seven years later, and (b) a patient who developed cor pulmonale at 36 weeks during an unplanned pregnancy. Figure 11.4 shows a patient with

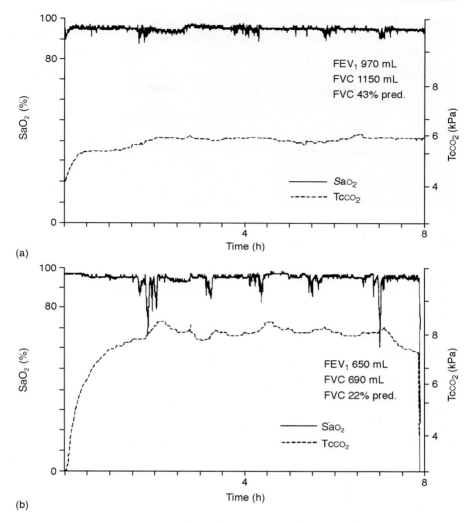

Figure 11.3 *Spirometry and overnight monitoring of Sao$_2$ and Tcco$_2$ in (a) a patient with Pott's kyphosis who underwent an uneventful pregnancy and (b) a patient with congenital scoliosis who developed cor pulmonale during the final trimester of an unplanned pregnancy.*

congenital scoliosis on nocturnal NIPPV before pregnancy (left) and when four months pregnant (right). Note the fall in nocturnal and diurnal Pco$_2$ despite no change in ventilator settings, which is likely to be attributable to the normal pregnancy-induced increase in minute ventilation. Mean Sao$_2$ is normal.

It can be seen that the use of NIPPV in some patients with restrictive disorders has increased the chances of a successful pregnancy in some patients. We have recently seen pregnancies without cardiorespiratory complications in two females with a vital capacity of 800 mL. Delivery was carried out electively at 34–36 weeks

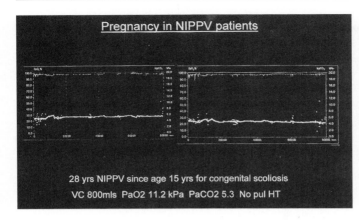

Figure 11.4
Overnight monitoring of Sao$_2$ and transcutaneous CO$_2$ in a patient with congenital scoliosis using domiciliary NIPPV before pregnancy (left) and when 4 months pregnant (right). Pul HT: pulmonary hypertension.

in both. One patient had Freiderich's ataxia, and the other with a presumed congenital idiopathic scoliosis and had been using nocturnal NIPPV for over 10 years before becoming pregnant (Figure 11.4). Providing arterial blood gas tensions can be maintained in the normal range by day and by night using nocturnal NIPPV, and there is no evidence of pulmonary hypertension or congenital heart disease at the outset, then a select number of patients with severe restrictive disorders may have a successful outcome from pregnancy.

Patients who present *de novo* to the respiratory physician with respiratory failure and cor pulmonale at an advanced stage of pregnancy pose a difficult problem. It is important to avoid the misdiagnosis of pre-eclampsia in this situation. NIPPV or negative pressure ventilation has been used successfully to salvage both mother and baby, and may avert premature labour. NIPPV has also been used semi-electively to support a woman through the last trimester, and throughout pregnancy in a patient with central hypoventilation syndrome. Caution is, however, advisable and it is unlikely that a pregnancy in a patient with a vital capacity of less than 800 mL will be viable, even with the use of ventilatory support. (See Chapter 13 for the use of NIPPV during pregnancy for cystic fibrosis patients.)

NIPPV DURING EXERCISE AND PULMONARY REHABILITATION PROGRAMMES

Pulmonary rehabilitation regimes containing an exercise component have been shown to reduce breathlessness and improve quality of life in patients with COPD[22,23] although evidence of benefit in COPD patients with ventilatory failure is lacking, and exertion in this situation may potentially worsen muscle fatigue and pulmonary hypertension. Reconditioning programmes in patients with restrictive chest wall disease may also be beneficial,[24] but there are few randomized controlled trials in this area. It has, however, been demonstrated that restrictive and obstructive patients using nocturnal NIPPV can have just as successful results from a rehabilitation programme as patients who did not require NIPPV (Figure 11.5). Wanke *et al.*[25] have shown that a respiratory muscle training (as opposed to general

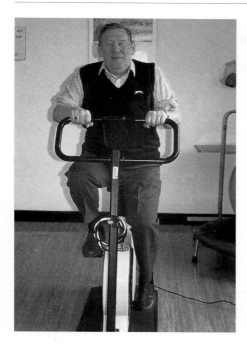

Figure 11.5 *Pulmonary rehabilitation to maximize respiratory function in a restrictive patient (previous thoracoplasty) after initiation of long-term NIPPV.*

training regime) can improve respiratory muscle strength in patients with Duchenne muscular dystrophy, but a subgroup who were already hypercapnic did not benefit, suggesting that the timing of introduction of the training programme is crucial. For patients with COPD or restrictive disorders resulting in severe ventilatory limitation, the use of ventilatory support such as NIPPV during exercise or pulmonary rehabilitation programmes offers the possibility that exercise tolerance may be increased and training benefit may be obtained without exhausting the respiratory muscles. It has been shown that the use of inspiratory pressure support during treadmill exercise reduces dyspnoea and prolongs the distance walks by successfully offloading the respiratory muscles.[26,27] It is possible that progressive dynamic hyperinflation generated during exercise in obstructive patients may be further offloaded by EPAP. The use of CPAP and proportional assist ventilation during exercise has also produced promising results and this area warrants further investigation. Several portable mini-ventilators have been developed, but so far the limited size has resulted in a poor triggering capability which is a major problem, as use of a ventilator during exercise requires an lightweight, extremely flexible, responsive device able to meet high and rapidly changing ventilatory needs.

T-IPPV IN RESTRICTIVE DISORDERS

Outcome information on T-IPPV in restrictive disorders is mainly available from French multicentre series dating from several decades ago. Robert *et al.*[29] have shown five-year survival rates of 95% in post-polio patients and 70% in those with TB sequelae. In a 20-year experience of T-IPPV in the home from 1962–1983

Splaingard et al.[30] report on 40 adults and children with neuromuscular disease, including spinal cord injury or central hypoventilation syndromes. Three-year survival was 63% for spinal cord injury patients and 74% for other neuromuscular diagnoses combined i.e. figures not dissimilar from NIPPV results. However, as discussed elsewhere patients prefer a non-invasive modes where these are feasible,[31] and certainly the practicalities of implementing NIPPV are simpler than those of T-IPPV. The possibility of weaning on to NIPPV should always be considered in any patient using T-IPPV long-term. Currently the main indications for T-IPPV in restrictive disorders are:

- Extreme ventilator dependency
- Upper airway problems e.g. in mucopolysaccharidoses
- Marked bulbar weakness with swallowing and cough difficulties
- Inability to use mask
- Neonatal ventilatory problems.

REFERENCES

1   Splaingard ML, Frates RC, Jefferson LS, Rosen CL, Harrison GM. Home negative pressure ventilation: report of 20 years experience in patients with neuromuscular disease. *Arch Phys Med Rehab* 1985; **66**: 239–42.

2   Baydur A, Layne E, Aral H, *et al*. Long term non-invasive ventilation in the community for patients with musculoskeletal disorders: a 46 year experince and review. *Thorax* 2000; **55**: 4–11.

3   Jackson M, Kinnear W, King M, Hockley S, Shneerson J. The effects of five years of nocturnal cuirass-assisted ventilation in chest wall disease. *Eur Respir J* 1993; **6**: 630–5.

4   Sawicka EH, Loh L, Branthwaite MA. Domicilary ventilatory support; an analysis of outcome. *Thorax* 1988; **43**: 31–5.

5   Bach JR, Penek J. Obstructive sleep apnea complicating negative pressure ventilatory support in patients with chronic paralytic/restrictive ventilatory dysfunction. *Chest* 1991; **99**: 1386–93.

6   Hill NS, Redline S, Carskadon M, Curran FJ, Millman RP. Sleep-disordered breathing in patients with Duchenne muscular dystrophy using negative pressure ventilators. *Chest* 1992; **102**: 1656–62.

7   Belman MJ, Soo Hoo GW, Kuei JH, Shadmehr R. Efficacy of positive vs negative pressure ventilation in unloading the respiratory muscles. *Chest* 1990; **98**: 850–6.

8   Simonds AK, Elliott MW. Outcome of domiciliary nasal intermittent positive pressure ventilation in restrictive and obstructive disorders. *Thorax* 1995; **50**: 604–9.

9   Thomson A. The role of negative pressure ventilation. *Arch Dis Child* 1997; **77**: 454–8.

10 Samuels MP, Southall DP. Negative extrathoracic pressure in the treatment of respiratory failure in infants and young children. *Brit Med J* 1989; **299**: 1253–7.

11 Jardine EJ, Wallis C. A survey of UK children receiving long-term ventilatory support at home. *Thorax* 1997; **52**(Suppl 6): A23.

12 Leger P, Bedicam JM, Cornette A, *et al*. Nasal intermittent positive pressure ventilation. Long term follow-up in patients with severe chronic respiratory insufficiency. *Chest* 1994; **105**: 100–105.

13 Fauroux B, Sardet A, Foret D. Home treatment for chronic respiratory failure in children: a prospective study. *Eur Respir J* 1995; **8**: 2062–6.

14 Piper AJ, Sullivan CE. Effects of long term nocturnal nasal ventilation on spontaneous breathing during sleep in neuromuscular and chest wall disorders. *Thorax* 1996; **9**: 1515–22.

15 Braun NMT, Marino WD. Effect of daily intermittent rest of respiratory muscles in patients with severe chronic airflow limitation. *Chest* 1984; **85**: 59S.

16 Elliott MW, Mulvey DA, Moxham J, Green M, Branthwaite MA. Domiciliary nocturnal nasal intermittent positive pressure ventilation in COPD: mechanisms underlying changes in arterial blood gas tensions. *Eur Respir J* 1991; **4**: 1044–52.

17 Annane D, Quera-Salva MA, Lofaso F, *et al*. Mechanisms underlying the effects of nocturnal ventilation on daytime blood gases in neuromuscular diseases. *Eur Respir J* 1999; **13**: 157–62.

18 Hill NS, Eveloff SE, Carlisle CC, Goff SG. Efficacy of nocturnal nasal ventilation in patients with restrictive thoracic disease. *Am Rev Respir Dis* 1992; **145**: 365–71.

19 Schonhofer B, Geibel M, Sonneborn M, Haidl P, Kohler D. Daytime mechanical ventilation in chronic respiratory insufficiency. *Eur Respir J* 1997; **10**: 2840–6.

20 Criner GJ, Brennan K, Travaline JM, Kreimer D. Efficacy and compliance with non-invasive positive pressure ventilation in patients with chronic respiratory failure. *Chest* 1999; **116**: 667–75.

21 Siegler D, Zorab PA. Pregnancy in thoracic scoliosis. *Br J Dis Chest* 1981; **75**: 367–70.

22 Ries AL, Kaplan RM, Limberg TM, Prewitt LM. Effects of pulmonary rehabilitation on physiologic and psychosocial outcomes in chronic obstructive pulmonary disease. *Ann Intern Med* 1995; **122**: 823–32.

23 Lacasse Y, Wong E, Guyatt GH, King D, Cook D, Goldstein RS. Meta-analysis of respiratory rehabilitation in chronic obstructive pulmonary disease. *Lancet* 1996; **348**: 1115–19.

24 Novitch RS, Thomas HM. Rehabilitation of patients with chronic ventilatory limitation from nonobstructive lung disease. In: Casaburi R, Petty TL (eds). *Principles and practise of pulmonary rehabilitation*. Philadelphia: W.B. Saunders, 1993: 416–23.

25 Wanke T, Toifl K, Merkle M, Formanek D, Lahrmann H, Zwick H. Inspiratory muscle training in patients with Duchenne muscular dystrophy. *Chest* 1994; **105**: 475–82.

26 Polkey MI, Kyroussis D, Mills GH, *et al*. Inspiratory pressure support reduces slowing of inspiratory muscle relaxation rate during exhaustive treadmill walking in severe COPD. *Am J Respir Crit Care Med* 1996; **154**: 1146–50.

27 Kyroussis D, Polkey MI, Hamnegard C-H, Mills GH, Green M, Moxham J. Respiratory muscle activity in patients with COPD walking to exhaustion with and without pressure support. *Eur Respir J* 2000; **15**: 649–55.

28 Polkey MI, Hawkins P, Kyroussis D, Ellum SG, Sherwood R, Moxham J. Inspiratory pressure support prolongs exercise induced lactataemia in severe COPD. *Thorax* 2000; **55**: 547–9.

29 Robert D, Gerard M, Leger P, *et al*. Domiciliary ventilation by tracheostomy for chronic respiratory failure. *Rev Fr Mal Resp* 1983; **11**: 923–36.

30 Splaingard ML, Frates FC, Harrison GM, *et al*. Home positive pressure ventilation. Twenty years experience. *Chest* 1983; **84**: 376–82.

31 Bach J. A comparison of long-term ventilatory support alternatives from the perspective of the patient and care-giver. *Chest* 1993; **104**: 1702–6.

12

Domiciliary non-invasive ventilation in chronic obstructive pulmonary disease

M W ELLIOTT

INTRODUCTION

Long-term oxygen therapy (LTOT) is the only therapy which has been shown to improve survival in patients with respiratory failure because of chronic obstructive pulmonary disease (COPD).[1,2] It is the first-line treatment for such patients, but it is reasonable to explore alternatives. Drug therapy has been disappointing, but with the excellent results of non-invasive positive pressure ventilation (NIPPV) in patients with neuromuscular disease and chest wall deformity[3,4] increasingly attention has focused on the numerically much larger group of patients with COPD. There are a number of theoretical reasons why NIPPV may be preferable to LTOT.

Firstly although compliance with LTOT was very good in the trials this is not always the case in routine clinical practice, the main reason being the restriction placed upon lifestyle by the need for 16 hours oxygen per day. Symptomatic patients, who gain subjective benefit from LTOT are more likely to comply with therapy, but asymptomatic patients tend to use oxygen for insufficient time to gain survival benefit.[5,6] NIPPV used only during sleep may prove more acceptable. However in the NOTT study the outcome was better in the continuously treated group than in those who received oxygen predominantly during sleep alone.[2]

Secondly hypercapnia is one factor which may indicate a poor prognosis and lack of benefit from LTOT. Connors et al.[7] found that patients with COPD with $PaCO_2 > 50$ mmHg at or just before admission to hospital had a 50% mortality at 2 years. In the Medical Research Council (MRC) Trial[1] no survival advantage from oxygen became apparent until 500 days' treatment had elapsed. The best predictor of death, and therefore a lack of benefit from oxygen, during this period was a combination of polycythaemia and hypercapnia. The NOTT study showed that a change in haematocrit was unrelated to survival and this therefore suggests that hypercapnia may be responsible for the worse prognosis and lack of response to oxygen therapy. Cooper et al.[8] found that, although the benefit from oxygen was apparent immediately, 29 of the 57 patients who were hypercapnic at entry, died during the course of the study compared with only three of 15 normocapnic patients. On the other hand a study of 4552 patients with COPD from Japan did not show any difference in outcome between patients with hypercapnia and those who were normocapnic.[9] NIPPV by improving oxygenation and reducing CO_2 may be advantageous compared with oxygen alone.

Impaired sleep quality is well recognized in COPD compared with age matched controls[10] and experience from patients with obstructive sleep apnoea (OSA) suggests that sleep disruption is associated with impaired neuropsychiatric functioning and reduced quality of life.[11] The effect of oxygen on sleep quality is contentious with some investigators showing an improvement[12] and others no benefit.[13] Carbon dioxide tension was not measured in either of these studies and although severe hypoxia ($SaO_2 < 70\%$) may not cause arousal in humans[14] acute hypercapnia, with a rise in $PaCO_2$ of 6–15 mmHg, has been shown to be a reliable and powerful arousal stimulus.[15] Alternatively sleep quality may be impaired by the increased respiratory effort associated with COPD, as seen in patients with increased upper airway resistance,[16] because of loading of respiratory muscles. Therefore assisted ventilation may improve sleep quality by reducing carbon dioxide or unloading respiratory muscles. It is of course equally possible that NIPPV could disrupt sleep further in some patients.

Table 12.1 *Possible advantages to NIPPV in chronic respiratory failure due to COPD*

- If needed only during sleep – ? more acceptable to patients
- Improvement in diurnal CO_2 may confer a survival advantage
- Possible beneficial effects upon sleep quality

MECHANICALLY ASSISTED VENTILATION IN COPD

The concept of mechanically assisted ventilation in COPD is not new. It was first tried by day using intermittent positive pressure breathing (IPPB) through a mouthpiece. The technique involves active inflation of the lungs under positive pressure and of passive deflation during expiration, produced by the elastic recoil of the lungs and the chest wall. Gas flow from the machine ceases when a predetermined pressure is reached, and the expiratory pathway is then open to atmosphere. Machines in use today, primarily as a physiotherapy adjunct, include The Bird (M and IE Dentsply, Sowton Industrial Estate, Exeter) and the Bennett (UK supplier: Puritan Bennett, 152–176 Great South West Road, Hounslow, Middlesex). IPPB has been shown to reduce $PaCO_2$[17] or abolish the rise of $PaCO_2$ associated with breathing 100% O_2,[18] usually as a result of an increase in tidal volume (V_T), and therefore MV. It has been said to decrease the work and oxygen cost of breathing.[17,19] but both of these claims have been disputed.[20,21] There are no data about its use during sleep. Studies of the chronic use of IPPB in COPD have shown no consistent benefit.[22–25] In the largest study 985 patients were randomized to IPPB or conventional therapy.[25] In the treatment group patients were asked to use IPPB for 10 minutes three times a day, during which time they inhaled a beta agonist generated by the machine's nebulizer. The control group had the same treatment administered by compressor over the same time. There were no statistically significant differences in mortality, need for hospitalization, change in lung function or quality of life during an average follow-up of 33 months. The main conclusion was that IPPB was no better than a compressor in providing nebulized bronchodilators. However in all the studies the duration of each treatment session was no more than 20 minutes, which is unlikely to be long enough to have a lasting physiological effect. Because the inspiratory phase is terminated as soon as the predetermined pressure is reached, it is unlikely that these machines will provide effective ventilation in most patients with COPD in whom the impedance to inflation is high and may change with time.

NEGATIVE PRESSURE VENTILATION

Various trials of in-hospital assisted ventilation, using negative pressure devices, in patients with COPD have been reported.[26–30] Ventilation has usually been assisted during wakefulness with the aim of reducing respiratory muscle activity and allowing recovery from 'respiratory muscle fatigue'. In these uncontrolled studies improvements, sometimes striking, in several variables have been attributed to relatively short periods of assisted ventilation. In many patients it is possible that the improvements seen simply reflected the natural recovery from an acute exacerbation. The use of negative pressure devices at home and during sleep in patients with COPD has been largely unsuccessful.[30–32] In these controlled trials patients were generally unable to sleep during negative pressure ventilation and most either failed to complete the protocol, because of lack of improvement or discomfort associated with the use of the equipment,[31] or did not wish to continue treatment after the study was completed.[30] In the largest trial Shapiro et al.[32] studied 184 patients randomized to active or sham negative pressure ventilation at home using a ponchowrap ventilator. They did not show any significant difference between the two groups, but compliance with treatment was much less than anticipated with most patients unable to sleep during negative pressure ventilation. The mean $PaCO_2$

of the patients studied was only 44 mmHg and a review of the literature[26,28–30,33] suggests that it is hypercapnic patients who are most likely to benefit from non-invasive ventilation. The conclusions from these studies are that negative pressure ventilation at home of patients with COPD is poorly tolerated, cannot usually be used during sleep and results in little benefit.

POSITIVE PRESSURE VENTILATION VIA TRACHEOSTOMY

In a retrospective study, survival in 50 patients with COPD ventilated at home via a tracheostomy[34] was little different from oxygen treated patients in the MRC study of long-term oxygen therapy.[1] However, survival was no worse, despite the presence of a tracheostomy, which may be associated with a significant morbidity and mortality.[35] Another retrospective study of 259 patients with COPD ventilated at home via tracheostomy showed similar results, but survival was better than the oxygen treated patients in the MRC study,[1] until the fourth year when the survival curves rejoined.[36] Positive pressure ventilation via tracheostomy is feasible, but the invasive nature is a significant disincentive to this approach.

NASAL POSITIVE PRESSURE VENTILATION

NIPPV has been used at home during sleep in patients with COPD with some success. Carroll and Branthwaite[37] included four patients with COPD who benefited from NIPPV, albeit to a lesser extent than those with extra-pulmonary restrictive disease. Marino[38] showed reduced respiratory rate, $Paco_2$ and heart rate in nine (eight with COPD) out of 13 patients with progressive chronic ventilatory failure when started on NIPPV in hospital. Of the eight patients with COPD, four found the system so uncomfortable that they did not wish to continue, but the remaining four continued using the ventilator at home daily for periods of 6 to 10 months. They had improved physical capacity and daytime $Paco_2$ at mean follow up of 20 months. Elliott et al.[39] showed some improvement in 8 of 12 patients with COPD and hypercapnic ventilatory failure receiving NIPPV at home during sleep. At 6 months, eight were continuing with NIPPV. One patient had died and three had withdrawn because they were unable to sleep with the equipment. Full polysomnography performed during NIPPV in patients continuing treatment at 6 months showed an increase in mean arterial oxygen saturation and lower mean transcutaneous carbon dioxide tension ($P_{tc}CO_2$) overnight compared with spontaneous breathing before starting NIPPV. Total sleep time increased during NIPPV, but sleep architecture and the number of arousals were unchanged. Quality of life did not change, but was no worse during NIPPV. Six patients showed a reduction and two an increase in $Paco_2$, and seven an improvement in Pao_2 during spontaneous breathing by day. Bicarbonate ion concentration fell in seven patients. At one year seven patients were still using the ventilator and $Paco_2$ and bicarbonate ion concentration during the day had improved further compared with values at 6 months.

Sivasothy et al.[40] retrospectively studied the effect of domiciliary NIPPV in 26 consecutive patients with hypercapnic ventilatory failure due to COPD in whom oxygen therapy caused worsening hypercapnia. Supplemental oxygen was added if it was not possible to increase $SaO_2 > 90\%$ with NIPPV despite a reduction in $PaCO_2$. After one year PaO_2 had increased by median 2.4 kPa and $PaCO_2$ fallen by median 1.4 kPa. The change in daytime $PaCO_2$ correlated with overnight $P_{tc}CO_2$. Haematocrit improved and there was an improvement in the 'role limitation physical' domain of the short form 36 health status questionnaire. Survival was comparable to oxygen treated patients in other studies and better than that in historical controls. Jones et al.[41] followed 11 patients with severe stable COPD and hypercapnic ventilatory failure for 2 years. In addition to sustained improvements in arterial blood gas tensions they also found that hospitalization rates and general practitioner consultation rates were halved in the year after starting NIPPV, compared with the previous year. These data suggest that there may be economic advantages to home ventilation, but these findings need to be confirmed in larger prospective studies.

There have been few controlled trials and most of these had small numbers of patients followed over a short period of time. Strumpf et al.[42] performed a randomized controlled crossover study in 19 patients with COPD and found that seven were unable to tolerate the nasal mask and a further five withdrew because of intercurrent illness. In the seven who did complete the study, there were significant differences only in neuropsychologic testing. Meecham Jones et al.[43] performed a similarly designed crossover study of the use of nasal pressure support ventilation and oxygen with oxygen alone and showed improved daytime arterial blood gas tensions, better quality sleep and improved quality of life during the pressure support limb of the study. The improvement in daytime $PaCO_2$ correlated with a reduction in overnight transcutaneous CO_2. Lin[44] studied 12 patients in a prospective randomized crossover study of oxygen alone, NIPPV alone and oxygen plus NIPPV each for 2 weeks. There were no differences in tidal volume, minute volume, spirometry, diurnal arterial blood gas tensions, mouth pressures or ventilatory drive. Sleep efficiency was worse during NIPPV than with oxygen alone.

In summary one study showed some benefit from the combination of NIPPV and LTOT with the other two failing to show any advantage to NIPPV. There are a number of possible explanations for this. Firstly there were differences in the way in which patients were acclimatized to NIPPV. In the study of Strumpf et al.[42] acclimatization was performed as an outpatient, but with regular visits from a respiratory therapist. Many patients do not find NIPPV easy initially and in uncontrolled studies a higher success rate was achieved when patients started NIPPV in hospital under close supervision.[37,38,45,46] In the study of Lin[44] patients only received NIPPV for two weeks; practical experience with both NIPPV and CPAP suggests that most patients requires several weeks of acclimatization before they are comfortable, and confident, with the delivery of ventilatory support during sleep.

Secondly the patients in the studies of Strumpf et al.[42] and Lin[44] were not particularly hypercapnic (mean $PaCO_2$ 46 mmHg and 50.5 mmHg respectively), whereas those in the study of Meecham-Jones et al.[43] had a mean $PaCO_2$ of 55.8 mmHg. In studies using negative pressure devices, where benefit has been seen, it has usually been in those with daytime hypercapnia.[26,28-30,33]

Thirdly there were differences in the type and settings of the ventilators. Meecham-Jones et al.[43] used pressure support ventilation with a mean IPAP of 18 cmH$_2$O. Strumpf et al.[42] used a timed mode because it is more likely to reduce inspiratory muscle effort than patient initiated ventilation, but noted that approximately 25% of the night was spent with the patient breathing out of synchrony with the ventilator. Asynchrony between the patient and ventilator may cause marked worsening of gas exchange with both negative and positive pressure devices. In the study of Lin[44] the maximum tolerated inspiratory pressure ranged from only 8 cmH$_2$O to a maximum of 15 cmH$_2$O. In the study of Strumpf et al.[42] carbon dioxide control during sleep was assessed on the basis of reduced spot measurements of EtCO$_2$. This may have missed periods of hypoventilation, for instance associated with asynchrony, and in addition EtCO$_2$ is an unreliable measure of PaCO$_2$ in patients with severe airways obstruction. In the study of Lin[44] no data were given about the effect of NIPPV on blood gas tensions during ventilation and there was no statistically significant improvement in sleep hypoventilation with NIPPV. By contrast in the study of Meecham-Jones et al.[43] a reduction in P$_{tc}$CO$_2$ was documented during sleep and correlated with the improvement in daytime PaCO$_2$ that was seen. Since a primary aim of non-invasive ventilation delivered during sleep is to control nocturnal hypoventilation, it can be argued that this was not achieved in the studies of Strumpf et al.[42] and Lin[44] and therefore it is not surprising that there was no evidence of any therapeutic effect with NIPPV in these studies. The fact that no patient could tolerate an inspiratory positive airway pressure (IPAP) of more than 15 cmH$_2$O in the Lin study is surprising since in the study of Meecham Jones et al..[43] the mean IPAP for the group was 18 cmH$_2$O. Further, in the study of Ambrosino et al.,[47] the mean IPAP was 22 cmH$_2$O and in the study of Elliott et al.,[39] in which volume cycled flow generators were used, most patients tolerated peak inflation pressures of 35–40 cmH$_2$O.

These data from short-term studies certainly do not justify the routine use of non-invasive ventilation in COPD. Two more long-term uncontrolled studies[3,4] have shown 5-year survival rates comparable to the oxygen treated patients in the NOTT and MRC studies.[1,2] It should be acknowledged that most of the patients recruited to these studies were hypercapnic and thus, on the basis of the MRC study, less likely to benefit from LTOT. Also at the time when NIPPV was started, the patients were deemed to have failed oxygen therapy. The results in a group of 'oxygen failures' were therefore encouraging. However what constituted 'oxygen failure' was not defined and it is inappropriate to make comparisons with historical controls from over 20 years ago. Preliminary results from two multicentre European trials comparing NIPPV with LTOT in COPD suggest that NIPPV does not improve survival, but may reduce the need for hospitalization.[48,49] Until further data are available a trial of NIPPV can only be justified in patients who have failed with or cannot tolerate the gold standard treatment, namely LTOT.

MECHANISMS OF IMPROVEMENT IN DAYTIME FUNCTION

The finding of improved arterial blood gas tensions during spontaneous breathing by day when ventilation has been assisted during sleep is perhaps surprising. It is helpful to consider the effects upon subsequent spontaneous ventilation in terms of changes in respiratory muscle function, the load against which the respiratory muscle pump is working and the central drive to breathe. An improvement in blood gas tensions may occur if capacity or central drive increases or load is reduced.

Improved respiratory muscle function

One difficulty in exploring this hypothesis is the lack of any objective test of chronic fatigue. Some studies of non-invasive ventilation have cited increased respiratory muscle strength as evidence for the resolution of chronic fatigue.[27] However, tests of respiratory muscle strength require maximum voluntary efforts and an improvement in general well-being may have been responsible for the enhanced performance. In other studies improved arterial blood gas tensions, but without increased respiratory muscle strength have been reported.[45] Secondly although accessory muscle and diaphragmatic electromyogram (EMG) activity can be reduced by both negative[50] and positive pressure devices,[51] in most cases this has not been documented during the study. Rodenstein and colleagues[52] have shown that accessory muscle and diaphragmatic EMG activity may not be reduced at all in naive patients and Ambrosino and colleagues,[29] who measured integrated EMG activity during ENPV, stated that activity was reduced by 50% only *temporarily*. The assumption that abolition of EMG activity occurring under ideal conditions, when ventilator controls have been adjusted to achieve this goal, also occurs during routine use may not be valid and it is therefore possible that the respiratory muscles were not rested at all in these studies. In some studies patients have been recruited during recovery from an acute exacerbation[28,33] and the changes seen may simply reflect the natural history of recovery, rather than any beneficial effect of assisted ventilation *per se*. Shapiro *et al.*[32] attempted to reduce respiratory muscle EMG activity using negative pressure devices in a randomized placebo controlled study. While this was not uniformly successful there was no evidence that respiratory muscle rest was of benefit. Further data are needed before the use of NIPPV to rest the respiratory muscles can be justified.

Restored chemosensitivity

There are some data to support the hypothesis that a restoration in central drive is important. Berthon Jones *et al.*[53] showed a left shift of the ventilatory response curve to progressive hypercapnia in patients with severe obstructive sleep apnoea after 90 days treatment with continuous positive airway pressure. Annane *et al.*[54] found that the improvement in diurnal $PaCO_2$ correlated with the improvement in the slope of the ventilatory response to carbon dioxide in patients with neuromuscular disease and chest wall deformity. In eight patients with severe COPD ventilated non-invasively during sleep for 6 months Elliott *et al.*[46] showed a reduction in bicarbonate ion concentration and base excess and a resetting of the ventilatory response to CO_2 at a lower level. However Appendini *et al.*[55] recorded a high P0.1, a measure of central drive, in eight ventilator dependent patients with COPD suggesting, in these patients, that an abnormality of respiratory centre output was unlikely.

Reduced load

The effect of domiciliary ventilation upon respiratory system load in COPD has not been addressed in many studies. A small (non-significant) improvement in dynamic compliance and a correlation between the reduction in $Paco_2$ during spontaneous breathing and a decrease in gas trapping (Spearman rank correlation coefficient (r_s) 0.85 $p < 0.05$) and in the residual volume (r_s 0.78; $p < 0.05$), suggesting reduced small airway obstruction and therefore a reduction in load, was seen in one study.[46] It was postulated that a reduction in lung water was one possible mechanism for these changes because if anything bronchodilator requirements were less following NIPPV. In most circumstances it is likely that any reduction in ventilatory load secondary to improved compliance is a relatively minor factor in the reversal of ventilatory failure.

Schonhofer et al.[56] have attempted to elucidate possible mechanisms of the improvement in physiological parameters. In a carefully designed study, patients with extra-pulmonary restrictive disorders were allocated to receive either NIPPV during sleep or during the day for a one month period. In the latter group, patients were prevented from sleeping by having to respond to intermittent prompts by pressing a button when a light came on. They were thus able to compare the effects of NIPPV during sleep and wakefulness. There were no differences between the two groups with each showing improved diurnal blood gas tensions, increased respiratory muscle strength, and a slight reduction in the P0.1. Overnight Sao_2 and transcutaneous CO_2 tensions were also improved in both groups at the end of the study during spontaneous breathing overnight. Sleep quality was also shown to improve in a small subgroup who underwent full polysomnography. The finding of a reduction in P0.1 and an improvement in respiratory muscle strength suggests that an improvement in muscle function rather than a restoration of central drive was the important mechanism. This study also shows that daytime ventilation is as effective as night-time NIPPV both in terms of effects upon arterial blood gas tensions during the day and also upon gas exchange and sleep quality overnight; clearly nocturnal support, if tolerated, is more convenient for the patient.

In summary, there are conflicting data about the mechanism of benefit from NIPPV. Further studies are needed, but on the basis of current knowledge NIPPV should be targeted to improve arterial blood gas tensions, reduce respiratory muscle activity and improve sleep quality; fortunately these goals are not mutually exclusive.

PRACTICAL PROBLEMS SPECIFIC TO PATIENTS WITH COPD

The technique of initiating NIPPV was discussed in detail in Chapter 5. However there are problems which may be specific to patients with obstructive airways disease. Firstly these patients may have intrinsic positive end-expiratory pressure ($PEEP_i$) because of premature airway closure and air trapping.[57] The presence of $PEEP_i$ increases the work of breathing during spontaneous or triggered ventilation by adding an inspiratory threshold load. In addition it decreases the effective trigger sensitivity because $PEEP_i$ must first be overcome before pressure change and flow occur and can be sensed at the nose.[58] This may result in asynchrony between the patient's inspiratory efforts and machine breaths, which is inefficient and uncomfortable for the patient, and can be improved by counterbalancing $PEEP_i$ with extrinsic PEEP. Some patients with COPD prefer to mouth breathe, particularly when acutely distressed. As well as promoting leaks, this effectively bypasses the ventilator, which is therefore not triggered in response to patient efforts and marked asynchrony occurs. The primary aim when starting NIPPV is the effective capture of ventilation, such that there is complete synchrony between patient and ventilator. In such circumstances full facemask ventilation may be successful. The acceptance of any medical treatment depends upon the patient's perception of whether it is beneficial or not. Medical intervention that is unpleasant and is not perceived as beneficial will be poorly tolerated. There is no doubt that the results of NIPPV in patients with COPD are not as good as in those with chest wall deformity and stable neuromuscular disease.[3,4] The balance towards benefit is less and adequate motivation is an essential ingredient for a successful outcome. Patients with COPD may need considerable encouragement to persist during the early stages of NIPPV.

Table 12.2 *Practical problems of NIPPV particular to patients with COPD*

Problem	Solution
$PEEP_i$	Counterbalance with extrinsic PEEP (EPAP)
Mouth breathing	Full facemask Chin strap
Less benefit than for patients with neuromuscular disease etc.	Motivation Encouragement ? in patient acclimatization

CONCLUSION (Table 12.3)

In conclusion NIPPV can be used effectively in some patients with COPD. Experience with ENPV has shown that, though feasible in small uncontrolled pilot studies, extension to a wider population has been disappointing. Published studies do show however that patients with COPD have difficulty acclimatizing to NIPPV, but if this can be

Table 12.3 *Recommendations for the use of NIPPV in chronic ventilatory failure due to COPD*

- Deterioration despite maximum conventional treatment or unable to tolerate oxygen therapy
- Hypercapnia during spontaneous breathing by day
- Not end-stage emphysema, i.e. moderately preserved transfer factor
- Well motivated patient
- Inpatient acclimatization and education
- Documented control of nocturnal hypoventilation by NIPPV

achieved there is some evidence to suggest that provided nocturnal hypoventilation is controlled, there is a therapeutic effect. Conversely, titration of ventilator settings to daytime physiological goals may result in no overall benefit.[59] In light of this, if NIPPV is to be tried in patients with COPD, the effective control of nocturnal hypoventilation should be targeted. Patient motivation is critical and hypercapnic patients are most likely to benefit from NIPPV. Adequate education and acclimatization to the technique are essential. In-hospital initiation of ventilation is probably preferable, though more costly. Although it cannot currently be recommended as first-line treatment for hypercapnic patients with COPD a trial of NIPPV should be considered in those cases deteriorating despite, or intolerant of, oxygen therapy.

Key points

- LTOT remains the gold standard for the treatment of chronic respiratory failure due to COPD.
- NIPPV may be an alternative for selected patients
  - Hypercapnic patients who continue to deteriorate despite maximal therapy, including LTOT
  - Those who cannot tolerate carefully titrated supplemental oxygen because of significant symptomatic hypercapnia
  - Motivation is key.
- Time should be spent on education and acclimatization to NIPPV.
- There are no controlled trial data to support the widespread use of NIPPV in this patient group.

REFERENCES

1   Medical Research Council Working Party Report. Long term domiciliary oxygen therapy in chronic hypoxic cor pulmonale complicating chronic bronchitis and emphysema. *Lancet* 1981; **1**: 681–5.
2   Nocturnal Oxygen Therapy Trial Group. Continuous or nocturnal oxygen therapy in hypoxaemic chronic obstructive lung disease, a clinical trial. *Ann Intern Med* 1980; **93**: 391–8.
3   Simonds AK, Elliott MW. Outcome of domiciliary nasal intermittent positive pressure ventilation in restrictive and obstructive disorders. *Thorax* 1995; **50**: 604–9.
4   Leger P, Bedicam JM, Cornette A, *et al*. Nasal intermittent positive pressure ventilation. Long-term follow-up in patients with severe chronic respiratory insufficiency. *Chest* 1994; **105**: 100–5.
5   Baudouin SV, Waterhouse JC, Tahtamouni T, Smith JA, Baxter J, Howard P. Long term domiciliary oxygen treatment for chronic respiratory failure reviewed. *Thorax* 1990; **45**: 195–8.
6   Walshaw MJ, Lim R, Evans CC, Hind CRK. Factors influencing compliance of patients using oxygen concentrators for long-term home oxygen therapy. *Respir Med* 1990; **84**: 331–3.

7   Connors AF, Jr., Dawson NV, Thomas C, *et al*. Outcomes following acute exacerbation of severe chronic obstructive lung disease. The SUPPORT investigators (Study to Understand Prognoses and Preferences for Outcomes and Risks of Treatments). *Am J Respir Crit Care Med* 1996; **154**: 959–67.

8   Cooper CB, Waterhouse J, Howard P. Twelve year clinical study of patients with hypoxic cor pulmonale given long term domiciliary oxygen therapy. *Thorax* 1987; **42**: 105–10.

9   Aida A, Miyamoto K, Nishimura M, *et al*. Prognostic value of hypercapnia in patients with chronic respiratory failure during long term oxygen therapy. *Am J Respir Crit Care Med* 1998; **158**: 188–93.

10   Arand DL, McGinty DJ, Littner MR. Respiratory patterns associated with hemoglobin desaturation during sleep in chronic obstructive pulmonary disease. *Chest* 1981; **80**: 183–90.

11   Singh B. Sleep apnea: a psychiatric perspective. In: Saunders NA, Sullivan CE (eds). *Sleep and breathing*. New York: Marcel Dekker, 1984: 403–22.

12   Calverley PMA, Brezinova V, Douglas NJ, Catterall JR, Flenley DC. The effect of oxygenation on sleep quality in chronic bronchitis and emphysema. *Am Rev Respir Dis* 1982; **126**: 206–10.

13   Fleetham JA, West P, Mezon B, Conway W, Roth T, Kryger M. Sleep, arousals, and oxygen desaturation in COPD. *Am Rev Respir Dis* 1982; **126**: 429–33.

14   Berthon-Jones M, Sullivan CE. Ventilatory and arousal responses to hypoxia in sleeping humans. *Am Rev Respir Dis* 1982; **125**: 632–9.

15   Hedemark L, Kronenberg R. Ventilatory responses to hypoxia and CO_2 during natural and flurazepam induced sleep in normal adults. *Am Rev Respir Dis* 1981; **123**: 190 (abstract).

16   Guilleminault C, Stoohs R, Duncan S. Snoring (I). Daytime sleepiness in regular heavy snorers. *Chest* 1991; **99**: 40–8.

17   Emmanuel GE, Smith WM, Briscoe WA. The effect of intermittent positive pressure breathing and voluntary hyperventilation upon the distibution of ventilation and pulmonary blood flow to the lung in chronic obstructive lung disease. *J Clin Invest* 1966; **45**: 1221–3.

18   Fraimow W, Cathcart RT, Goodman E. The use of intermittent positive pressure breathing in the prevention of carbon dioxide narcosis associated with oxygen therapy. *Am Rev Respir Dis* 1960; **81**: 815–22.

19   Ayres SM, Kozam RL, Lukas DS. The effects of intermittent positive pressure breathing on intrathoracic pressure, pulmonary mechanics and the work of breathing. *Am Rev Respir Dis* 1963; **87**: 370–9.

20   Sukulmalchantra Y, Park SS, Williams MH. The effects of intermittent positive pressure breathing (IPPB) in acute ventilatory failure. *Am Rev Respir Dis* 1965; **92**: 885–93.

21   Kamat SR, Dulfano MJ, Segal MS. The effects of intermittent positive pressure breathing (IPPB/I) with compressed air in patients with severe chronic nonspecific obstructive pulmonary disease. *Am Rev Respir Dis* 1962; **86**: 360–80.

22   Curtis JK, Liska AP, Rasmussen HK, Cree EM. IPPB therapy in chronic obstructive pulmonary disease. *JAMA* 1968; **206**: 1037–40.

23   Thornton JA, Darke CS, Herbert P. Intermittent positive pressure breathing (IPPB) in chronic respiratory disease. *Anaesthesia* 1974; **29**: 44–9.

24 Emirgil C, Sobol BJ, Norman J, Moskowitz E, Goyal P, Wadwhani B. A study of the long-term effect of therapy in chronic obstructive pulmonary disease. *Am J Med* 1969; **47**: 367–77.

25 The Intermittent Positive Pressure Breathing Trial Group. Intermittent positive pressure breathing therapy of chronic obstructive pulmonary disease. *Ann Int Med* 1983; **99**: 612–20.

26 Gutierrez M, Beroiza T, Contreras G, *et al.* Weekly cuirass ventilation improves blood gases and inspiratory muscle strength in patients with chronic airflow limitation and hypercarbia. *Am Rev Respir Dis* 1988; **138**: 617–23.

27 Cropp A, Dimarco AF. Effects of intermittent negative pressure ventilation on respiratory muscle function in patients with severe chronic obstructive pulmonary disease. *Am Rev Respir Dis* 1987; **135**: 1056–61.

28 Scano G, Gigliotti F, Duranti R, Spinelli A, Gorini M, Schiavina M. Changes in ventilatory muscle function with negative pressure ventilation in COPD. *Chest* 1990; **97**: 322–7.

29 Ambrosino N, Montagna T, Nava S, *et al.* Short term effect of intermittent negative pressure ventilation in COPD patients with respiratory failure. *Eur Respir J* 1990; **3**: 502–8.

30 Celli B, Lee H, Criner G, *et al.* Controlled trial of external negative pressure ventilation in patients with severe chronic airflow limitation. *Am Rev Respir Dis* 1989; **140**: 1251–6.

31 Zibrak JD, Hill NS, Federman EC, Kwa SL, O'Donnell C. Evaluation of intermittent long term negative-pressure ventilation in patients with severe COPD. *Am Rev Respir Dis* 1988; **138**: 1515–18.

32 Shapiro SH, Ernst P, Gray-Donald K, *et al.* Effect of negative pressure ventilation in severe chronic obstructive pulmonary disease. *Lancet* 1992; **340**: 1425–9.

33 Corrado A, Bruscoli G, De Paola E, Ciardi-Dupre GF, Baccini A, Taddel M. Respiratory muscle insufficiency in acute respiratory failure of subjects with severe COPD: treatment with intermittent negative pressure ventilation. *Eur Respir J* 1990; **3**: 644–8.

34 Robert D, Gerard M, Leger P, *et al.* Domiciliary ventilation by tracheostomy for chronic respiratory failure. *Rev Fr Mal Resp* 1983; **11**: 923–36.

35 Stauffer JL, Olson DE, Petty TL. Complications and consequences of endotracheal intubation and tracheostomy. *Am J Med* 1981; **70**: 65–75.

36 Muir J, and Cooperative Group. Multicentre study of 259 severe COPD patients with tracheostomy and home mechanical ventilation. In: *Proceedings of the World Congress on Oxygen Therapy and Pulmonary Rehabilitation*. Denver: 1987.

37 Carroll N, Branthwaite MA. Control of nocturnal hypoventilation by nasal intermittent positive pressure ventilation. *Thorax* 1988; **43**: 349–53.

38 Marino W. Intermittent volume cycled mechanical ventilation via nasal mask in patients with respiratory failure due to COPD. *Chest* 1991; **99**: 681–4.

39 Elliott MW, Simonds AK, Carroll MP, Wedzicha JA, Branthwaite MA. Domiciliary nocturnal nasal intermittent positive pressure ventilation in hypercapnic respiratory failure due to chronic obstructive lung disease: effects on sleep and quality of life. *Thorax* 1992; **47**: 342–8.

40 Sivasothy P, Smith IE, Shneerson JM. Mask intermittent positive pressure ventilation in chronic hypercapnic respiratory failure due to chronic obstructive pulmonary disease. *Eur Respir J* 1998; **11**: 34–40.

41 Jones SE, Packham S, Hebden M, Smith AP. Domiciliary nocturnal intermittent positive pressure ventilation in patients with respiratory failure due to severe COPD; long term follow up and effect on survival. *Thorax* 1998; **53**: 495–8.

42 Strumpf DA, Millman RP, Carlisle CC, *et al*. Nocturnal positive-pressure ventilation via nasal mask in patients with severe chronic obstructive pulmonary disease. *Am Rev Respir Dis* 1991; **144**: 1234–9.

43 Meecham Jones DJ, Paul EA, Jones PW, Wedzicha JA. Nasal pressure support ventilation plus oxygen compared with oxygen therapy alone in hypercapnic COPD. *Am J Respir Crit Care Med* 1995; **152**: 538–44.

44 Lin CC. Comparison between nocturnal nasal positive pressure ventilation combined with oxygen therapy and oxygen monotherapy in patients with severe COPD. *Am J Respir Crit Care Med* 1996; **154**: 353–8.

45 Gay PC, Patel AM, Viggiano RW, Hubmayr RD. Nocturnal nasal ventilation for treatment of patients with hypercapnic respiratory failure. *Mayo Clin Proc* 1991; **66**: 695–703.

46 Elliott MW, Mulvey DA, Moxham J, Green M, Branthwaite MA. Domiciliary nocturnal nasal intermittent positive pressure ventilation in COPD: mechanisms underlying changes in arterial blood gas tensions. *Eur Respir J* 1991; **4**: 1044–52.

47 Ambrosino N, Nava S, Bertone P, Fracchia C, Rampulla C. Physiologic evaluation of pressure support ventilation by nasal mask in patients with stable COPD. *Chest* 1992; **101**: 385–91.

48 Muir JF, de la Salmoniere P, Cuvelier A, *et al*. Survival of severe hypercapnic COPD under long term home mechanical ventilation with NIPPV + oxygen versus oxygen therapy alone: preliminary results of a European multicentre study. *Am J Respir Crit Care Med* 1999; **159**: A295 (abstract).

49 Clini E, Sturani C, on behalf of AIPO. The Italian multicentric study of non-invasive nocturnal pressure support ventilation (NPSV) in COPD patients. *Am J Respir Crit Care Med* 1999; **159**: A295 (abstract).

50 Rochester DF, Braun NM, Laine S. Diaphragmatic energy expenditure in chronic respiratory failure. *Am J Med* 1977; **63**: 223–31.

51 Carrey Z, Gottfried SB, Levy RD. Ventilatory muscle support in respiratory failure with nasal positive pressure ventilation. *Chest* 1990; **97**: 150–8.

52 Rodenstein DO, Stanescu DC, Cuttita G, Liistro G, Veriter C. Ventilatory and diaphragmatic EMG responses to negative-pressure ventilation in airflow obstruction. *J Appl Physiol* 1988; **65**: 1621–6.

53 Berthon-Jones M, Sullivan CE. Time course of change in ventilatory response to CO_2 with long-term CPAP therapy for obstructive sleep apnea. *Am Rev Respir Dis* 1987; **135**: 144–7.

54 Annane D, Quera-Salva MA, Lofaso F, *et al*. Mechanisms underlying effects of nocturnal ventilation on daytime blood gases in neuromuscular diseases. *Eur Respir J* 1999; **13**: 157–62.

55 Appendini L, Purro A, Patessio A, *et al*. Partitioning of inspiratory muscle workload and pressure assistance in ventilator-dependent COPD patients. *Am J Respir Crit Care Med* 1996; **154**: 1301–9.

56 Schonhofer B, Geibel M, Sonnerborn M, Kohler D. Daytime mechanical ventilation in chronic respiratory insufficiency. *Eur Respir J* 1997; **10**: 2840–6.

57 Pepe PE, Marini JJ. Occult positive end expiratory pressure in mechanically ventilated patients with airflow limitation. *Am Rev Respir Dis* 1982; **126**: 166–70.

58 Smith TC, Marini JJ. Impact of PEEP on lung mechanics and work of breathing in severe airflow obstruction. *J Appl Physiol* 1988; **65**: 1488–99.

59 Casanova C, Celli BR, Tost L, Soriano E, Abreu J, Velasco V, Santolaria F. Long-term controlled trial of nocturnal nasal positive pressure ventilation in patients with severe COPD. *Chest* 2000; **118**: 1582–90.

13

Non-invasive ventilation in cystic fibrosis, bronchiectasis and diffuse interstitial lung disease

A K SIMONDS

Unlike neuromuscular and chest wall disorders, advanced diffuse interstitial lung disease, bronchiectasis and cystic fibrosis (CF) are characterized by marked ventilation perfusion mismatch and diffusion problems, although the work of breathing is also increased by airflow obstruction and hyperinflation in CF and bronchiectasis, and reduced lung compliance in interstitial lung disease patients. Chronic CO_2 retention is an end-stage phenomenon.

NIPPV IN CF

The majority of CF patients die of respiratory complications. Important predictive factors for mortality are FEV_1 and Pao_2, but in patients with a $Paco_2$ of >6.7 kPa two-year mortality is in excess of 50%.[1]

Piper *et al.*[2] reported the use of domiciliary NIPPV for up to 18 months in four CF patients with chronic ventilatory failure who had failed to respond to optimal conventional measures. Average FEV_1 was 0.5 L (14% predicted) and most had a

Paco$_2$ level on O$_2$ 2 L/minute of > 8 kPa. A volume cycled ventilator was used and within a few days of starting NIPPV, Paco$_2$ fell (although did not normalize), sleep quality improved, and respiratory muscle strength increased.

Gozal[3] compared nocturnal NIPPV with LTOT in six patients (mean age 22 years) with FEV$_1$ 29% predicted. NIPPV and oxygen therapy both improved overnight Sao$_2$, but a marked increase in transcutaneous CO$_2$ was only seen on oxygen therapy. Sleep stage, arousals and sleep efficiency did not differ between treatments, so overall benefit is not yet clear.

As hypercapnia is a poor prognostic feature, NIPPV has been suggested as a means of 'bridging' patients to heart/lung or lung transplantation. Hodson et al.[4] used volume preset NIPPV in preference to conventional intubation and ventilation in a cohort of six patients awaiting heart–lung transplantation with successful outcome in four patients. In those who were transplanted the post-operative course was no different from patients who had not required pre-operative ventilatory support. Other groups have also used NIPPV to bridge children with CF to transplantation. Caronia et al.[5] report nine consecutive children with end-stage CF treated with nocturnal bilevel pressure support. Oxygen requirements for the group fell from a mean (SD) of 4.6 (1.1) L/minute to 2.3 (1.5) L/minute while diurnal Sao$_2$ rose from 80% to 91%. All families coped well with NIPPV at home. Bilevel ventilatory settings were IPAP 14–18 cmH$_2$O, EPAP 4–8 cmH$_2$O. Further applications of NIPPV in children with CF are discussed in Chapter 15. Some units advocate the use of NIPPV in all patients awaiting transplantation. Hill et al.[6] used NIPPV in 12 CF transplant candidates with an FEV$_1$ 15% predicted and mean (SD) Paco$_2$ 8.7 (0.6) kPa. Ten of the 12 tolerated NIPPV well and reported improvement in morning headache and sleep quality. After 3 months of domiciliary NIPPV, there was a significant decrease in Paco$_2$ and HCO$_3$ concentration. Days spent in hospital also fell ($p < 0.05$). At the time of the report, three individuals had received a transplant, four died while waiting for surgery, and three were still on the active transplant list. Two failed to tolerate NIPPV long-term.

USE OF NIPPV IN PREGNANCY IN CF

In some patients, particularly those with an FEV$_1$ of less than 80% predicted, a serious deterioration in lung function can occur during pregnancy resulting in ventilatory decompensation. Case reports have detailed both successful[2] and unsuccessful[7] applications of NIPPV in these difficult circumstances. If the situation allows, it seems sensible to try NIPPV before conventional ventilation in hypercapnic pregnant patients.

NIPPV AS AN ADJUNCT TO PHYSIOTHERAPY IN CF

Chest physiotherapy using the forced expiration technique is a vital part of the treatment regime in CF patients. However, adults and children with poor lung function may tire quickly, reducing the efficacy of the physiotherapy session. The use of NIPPV as an adjunct to physiotherapy has been explored in a controlled study.[8] Respiratory rate fell and SaO_2 was higher after physiotherapy sessions using pressure support ventilation compared with control sessions with no respiratory support. In addition, respiratory mouth pressures fell during the unassisted session, but rose after the session using pressure support ventilation. Patients reported less fatigue after the assisted session, but the volume of sputum produced did not differ between the groups.

CPAP OR NIPPV IN CF?

In CF patients with nocturnal hypoventilation, nocturnal CPAP therapy has been shown to reduce the respiratory disturbance index and REM-related desaturation, without causing a rise in transcutaneous CO_2.[9] CPAP may therefore be of value in a proportion of patients, but it should be noted that the respiratory disturbance index in this study was relatively low (25/hour), and those with more severe nocturnal hypoventilation are more likely to benefit from NIPPV.

Henke et al.[10] have investigated the use of CPAP during exercise in CF patients. Compared with bicycle ergometry when breathing spontaneously, exercise carried out with CPAP assistance produced less dyspnoea, and a decrease in transdiaphragmatic pressure level indicating a reduction in the work of breathing. Further work is needed to assess the benefits of CPAP during exercise and during pulmonary rehabilitation schemes.

BRONCHIECTASIS

In a French cohort study[11] patients with bronchiectasis (mean age 55 years) had 3-year probability of continuing NIPPV of 48%. Overall the number of days of hospitalization for the group decreased compared with pre-NIPPV admissions, but numbers included in this analysis were small. Sixteen per cent of NIPPV recipients with bronchiectasis died of respiratory disease during the 3-year study period, a percentage similar to those with COPD. Benhamou et al.[12] examined the long-term outcome of NIPPV in diffuse bronchiectasis using a comparative case–control study. Fourteen cases treated with NIPPV and LTOT were compared with matched patients using LTOT only. Mean FEV_1 on entry to the study was 700 mL and it was notable that NIPPV was initiated in most cases at the time of an acuté infective exacerbation. Volume preset ventilators were used and long-term compliance was reported as satisfactory in 11/14 patients. Compared with the LTOT group, those using the combination of NIPPV + LTOT spent fewer days in hospital, but there was no significant impact on survival or PaO_2 level. Median survival was 45 months.

In the UK cohort study[13] bronchiectasis patients showed the worst survival of all NIPPV recipients, with a 2-year probability of continuing NIPPV of < 20%. However, lung function and arterial blood gas tensions at the initiation of NIPPV was far worse than in three French series (Table 13.1). It is probably not surprising that patients started on NIPPV earlier in the course of the disease, do better

Table 13.1 *Comparison of outcome in bronchiectasis patients receiving long-term NIPPV*

Reference	Pao$_2$ at start of NIPPV	Paco$_2$ (kPa)	Probability of continuing NIPPV at 3 years	Other outcome
Leger[11]	6.1	6.8	48%	Decrease hospital days
Benhamou[12]				
NIPPV	6.4	7.6	55%	Decrease hospital days
Controls	6.7	7.2	55%	No decrease hospital days
Simonds[13]	5.6	9.1	< 20%	

than those in whom NIPPV is begun in an end-stage phase As with CF patients, individuals with bronchiectasis due to other causes can be successfully bridged to transplantation. The chest X-ray of a 15-year-old boy with idiopathic bronchiectasis who was bridged to double lung transplantation by using 24-hour NIPPV for 8 weeks is shown in Figure 13.1.

DIFFUSE INTERSTITIAL LUNG DISEASE

At first sight NIPPV would appear of limited value in patients with interstitial lung disease. To a large extent this is true, although patients in the terminal stage of the disease develop CO_2 retention which may be helped symptomatically by NIPPV. In general, however, nocturnal hypoventilation is not a feature unless the interstitial process is accompanied by respiratory muscle weakness (e.g. systemic lupus erythematosis, polymyosistis) or chest wall involvement (scleroderma, systemic sclerosis).

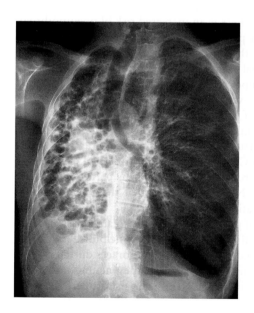

Figure 13.1 *Pre-operative chest X-ray in a 15-year-old patient with idiopathaic bronchiectasis successfully bridged to double lung transplantation using 24-hour NIPPV.*

12 Benhamou D, Muir J-F, Raspaud C, *et al*. Long-term efficiency of home nasal mask ventilation in patients with diffuse bronchiectasis and severe chronic respiratory failure. *Chest* 1997; **112**: 1259–66.
13 Simonds AK, Elliott MW. Outcome of domiciliary nasal intermittent positive pressure ventilation in restrictive and obstructive disorders. *Thorax* 1995; **50**: 604–9.
14 Nava S, Rubini F. Lung and chest wall mechanics in ventilated patients with endstage idiopathic pulmonary fibrosis. *Thorax* 1999; **54**: 390–5.
15 Freiberg DB, Young IH, Laks L, Lehrhaft B, Sullivan CE. Improvement in gas exchange with nasal continuous positive airway pressure in pulmonary alveolar microlithiasis. *Am Rev Respir Dis* 1992; **145**: 1215–16.
16 Haworth CS, Dodd ME, Atkins M, Woodcock AA, Webb AK. Pneumothorax in adults with cystic fibrosis dependent on nasal intermittent positive pressure ventilation (NIPPV): a management dilemma. *Thorax* 2000; **55**: 620–2.

14

Non-invasive ventilation in progressive neuromuscular disease and quadriplegia

A K SIMONDS

INTRODUCTION

Respiratory failure, often exacerbated by a chest infection, is the terminal event in many patients with progressive neuromuscular disease. Motor neurone disease, MND (or amyotrophic lateral sclerosis, ALS) is the most prevalent of these disorders; other progressive conditions such as Duchenne muscular dystrophy (DMD) and spinal muscular atrophy are considered in Chapter 15. It is clear that assisted ventilation may extend the life of patients and alter the natural history of these disorders; however the effects of the intervention on quality of life have not been systematically studied and data are mainly derived from uncontrolled studies. Conditions such as quadriplegeia due to cervical cord injury, and spina bifida comprise another area where the use of non-invasive ventilatory support is growing but has not yet been well evaluated. Some information on prognostic factors and the outcome of NIPPV is, however, available. The possible indications for NIPPV and the practical challenges which are associated will be considered.

MOTOR NEURONE DISEASE (MND)

There are approximately 5000 individuals with MND in the UK. The incidence is 1 in 50,000 per year, with a mean age at onset of 56 years. The commonest presentation is with a constellation of progressive upper and lower motor neurone signs in the spinal and bulbar territory ('classical ALS') although diagnosis may be problematical, and up to 40% of patients are initially misdiagnosed.[1] Most texts suggest that respiratory symptoms in MND patients appear late and can be identified by simple spirometric monitoring. However, an acute presentation with overt respiratory failure,[2] or features of nocturnal hypoventilation is not uncommon,[3,4] and we have seen an increasing number of referrals for ventilatory support in the last 5 years. Bulbar involvement affects up to 30% of individuals at the onset of the disease[5] and is not related to prognosis. However bulbar symptoms are virtually inevitable by the terminal phase. Median survival is around 2.5 years, but 25% of affected individuals may live for 5 years or more. Prognosis tend to be more favourable in younger patients. The cause of nerve degeneration in MND is unknown, but it may be related to the excessive stimulation of glutamate receptors on the motor neurone. The only available pharmacological therapy, riluzole (Rilutek, Rhone-Poulenc Rorer), was introduced in the Europe in 1996 as an anti-excitogenic agent, and is known to inhibit glutamate release. Two randomized controlled trials[6,7] using the primary endpoints of death or the need for tracheostomy have suggested that riluzole may extend tracheostomy-free survival in MND/ALS patients after a year of therapy. However, this advantage seems greater in a small subgroup with bulbar onset disease and may be lost by 18 months. There have also been methodological criticisms of the studies,[8] and neither assessed quality of life.

Box 14.1 *The key respiratory problems in MND patients*

Dyspnoea
Alveolar hypoventilation
Sleep disturbance, morning headaches, daytime sleepiness
Ineffective cough, resulting in chest infections
Aspiration and choking episodes secondary to bulbar involvement

---

Dyspnoea is unusual if vital capacity (VC) exceeds 50% predicted, but respiratory muscle function should be closely monitored if the VC falls below this value as respiratory decompensation commonly ensues within the next 12 months. Respiratory failure is virtually inevitable if VC falls below 30% predicted. Analysis of flow-volume loops will demonstrate abnormalities suggestive of upper airway dysfunction in many patients with MND. Not surprisingly these findings occur more often, but not exclusively, in patients with bulbar involvement. Bulbar insufficiency can worsen respiratory function by causing recurrent clinical and subclinical episodes of aspiration pneumonia. In addition to testing the gag reflex, swallowing ability can be easily assessed at the bedside by watching the patient drink a glass of water as rapidly as possible. A more accurate evaluation of bulbar function can be obtained by video-fluoroscopy.

The development of respiratory failure early in the course of the disease denotes phrenic nerve involvement, often in conjunction with weakness of other respiratory muscles. Recent work has shown that respiratory muscle strength can be accurately measured using manoeuvres such as maximal sniff pressure[9,10] with minimal discomfort to patients. It is this subgroup of patients with early respiratory muscle involvement, but normal or only mildy impaired bulbar function and preserved limb strength, which responds best to non-invasive ventilation.

CHOICE OF VENTILATORY TECHNIQUE

Tracheostomy-IPPV (T-IPPV) has been used quite extensively in ALS/MND in the USA to circumvent progressive bulbar problems. In practice, selection of patients is often heavily influenced by the degree of insurance cover, the extent of independent financial resources, and the availability of carers. Salamand et al.[11] report a 1-year survival of 24% in 24 MND patients receiving home T-IPPV. However, Oppenheimer and colleagues[12] have demonstrated an improved outcome with up to 85% 1-year survival. In this series more than 50% of patients survived for 3 years or more using T-IPPV at home. A French group of patients using nasal/mouth ventilation or T-IPPV showed a transient improvement in pulmonary function, and it was possible to discharge all patients home.[13] Clearly T-IPPV is the only ventilatory option in patients with severe bulbar disease.

Negative pressure techniques are unlikely to be helpful in MND as they may exacerbate upper airway dysfunction during sleep and worsen aspiration. NPV has been shown to reduce the symptoms of dyspnoea in several studies, however.[14,15]

On theoretical grounds NIPPV should be helpful in patients with MND and early respiratory muscle involvement as it may help stabilize the upper airway during sleep. In the only controlled study of NIPPV in ALS/MND Pinto et al.[16] showed a significant increase in survival in patients with respiratory insufficiency using bilevel ventilatory support compared with a non-ventilated control group. However, the quality of life tool used in this study showed no improvement. Aboussouan et al.[17] also found that prognosis was improved in patients who could tolerate NIPPV. We have seen excellent control of symptoms, increased confidence levels in the patient and family, and a relatively stable clinical state maintained for up to a year in patients with nocturnal hypoventilation started on NIPPV. Our practice is to treat symptomatic patients and keep asymptomatic individuals with hypoventilation under close review. Recent research[18] has shown an increase in energy and vitality in patients after starting NIPPV. It is crucial to note that once daytime $PaCO_2$ rises above 6.0 kPa, severe ventilatory decompensation is imminent. Bulbar symptoms are not a contraindication to NIPPV if they are mild or moderate, but may make tolerance of NIPPV more difficult for the patient (see Box 14.2).[17]

Occasionally, it may be difficult to separate out nocturnal symptoms related to hypoventilation and those due to upper airway obstruction and aspiration. For this reason monitoring of respiration during sleep is essential before starting assisted ventilation. Oximetry alone may be misleading in mild hypoventilation as individuals with MND/ALS usually have a brisk arousal response, leading to profound

Box 14.2 *Favourable features for successful use of NIPPV in the home in ALS/MND*

- Early respiratory muscle involvement
- Symptomatic nocturnal hypoventilation (morning headaches, poor sleep quality, daytime somnolence)
- Some independent breathing capacity
- Bulbar involvement not marked
- Strong patient motivation
- Adequate resources: caregivers, ventilatory equipment, aids to daily living
- Experienced homecare team
- Agreed plan for terminal care/advance directives
- Good liaison between hospital, GP, carers, and hospice

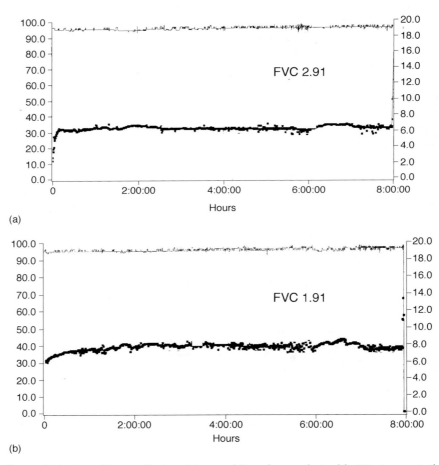

Figure 14.1 *Overnight monitoring of SaO$_2$ and TccO$_2$ in a patient with ALS at presentation (a) and 6 months later (b) when symptoms of nocturnal hypoventilation had developed. Note the fall in vital capacity and rise in nocturnal TccO$_2$.*

sleep fragmentation but only minor changes in SaO_2 and $TcCO_2$. Progression in overnight hypercapnia from trace (a) to (b) is seen in an ALS patient in Figure 14.1 in whom vital capacity fell by 1 litre over 6 months, although daytime arterial blood gas tensions remained normal. Sleep symptoms including restlessness and morning headache had developed by trace (b). There is no evidence that NIPPV will reduce dyspnoea in patients who are normocapnic. Similarly, although continuous positive airway pressure (CPAP) might be predicted to help patients with nocturnal choking in the absence of hypoventilation, in practice it is often unhelpful and may only serve to burden the patient further.

The combination of NIPPV and percutaneous gastrostomy feeding (PEG) may be suitable in patients with fairly severe bulbar weakness and symptoms of aspiration. Providing close peri- and post-operative monitoring is carried out, it is possible to safely insert a PEG feeding tube in a patient reliant on NIPPV (see also Chapter 8).

DECISION-MAKING IN MND/ALS

Patients and their families cannot make informed decisions unless they are provided with information about treatment options and their outcome in an understandable form. It is often assumed that presenting the individual with details of the progressive nature of the disease and its complications will be burdensome and cause undue depression. Clinical experience and research has shown that this paternalistic approach is over-protective and denies the individual an active part in decision-making, and therefore control over his or her future. Clearly, the discussions need to be sensitively handled and patients should not be overwhelmed with information – so-called 'truth dumping'.[19,20] Moss et al.[21] have shown that 96% of ALS/MND patients are in favour of making advance directives. A majority are able to place limits on the application of long-term mechanical ventilation e.g. they would wish ventilatory support to be discontinued if they had cardiac arrest or developed a permanent coma.

Oppenheimer[12] found that less than 25% of ALS/MND patients decided to use mechanical ventilation in advance of an emergency admission, but having started ventilatory support nearly all wished to continue this. In a further study[22] 100% of those using NIPPV were glad they had chosen this mode of support. From the family perspective 42% of familes who cared for a ALS/MND patient requiring ventilatory support at home felt this to be a major burden,[21] but 83% would encourage that individual to choose mechanical ventilation again, although they were less sure about receiving this treatment themselves if the need arose. The situation has changed somewhat with the introduction of NIPPV and some patients, for example, choose to limit ventilatory support to non-invasive methods. These issues are considered further in Chapter 20.

TERMINAL CARE

In some units NIPPV is used as an intermediate phase before proceeding to T-IPPV when bulbar symptoms become severe. This progressive care plan is less frequently seen in the UK as few centres carry out a tracheostomy in MND patients. All concerned should understand that if assisted ventilation is offered and accepted, patients should be able to opt to discontinue supportive therapy at any point. In practice it is easier to discontinue non-invasive methods than T-IPPV. In our experience it is more usual for the patient to want to continue with NIPPV in the terminal phase to maintain symptom relief. Increasing ventilator dependence is a certain accompaniment to this phase, and as weakness progresses many patients find the transition period from ventilatory support to self-ventilation increasingly difficult. In this situation a deliberate reduction in the ventilator pressure or flow settings so that overnight CO_2 rises to between 6 and 7 kPa may help, without leading to a recurrence of symptoms of nocturnal hypoventilation. Anxiolytic medication, including morphine derivatives, and anticholinergic preparations to reduce secretions may also be of value. In the UK the Motor Neurone Disease Association, in conjunction with the general practitioner, can provide a 'breathing space' kit. Its contents are titrated to the individual but may contain rectal diazepam for administration by a carer, and opiates for administration by a home nurse or doctor. Physiotherapy advice on control of breathing and the forced expiration technique ('huffing') often helps. Each case should however be managed on an individual basis. The needs and feelings of carers should not be overlooked at this difficult time, and respite care made available. Some hospices are not familiar with the use of ventilators, and careful liaison regarding the uses and limitations of nasal ventilation with the patient's general practitioner and the hospice team is essential. The final event is still likely to be a chest infection. Use of opiates to relieve dyspnoea will allow the ventilator to be withdrawn without distress in the last days or hours of the patient's life, or earlier in the terminal phase if this is in accordance with the individual's wishes.

QUADRIPLEGIA

Patients with high cervical cord or bulbar lesions with no independent ventilatory capacity and an inability to clear secretions require tracheostomy assisted ventilation. Expertise in managing these patients has been gained in many spinal injuries centres.

In recent years it has been demonstrated that a proportion of quadriplegic patients with minimal respiratory reserve may cope with long-term non-invasive methods and where this is feasible, the option of non-invasive support should be pursued as it simplifies care and is preferable to patients and carers.[23] Patients with unrecordable vital capacity may be able to self-ventilate for periods using glossopharyngeal ('frog') breathing. This involves the patient gulping a series of breaths in succession so that he effectively breath stacks. Few respiratory therapists or physiotherapists are experienced in teaching this technique, but educational videos are available (e.g. glossopharygeal breathing – what, when and how? by BA Webber and J Higgens – see Appendix II).

The aetiology of quadriplegia ranges from traumatic cervical cord injury to stable neurological disorders (e.g. spina bifida – see below) and progressive neuromuscular disease. An individual with a cervical cord lesion rostral to C4 is likely to need ventilation immediately. Those with a C4/5 injury may be able to support ventilation independently, but will decompensate in the presence of underlying chronic lung disease, spinal shock or the development of a chest infection. Delayed progression to ventilatory failure may occur in others. Critical to the well-being of these patients is physiotherapy and assisted coughing. Hyperinflation of the chest may be helpful in reducing the tendency to atelectasis and perhaps improving chest wall and pulmonary compliance, but there is little in the way of controlled trials in this area.

Assessment should include measurement of lung volumes, mouth pressures and overnight monitoring of respiration when symptoms of nocturnal hypoventilation are present, or vital capacity is less than 50% predicted. Sortor[24] has described the evaluation cough efficacy by separating the action into several components – see Box 14.3.

Box 14.3 Components of an effective cough

1 The ability of the airway to respond to irritation
2 Maximum inspiration: which may be reduced due to inspiratory muscle weakness
3 Glottic closure: which is not usually a problem
4 Contraction of the expiratory muscles against a closed airway: often markedly impaired due to expiratory muscle weakness
5 Opening of the airway: not usually a problem

Assistance with coughing is required if the patient's inspiratory capacity is less than 50% predicted. This can be achieved by teaching the individual to stack spontaneous breaths by using glossopharyngeal breathing as above, a hyperinflation device (e.g. Bird IPPB machine, Cape TC50) or increasing volume or flow settings during physiotherapy with the patient receiving NIPPV. The forced expiratory phase can be augmented by an abdominal thrust. Carers should be taught these techniques. The cough insufflator/exsufflator (Emerson) is widely used in some centres (see Chapters 15 and 17).

In a series[24,25] of 62 quadriplegic patients treated at the Dallas Rehabilitation Institute from 1984, 22 had a traumatic cervical cord lesion and 40 had neuromuscular disease (20 poliomyelitis, nine muscular dystrophy, six spinal muscular atrophy, three motor neurone disease and two spina bifida). Of the cervical cord trauma group, 15 had lesions at C3 and above, four at C4 and three at C5. Nearly all were admitted with a tracheostomy and requiring ventilatory support, but it was possible to discharge 15 patients (68%) without a tracheostomy. Nine of these patients were transferred to nocturnal mask ventilation and five used negative pressure pneumojackets. Some employed mouth ventilation or a pneumobelt as a ventilatory adjunct during the day.

In the neuromuscular group, only three (7.5%) required a long-term tracheostomy (two with MND and one with muscular dystrophy). Of the remainder, 30 (were supported with mask ventilation and seven (including five children with spinal muscular atrophy) received negative pressure ventilation.

SPINA BIFIDA

Individuals with this condition require special consideration. Most spina bifida patients with severe lesions in the thoracic or lumbar region are wheelchair bound, scoliotic and have impaired bladder function. A proportion have hydrocephalus, usually well-controlled by CSF shunt, and some have learning disabilities. While the long-term outlook in those with lumbar/sacral defects may be good, death from respiratory failure in the second or third decade is common in those with thoracic spinal defects.

Respiratory function in spina bifida patients may be compromised by multiple factors including thoracic scoliosis, respiratory muscle weakness and central drive defects. In a series of six spina bifida patients seen at the Royal Brompton Hospital ventilatory failure was associated with a thoracic spinal defect and vital capacity of less than 1000 mL.[26] Respiratory muscle strength and Cobb angle were not related to the degree of hypercapnia, but marked obesity was a potentially reversible factor in all patients with respiratory insufficiency. Sleep disordered breathing comprising a combination of hypoventilation and obstructive apnoea was seen in all patients and contributed to the progression of respiratory failure. It was corrected with nocturnal NIPPV which reversed respiratory failure effectively.[27] Despite the level of physical disability, the quality of life in spina bifida patients receiving domiciliary NIPPV did not differ from other groups including those with idiopathic scoliosis and previous poliomyelitis,[27] and long-term survival was achieved.

CONCLUSIONS

Non-invasive ventilatory support is feasible in patients with progressive neuro-muscular disease and may facilitate discharge from hospital and simplify care. The key aims are relief of symptoms, and an improvement in quality of life, while maintaining patient autonomy. Discussion of the advantages and disadvantages of ventilatory support *before* the development of ventilatory failure, and the use of advance directives should be encouraged. Applied appropriately, NIPPV may extend a life which is judged worthwhile by the recipient, rather than merely protract his/her death. Medical teams have a duty to use these techniques cost-effectively. There are little controlled data in this area and further work on quality of life in both patients and carers, the most appropriate time to initiate NIPPV, and long-term outcome is required. Wider public debate on the ethical aspects of respiratory support in these conditions should be promoted. Ethico-legal considerations are explored in more detail in Chapter 20.

REFERENCES

1   Hardiman O. Pitfalls in the diagnosis of motor neurone disease. *Hosp Med* 2000; **61**: 767–71.

2   Al-Shaikh B, Kinnear W, Higenbottam TW, Smith HS, Shneerson JM. Motor neurone disease presenting as respiratory failure. *BMJ* 1986; **292**: 1325–6.

3   Polkey MI, Lyall RA, Davidson AC, Leigh PN, Moxham J. Ethical and clinical issues in the use of home non-invasive ventilation for the palliation of breathlessness in motor neurone disease. *Thorax* 1999; **54**: 367–71.

4   Simonds AK. Non-invasive ventilation in neuromuscular disease. *Br J Hosp Med* 1997; **57**: 87–90.

5   Haverkamp LJ, Appel V, Appel SH. Natural history of amyotrophic lateral sclerosis in a database population. Validation of a scoring system and a model for survival prediction. *Brain* 1995; **118**: 707–19.

6   Bensimon G, Lacomblez L, Meninger V, the ALS/Riluzole Study Group. A controlled trial of riluzole in amyotrophic lateral sclerosis. *N Engl J Med* 1994; **330**: 585–91.

7   Lacomblez L, Bensimon G, Leigh PN, Guillet P, Meninger V, the ALS/Riluzole Study Group. Dose-ranging study of riluzole in amyotrophic lateral sclerosis. *Lancet* 1996; **347**: 1425–31.

8   AnonymousRiluzole for amyotrophic lateral sclerosis. *Drug Therapeut Bull* 1997; **35**: 11–12.

9   Lyall RA, Green M, Leigh PN, *et al.* Maximum sniff pressure in the assessment of patients with amyotrophic lateral sclerosis. *Am J Respir Crit Care Med* 1998; **157**: A (abstract).

10 Polkey MI, Lyall RA, Green M, Leigh PN, Moxham J. Expiratory muscle function in amyotrophic lateral sclerosis. *Am J Respir Crit Care Med* 1998; **158**: 1–8.

11 Salamand J, Robert D, Leger P, Langevin B, Barraud J. Definitive mechanical ventilation via tracheostomy in end-stage amyotrophic lateral sclerosis. *3rd International Conference on Pulmonary Rehabilitation and Home Ventilation* 1991; Denver: 50 (abstract).

12 Oppenheimer EA. Amyotrophic lateral sclerosis. *Eur Respir Rev* 1992; **2**(10): 323–9.

13 Goulon M, Goulon-Goeau C. Sclerose lateral amyotrophique et assistance respiratoire. *Rev Neurol* 1989; **145**: 293–8.

14 Sawicka EH, Loh L, Branthwaite MA. Domiciliary ventilatory support; an analysis of outcome. *Thorax* 1988; **43**: 31–5.

15 Howard RS, Wiles CM, Loh L. Respiratory complications and their management in motor neuron disease. *Brain* 1989; **112**: 1155–70.

16 Pinto AC, Evangelista T, Carvalho M, Alves MA, Sales Luis ML. Respiratory assistance with a non-invasive ventilator (BiPAP) in MND/ALS patients: survival rates in a controlled trial. *J Neurol Sci* 1995; **129** Suppl: 19–26.

17 Aboussouan LS, Khan SU, Meeker DP, Stelmach K, Mitsumoto H. Effect of noninvasive positive-pressure ventilation on survival in amyotrophic lateral sclerosis. *Ann Intern Med* 1997; **127**: 450–3.

18 Lyall RA, Donaldson N, Fleming T, *et al.* A prospective study of quality of life in ALS patients treated with non-invasive ventilation. *Neurology* 2001 (in press).

19 Muskin PR. The request to die: a role for a psychodynamic perspective on physician-assisted suicide. *JAMA* 1998; **279**: 323–8.

20 Rowland LP. Assisted suicide and alternatives in amyotrophic lateral sclerosis. *N Engl J Med* 1998; **339**: 987.

21 Moss AH, Oppenheimer EA, Casey P, *et al.* Patients with amyotrophic lateral sclerosis receiving long-term mechanical ventilation. Advance care planning and outcomes. *Chest* 1996; **110**: 249–55.

22 Cazzolli PA, Oppenheimer EA. Home mechanical ventilation for amyotrphic lateral sclerosis: nasal compared to tracheostomy intermittent postive pressure ventilation. *J Neurol Sci* 1996; **139**: 123–8.

23 Bach J. A comparison of long-term ventilatory support alternatives from the perspective of the patient and care-giver. *Chest* 1993; **104**: 1702–6.

24 Sortor S. Pulmonary issues in quadriplegia. *Eur Respir Rev* 1992; **2**(10): 330–4.

25 Viroslav J, Rosenblatt R, Tomazevic SM, Sortor-Leger S. Care, life expectancy and quality of life in respiratory tetraplegics. In: Robert D, Make BJ, Leger P, *et al.* (eds). *Home mechanical ventilation*, 1st edn. Paris: Arnette Blackwell, 1995: 241–7.

26 Varnava A, Woodhead M, Steven MH, Simonds AK. Respiratory failure in spina bifida: aetiology and prognostic features. *Am Rev Respir Dis* 1991; **145**: A863.

27 Dilworth JP, Potter N, Simonds AK. Outcome of nasal ventilation in spina bifida patients with hypercapnic respiratory failure. *Eur Respir J* 1994; **7**: 415s.

15

Paediatric non-invasive ventilation

A K SIMONDS

INTRODUCTION

The number of children receiving assisted ventilation at home is increasing. Regional surveys[1] of domiciliary ventilation in the USA in 1986 and 1992 showed that the largest subgroup of recipients consisted of children under the age of 11 years and this category demonstrated the most rapid growth over the intervening years. A follow-up study in 1997[2] found a further 42% increase in ventilator dependent patients, with those under 11 years and those above 70 years comprising the largest subgroups. Over half the increase in numbers was attributable to the use on non-invasive ventilatory modes. In 1997, 20% (60/306) of ventilator-assisted individuals in the state of Minnesota were in the paediatric age range.[1]

A study[3] of French children registered on the national ANTADIR scheme for home support in a 12-month period between 1992 and 1993 found that 158 children received mechanical ventilation. A small proportion (13%) of these used nasal CPAP or pneumobelt ventilation, and 12 had a tracheostomy but did not require ventilation. The majority used NIPPV, and the predominant diagnoses were neuromuscular and chest wall disease. Earlier, Robinson[4] examined the care of long-term ventilator dependent children in the UK during the period 1983–88. Only 24 chidren were identified, but this study focused on children receiving ventilation 24 hours/day (usually due to cervical cord injury, neuromuscular or parenchymal lung disease), and excluded a far larger group of individuals treated with non-invasive methods predominately at night. The main underlying diagnosis in this latter group was neuromuscular disease.

By the early 1990s more accurate UK figures were clearly required and a Working Party on Paediatric Home ventilation was established, funded by a Department of Health grant. This group identified around 150 children requiring long-term ventilatory support.[5] Twenty-eight per cent had neuromuscular disorders, 15% central hypoventilation syndromes, and 13% spinal cord injury. Approximately a third of children remained in hospital because of obstacles to home discharge[5] – this area is considered in Chapter 18.

Patients with parenchymal lung disease such as bronchopulomary dysplasia are likely to require tracheostomy-IPPV (T-IPPV), as are those with high cervical lesions who need 24-hour ventilatory support. Non-invasive methods of ventilation are suitable in other subgroups especially for night-time support, and there is now a growing body of experience in this area. In some situations T-IPPV is preferable because of the age of the child; in other instances T-IPPV was previously the standard treatment but has been superceded by nasal ventilation. Where available outcome data and the practical problems associated with these applications will be compared. Most information exists on domiciliary ventilation in childhood spinal muscular atrophy, Duchenne muscular dystrophy (DMD), congenital myopathies and chest wall disease and so these areas will be covered in detail. To set ventilatory activity in neuromuscular disease in perspective, the European Alliance of Muscular Dystrophy Associations estimates that the prevalence of cases of spinal muscular atrophy (types 1 and 2), DMD and congenital myopathies in Europe is approximately 6000, 18,000 and 15,000, respectively.

PHYSIOLOGICAL CONSIDERATIONS

Although treatment may be similar, there are important differences between adults and children in the pathogenesis of ventilatory failure. These need to be taken into account as they affect the vulnerability of the individual to decompensation, and may also act as a guide to the most appropriate time to introduce ventilatory support. The situation is always likely to be more dynamic in children as maturation of ventilatory responses with age and lung growth may improve overall ventilation, whereas the adolescent growth spurt and gain in weight in the teenage years may be sufficient to overload weak respiratory muscles in patients with non-progressive disorders. These differences are summarized in Box 15.1.

> **Box 15.1** *Physiological diffferences in ventilation between paediatric and adult patients*
>
> - Smaller lung volumes
> - Difference in sleep architecture: greater proportion of REM sleep
> - Immature ventilatory and arousal responses in babies and early childhood
> - High chest wall compliance
> - Lower relative strength and endurance of respiratory muscles
> - Nasal resistance a greater proportion of total respiratory resistance
> - Greater airway reactivity
> - Higher metabolic rate
> - Increased sensitivity of pulmonary vascular bed to hypoxaemia
> - Effects of chest wall deformity on lung and chest wall growth
> - Effects of pubertal growth spurt on ventilatory load

VENTILATORY SUPPORT IN NEUROMUSCULAR DISEASE

Spinal muscular atrophy (SMA)

This anterior horn cell disease is inherited as an autosomal recessive trait. Chromosome mapping has shown that the defective gene is located on the long arm of chromosome 5.[6] On developmental grounds SMA can be classified into Types I–III as illustrated in Box 15.2.

It is particularly important to note that division into Types I–III SMA is fairly arbitrary and a continuum exists from extremely floppy Type I neonates to Type

> **Box 15.2** *Classification of spinal muscular atrophy (SMA)*
>
> | Type I | Clinical features | Inheritance |
> |---|---|---|
> | Werdnig–Hoffman's disease | Hypotonic at birth. Unable to hold head up. May be accompanying brainstem stem abnormality and pulmonary aplasia Death before the age of 4 years in > 95% of cases | Autosomal recessive |
> | Type I Intermediate | Able to hold head up, unable to sit. Usually diagnosed in first year. Often recurrent respiratory tract infections | Autosomal recessive and dominant |
> | Type II Kugelberg–Welander | Able to sit up, unable to walk Proximal and intercostal muscle involvement. Diaphragm often spared. Scoliosis | Autosomal recessive |
> | Type III | Symmetrical proximal weakness. Scoliosis. Respiratory insufficiency possible in young adulthood | Autosomal recessive |

III adults with only minor motor limitation. Dubowitz[7] has subdivided the categories into: Severe Type 1.1–1.9, Intermediate Type 2.1–2.9, and Mild Type 3.1–3.9. SMA of 4.0 is defined as normal. Clearly a child with 1.9 SMA will have a disability level which has more in common with a child categorized as Type 2.1, than an individual with Type 1.1 SMA. This means that a careful individual assessment of functional performance is extremely important when considering management decisions, rather than making an assumption of poor outcome based on a diagnostic label.

Individuals with all forms of SMA are at risk from nocturnal hypoventilation, and ultimately diurnal respiratory failure. While infants with Type I SMA may require ventilation at or within several months of birth, those in the Type I intermediate and Type II groups often require ventilatory support in the first two years of life, and individuals with Type III SMA develop respiratory insufficiency in the second, third or fourth decades, depending on the extent of respiratory muscle involvement and the severity of scoliosis. Extensive experience in providing ventilatory support for SMA children has been reported by Barois[8] and colleagues, and from the USA.[13] Clearly the logistical and ethical problems are most complex in providing ventilatory assistance to children with Type I SMA, and this is a difficult and controversial area. However, Barois[8] has demonstrated favourable results in 22 children with Wernig–Hoffmann disease discharged home using TIPPV. This team advocate the use of home nasal ventilation where more than 4 hours a day ventilatory assistance is required, in the absence of swallowing problems and/or marked bronchial secretions. Fourteen children with SMA over the age of 2 years have been treated with NIPPV (mean age 10 years) and nine children under the age of 2 years (mean age 15.5 months). A tracheostomy was subsequently performed in a minority of patients.[9] A combination of mask ventilation and augmented coughing techniques (e.g. cough insufflator/exsufflator) may be sufficient to support children in the grey area between non-invasive and invasive ventilatory support say, say categories 1.7–2.5.

For untreated children with Type I SMA, the prognosis is poor. Death is almost inevitable by the age of 2 years, and 80% die by the age of one year[10] without respiratory support. Two groups have recently examined the value of a non-invasive ventilatory approach in Type I children. Birnkrant et al.[11] used non-invasive bilevel pressure support and medical management of gastro-oesphageal reflux (including gastrostomy) in four children diagnosed with Type I SMA between one and 5 months of age. Respiratory insufficiency occurred at the age of 2 to 7 months. Despite the application of bilevel pressure support ventilation, survival after the development of respiratory insufficiency was only 1 to 3.5 months. More favourable results have been reported by Bach et al.[12] In this retropsective analysis 11 Type I SMA children were treated with a non-invasive respiratory management protocol consisting of bilevel pressure support and mechanical insufflation–exsufflation to augment cough. The average age of the children at the first episode of ventilatory decompensation was 14.6 months (range 3–28 months). Parents of all children had refused tracheostomy. The outcome of episodes of acute respiratory failure (ARF) using a defined protocol (intubation followed by extubation on to NIPPV) versus conventional management was compared. Extubation was not attempted until arterial SaO$_2$ was > 90% breathing air. Successful extubation was defined as no

requirement to reintubate during the current hospital admission. Using the protocol nine children required multiple intubations for infective episodes, but were
successfully extubated back to the non-invasive regime without recourse to
tracheostomy on 23 out of 28 occasions. Two children survived for 37 and 66
months without intubation, although they required 24-hour non-invasive ventilation from the ages of 5 and 7 months. Two children were ultimately treated with
tracheostomy, one was lost to follow-up and the remaining six have continued at
home on intermittent mask ventilation for a mean of 30.4 months. This experince
shows that it is possible to avoid tracheostomy in some children with Type I SMA,
but it is clear that episodes of acute respiratory failure still occur, frequently requiring intensive care. These repeated admissions may be burdensome for the child and
family, and have major implications for paediatric ICU resources, despite the fact
that most children were successfully treated. It is important to note a tracheostomy
was not performed in accordance with the parent's wishes in 9/11 cases, but the
authors give no information on quality of life of the child and family. It is also
notable that the average age of the patients in the Birnkrant et al.[11] study (4.6
months) was much younger than the Bach et al.[12] cohort suggesting a greater severity of disease. A lower level of pressure support was also employed. Taken as the
whole, these studies suggest that a non-invasive approach may be of value in some
profoundly weak children with SMA Type I, but clearly a spectrum of problems
exists and in some cases little in the way of survival advantage is achieved. In other
cases NIPPV may reduce the need for hospitalization and allow the child to remain
at home, but this needs to be confirmed and data on quality of life are urgently
required.

Good quality of life has been reported[13] anecdotally in adolescence and beyond
in Type I intermediate and Type II forms, although detailed health status/quality
of life studies are rare, and insufficient time has elapsed to judge long-term results
with NIPPV. Long-term survival using nocturnal NIPPV has been recently demonstrated in a group of children with Type I Intermediate SMA (average age at developing respiratory insufficiency 5.7 ± 4.2 years), and all children were able to take
part in normal schooling.[14] Learning disabilities are not a feature of SMA. In

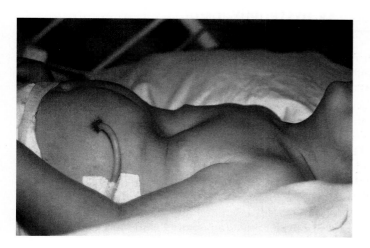

Figure 15.1 *Chest
wall recession in
Type I intermediate
SMA.*

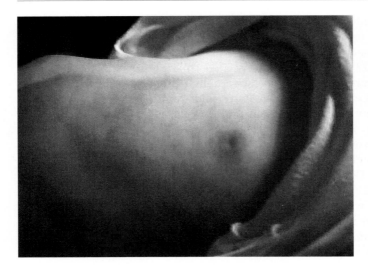

Figure 15.2 *Chest wall configuration in SMA patient from Figure 15.1 four years after starting nocturnal NIPPV.*

addition to symptom control and normalization of arterial blood gas tensions, positive pressure ventilation may be particularly helpful in fostering the normal development of alveoli and the chest wall as indicated by a progressive fall in vital capacity/total lung capacity ratio in untreated SMA patients and stable/increasing lung volumes in cases receiving assisted ventilation.[8] Severe chest wall recession is a characteristic feature of SMA as shown in a child with Type I intermediate disease in Figure 15.1. Chest wall configuration in the same child after 4 years' nocturnal NIPPV is shown in Figure 15.2, so it is possible that these deformities may be modified by adequate ventilation. Careful attention also needs to be paid to the development of scoliosis and contractures which compromise respiration and limit mobility. Use of NIPPV in the perioperative period may allow a child to undergo scoliosis surgery in whom surgery was previously contraindicated because of respiratory insufficiency.

DUCHENNE MUSCULAR DYSTROPHY (DMD)

This most common muscular dystrophy in childhood is inherited as an X-linked recessive disorder with an incidence of around 1 in 3500 live male births. The gene responsible for DMD and its milder variant Becker muscular dystrophy has been identified and its gene product (dystrophin) characterized. Lack of dystrophin appears to lead to the most severe forms of DMD, probably by causing muscle membrane dysfunction, fibrotic and fatty change and ultimately muscle atrophy.

Dubowitz[15] found that 20% of DMD cases were diagnosed by the age of 2 years and around 75% had presented by the age of 4 years with signs of motor delay. In a French series, Rideau *et al.*[16] showed that on average patients become wheelchair-bound by the age of 10 years and 50% develop a significant scoliosis. Without ventilatory support the mean age at death is around 19 years, with 73% of deaths occurring as a consequence of hypercapnic respiratory failure. Just under 20% of

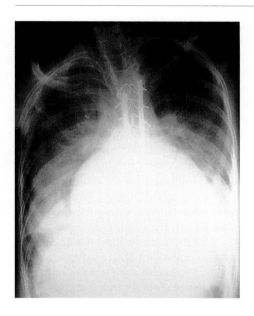

Figure 15.3 *Dilated cardiomyopathy in Duchenne muscular dystrophy.*

patients died during an acute infective exacerbation and 9% of deaths were attributed to cardiac disease.

The evolution of lung function changes in DMD has been divided into three stages: an initial phase during the first 10 years where forced vital capacity (FVC) increases as predicted, a second phase during which lung volumes plateau as muscle weakness +/- scoliosis becomes manifest, and a final phase in which FVC initially falls slowly, but may decline by as much as 250 mL/year in the last few years of life.[17] Peak vital capacity is a prognostic factor as Rideau *et al.*[16] showed that a peak VC of less than 1200 mL was associated with an average age at death of 15.3 years, while values in excess of 1700 mL resulted in survival to 21 years. Cardiac involvement takes the form of conduction defects and a dilated or hypertrophic cardiomyopathy. Dilated cardiomyopathy as evidenced by cardiomegaly and left ventricular dysfunction is the commonest abnormality (Figure 15.3). Nigro and coworkers[18] found pre-clinical evidence of cardiac disease in 25% of DMD patients under the age of 6 years and 59% between the ages of 6 and 10 years. Clinically apparent cardiac involvement was present in all patients by the age of 18 years, and about 72% of these patients were symptomatic. This is important as breathlessness and fatigue due to cardiac failure may be erroneously attributed to respiratory insufficiency.

The first signs of respiratory compromise occur during sleep. REM sleep related hypoventilation is common when vital capacity is less than 30% predicted and increases with age.[19,20] Obstructive apnoeas occur in a proportion of patients and may predate the development of hypoventilation.[20] A Cheyne–Stokes pattern of breathing may been seen in DMD patients with severe cardiomyopathy. Patients with mild to moderate nocturnal hypoxaemia often remain asymptomatic, symptoms tend to ensue when sleep disordered breathing progresses to non-REM sleep. Features of nocturnal hypoventilation should be sought carefully and a sleep study carried if these are present or in high risk cases (see Chapter 10)

Long-term ventilatory assistance in DMD is still not universally accepted despite the fact that various forms of ventilatory assistance have been employed and shown to be effective for over 20–30 years.[16,21] Concerns focus on the fact that DMD may progress rapidly with a marked reduction in general muscle strength as well as respiratory muscle involvement, so that the individual may end up ventilator dependent and immobile, with an unacceptable quality of life.

Before the mid-1980s the options available for ventilatory support were TIPPV, mouth-piece ventilation, negative pressure devices, the pneumobelt and rocking bed. Alexander et al.[21] report a series of patients with late stage DMD who received ventilatory assistance for up to 7 years. Patients used a variety of techniques including mouthpiece-IPPV, cuirass, pneumowrap and rocking bed, with the aim of continuing non-invasive methods long-term and avoiding tracheostomy. Treatment was begun in response to symptomatic hypercapnia and ventilatory support was continued for an average of 3.4 years. Care was delivered in the community and patients were reported to have a meaningful quality of life. By contrast, Rideau and coworkers[16] used IPPV via a fenestrated tracheostomy in a series of DMD patients following the development of acute on chronic respiratory failure or symptoms of nocturnal hypoventilation. All subjects had a moderate to severe scoliosis and vital capacity of less than 550 mL. A tracheostomy was performed between the ages of 16 and 23 years and none of the patients required daytime ventilatory support allowing them to complete schooling and carry on with other activities. It is notable that several patients died of complications related to the tracheostomy.

Mouth intermittent positive pressure ventilation has also been employed effectively in DMD[22], and may be used in addition to other modes as a ventilatory adjunct during the day.

Hill[23] examined the effects of negative pressure in DMD patients aged around 23 years with an average vital capacity of approximately 300 mL. Monitoring of respiration during sleep confirmed that nearly all patients experienced more than five episodes/hour of sleep disordered breathing accompanied by sleep disruption and destauration during negative pressure ventilation. These episodes were predominantly obstructive apnoeas or hypopnoeas. Supplemental oxygen was not helpful in alleviating respiratory disturbances, and tended to prolong the duration of events. The authors found it necessary to use nasal CPAP in two patients and a tracheostomy in another as an adjunct to NPV. This combination adds considerably to the complexity of treatment. Several groups have demonstrated desaturation precipitated by upper airway obstruction in patients using NPV and have shown that a switch to NIPPV can eliminate the problem.[24,25]

Recurrent aspiration during NPV may be a particular problem in individuals with reduced bulbar reflexes,[17] although patients with mild to moderate bulbar weakness can be effectively treated with NIPPV. For all these reasons NIPPV is almost certainly the treatment of choice in DMD, although a preliminary study comparing different ventilatory modes in DMD produced inconclusive results,[26] and some centres (particularly in France) follow a stepped care programme. Here patients are initially treated with NIPPV but progress to T-IPPV if extreme ventilator dependency or severe bulbar problems develop.[27]

There has been no controlled study of the use of assisted ventilation in DMD patients with nocturnal and diurnal hypercapnia. However, the long-term effects or NIPPV have been explored by comparing the clinical course and pulmonary function in five hypercapnic patients who received NIPPV and a control group of five patients who did not receive ventilatory support.[28] Over a 2-year period all the subjects receiving NIPPV survived, whereas four out of five of the control subjects died (mean survival 9.7 months). After 6 months mean loss of vital capacity and maximal voluntary ventilation was significantly greater in the control group. Although these subjects were not randomized to treatment and there was a trend to older age, higher $PaCO_2$ and smaller tidal volumes in the control group, these results strongly suggest NIPPV is of value in prolonging survival in some DMD patients. Hill[29] has concluded that the evidence for nocturnal NIPPV in sympto-matic, hypercapnic patients with DMD is now so persuasive that research activity should be focused on *how* it works, rather than *whether* it works.

Recent work tends to support this message. In a Royal Brompton Hospital, UK series of 23 consecutive DMD patients, who presented in hypercapnic ventilatory failure, all were successfully treated with NIPPV as the sole mode of ventilatory support.[30] Survival at 1 year was 85% and at 5 years 73% (Figure 15.4). This compares with a survival of 36% at 3 years in patients from an earlier French cohort,[27] suggesting that outcome is improving. Most UK patients needed only nocturnal NIPPV for the first 3 to 5 years and only subsequently became more ventilatory dependent during the day. Bulbar involvement was a late stage phenom-enon. Quality of life scores, measured using the SF 36 questionnaire, were compa-rable to other ventilator dependent patient groups.[30] Unfortunately information on the impact of NIPPV in DMD does not yet seem to have filtered through to all centres who manage such patients.[31]

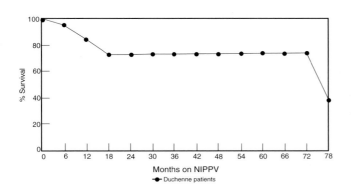

Figure 15.4 *Survival in Duchenne muscular dystrophy patients treated with NIPPV (from Ref. 29).*

Bach[32] has investigated 'life satisfaction' in ventilator dependent Duchenne patients. Using a postal survey, life satisfaction was assessed in 82 DMD patients and 273 physically intact healthcare professionals (nurses, physicians and thera-pists). These health professionals were also asked to estimate the quality of life of Duchenne patients known personally to them. On a scale of 1 (completely dissat-isfied) to 7 (completely satisfied), the average score for Duchenne patients was 4.9 and only 12.5% admitted to dissatisfaction with their lives, despite the fact that 32 patients were receiving 24-hour ventilatory support. The average score for healthcare workers was not markedly different at 5.4, and 9% expressed dissatisfaction with their lives. Importantly, the healthcare workers consistently underestimated the quality of life of the DMD patients. They also judged that the patients' main area of concern would be their inability to breathe spontaneously, whereas the DMD patients rated their most important concern as loss of upper limb function. Every single Duchenne patient felt that ventilatory assistance should be available to all DMD patients who required this, and would opt for ventilatory support applied in same manner, if they had their lives over again.

As a comparison, some investigators[33] have assessed the quality of life in a general group of muscular dystrophy patients, the majority of whom did not need ventilatory support. Once again, upper limb function was an important explanatory variable, as was mobility.

It should also be remembered that nocturnal ventilation is just one component of the management of patients with neuromuscular disease. Advice regarding physiotherapy, sputum clearance, nutrition, assessment of scoliosis, mobility, transportation, education and work opportunities, together with the provision of aids to daily living all form an essential part of a comprehensive care plan.

MANAGEMENT OF CARDIOMYOPATHY IN DMD

It is possible that the use of NIPPV in DMD may have a benficial effect on cardiac function, but this has not been proven. In theory, the addition of EPAP may reduce left ventricular workload. Cardiac failure should be treated with diuretic and ACE inhibitor therapy. In many patients receiving ventilatory support cardiac function is now a more consistent predictor of outcome than respiratory function. Factors affecting outcome in a series of Royal Brompton/Hammersmith Hospital patients with DMD are shown in Box 15.3.

Box 15.3 *Determinants of outcome in DMD*

- Early loss of ambulation
- Vital capacity
- Left ventricular function
- Nutritional state
- Age

PHYSIOTHERAPY AND SPUTUM CLEARANCE TECHNIQUES

In DMD expiratory muscle weakness tends to progress in tandem with inspiratory muscle weakness, whereas in SMA patients expiratory muscle involvement may occur before significant inspiratory limitation. Vital capacity and inspiratory mouth pressures can be used to assess inspiratory muscle strength (see Chapter 10), while expiratory muscle strength can be measured by maximum expiratory mouth pressure or cough peak flow rates. In small children and those unable to perform

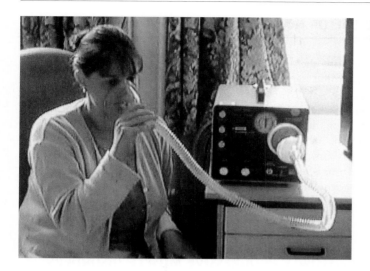

Figure 15.5 *Cough In-exsufflator (JH Emerson Co.).*

the measurement techniques, the sound generated by a cough effort is a rough guide to its effectiveness at clearing bronchial secretions.

Parents and carers need to be taught how to perform chest physiotherapy (see also Chapter 17). In nasal ventilator dependent patients it is helpful to carry out physiotherapy while the individual is using the ventilator. This will enhance vital capacity and aid expiratory flow, hence improving sputum clearance. Providing a slight increase in tidal volume or IPAP (e.g. by 2 cmH$_2$O) during the physiotherapy session and swapping from a full facemask to nasal mask may all aid expectoration.

Insufflator exsufflator machines (JH Emerson Co., Cambridge, Mass, USA) (Figure 15.5) have been advocated to augment cough. These machines provide a deep positive pressure insufflation followed by a swing to negative pressure to generate a forced expiration, applied via a facemask. In one comparison[34] of sputum clearance techniques, cough expiratory peak flow was higher using the insufflator/exsufflator compared with values obtained using manual assistance, or breath stacking (glossopharyngeal breathing). Normal values for peak cough expiratory flow rate should excede 6 L/second. Although the device might theoretically cause barotrauma, or haemodynamic compromise no complications were seen in 2000 courses of insufflator/exsufflator use.[35] It is important to note that at present the insufflator/exsufflator has not been subject to extensive controlled studies or detailed assessment in the paediatric age range, and has previously has been difficult to obtain in Europe. However, ongoing studies are encouraging and availability is likely to improve.

It is becoming clearer that use of a combination of non-invasive techniques with efficient physiotherapy is at least as effective as invasive tracheostomy ventilation in some patients providing there is reasonable preservation of bulbar function. Bach *et al.*[36] in a retrospective comparison have shown that a non-invasive protocol of inspiratory and expiratory aids significantly reduced pulmonary morbidity and hospitalization rates compared to conventional tracheostomy ventilation in DMD patients.

PROPHYLACTIC USE OF NON-INVASIVE VENTILATION IN DMD

The above reports describe the use of assisted ventilation in individuals with established, *symptomatic* chronic hypoventilation. As an extension of this work it has been suggested that the employment of non-invasive ventilation earlier in the course of the disease before the development of overt symptoms may have an even more beneficial effect on the natural history of the condition, by reducing the decline in lung function. A French study[37] has addressed this issue and shown *no* evidence that the early introduction of NIPPV in normocapnic DMD patients improves lung function or offers a survival advantage, and indeed harm may result if ventilation is not adequately monitored. Not surprisingly, the treatment was poorly tolerated.[38] *Prophylactic* use of NIPPV in DMD therefore *cannot* be recommended.

NON-PROGRESSIVE/SLOWLY PROGRESSIVE MUSCLE DISORDERS

Limb girdle muscular dystrophy (LGMD)

Generalizations are inadvisable in this condition as problems with diagnosis have lead to cases of Becker muscular dystrophy, spinal muscular atrophy and congenital muscular dystrophy being misclassified as limb girdle muscular dystrophy in the past. The course of the disease can also be variable. Although many patients remain ambulant until adulthood, a rapidly progressive form of the LGMD mimicking DMD can occur in childhood. LGMD is inherited as an autosomal recessive disorder and overall progression in members of an affected family usually follows a similar pattern with onset of respiratory failure at roughly the same age. Disproportionate early involvement of the respiratory muscles appears relatively common, so that some individuals remain ambulant but dependent on nocturnal hypoventilation. Cardiac complications are rare.[15]

Congenital muscular dystrophy (CMD)

This diagnostic category is used to define a group patients with weakness +/-hypotonia at birth, in whom a muscle biopsy shows features compatible with a dystrophic process.[15] The degree of weakness is highly variable, but respiratory and facial muscles can be involved, and contractures plus scoliosis are consistent features. Pulmonary hypolasia may complicate the picture (Figure 15.6). Although generalized weakness may be static, respiratory decompensation can occur during childhood or adolescence due to a progressive scoliosis and fall in respiratory muscle strength. In a series of CMD children treated by Barois *et al.*[9] one third had sufficient limb strength to continue walking, but diaphragm weakness was common. NIPPV was used in the majority of cases aged 2–10 years, a few patients required tracheostomy. In a series of patients with CMD seen at the Royal Brompton/Hammersmith Hospital, respiratory failure occurred at an average age

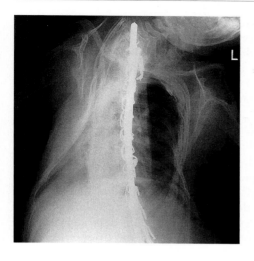

Figure 15.6 *Pulmonary hypoplasia and corrected thoracic scoliosis in congenital muscular dystrophy.*

of 11.6 years years. Symptoms and arterial blood gas tensions were controlled using nocturnal ventilatory support, allowing the individuals to continue normal activities during the day.

Myopathies

Congenital myopathies are listed in Box 15.4.

Box 15.4 *Congenital myopathies*

- Central core disease
- Minicore disease
- Nemaline myopathy
- Congenital fibre type disproportion
- Mitochondrial myopathy
- Minimal change myopathy

Respiratory muscle weakness appears to be particularly associated with nemaline and mitochondrial myopathies.

Of the metabolic myopathies, Pompe's disease (acid maltase deficiency) can produce classic features of diaphragm weakness as the most early manifestation of the disease. A severe form in childhood may resemble spinal muscular atrophy.

CENTRAL HYPOVENTILATION DISORDERS

Congenital central hypoventilation syndromes (CCHS) are relatively rare, but these patients do comprise a significant proportion of the children receiving ventilatory support worldwide. In affected individuals the metabolic control of ventilation is abnormal, but behavioural control is retained. Infants usually present in the first few days of life with apnoeic episodes and cyanosis. Acquired central hypoventilation can occur as a consequence of encephalitis, following trauma or due to brainstem lesions. A further group may develop hypoventilation as a result of hypothalamic/pituitary disease. In a Royal Brompton Hospital series of patients with congenital and acquired central hypoventilation disorders the sensation of dyspnoea, and hypercapnic ventilatory drive were both absent, and respiratory failure occurred in childhood or adolescence. Obesity, anterior and posterior pituitary deficiency and, in some cases, aberrant temperature and pain sensation may complicate the picture. Whereas in some cases ventilation may remain adequate during the day, profound hypoventilation usually occurs during sleep, so these individuals can derive benefit from nocturnal non-invasive ventilation. In one patient a progressive deterioration in respiratory control during the day was seen after 7 years of nocturnal ventilation. Conversely in one child who developed 24-hour ventilatory dependency at the age of one year following an episode of herpes simplex encephalitis, a gradual improvement in ventilatory response occurred so that by the age of 3 years she required only nocturnal support and could be switched from tracheostomy ventilation to NIPPV. In most patients, however, the level of ventilatory dependency does not change over time.

Diaphragm pacing (see Chapter 1) has been used in central hypoventilation disorders. In children bilateral phrenic nerve stimulation is usually needed to avoid mediastinal displacement with each respiratory cycle caused by unopposed unilateral phrenic nerve stimulation. Most adults and children using diaphragm pacing need additional ventilatory support during sleep or at the time of an intercurrent chest infection. A tracheostomy is generally retained to reduce the tendency to upper airway collapse during inspiration. Effective diaphragm pacing requires an experienced team, and is expensive. An American Thoracic Society Consensus statement on the diagnosis and management of CCHS has recently been published.[39]

CHEST WALL DISORDERS

Early onset scoliosis

Although congenital and juvenile scoliosis are risk factors for the development of respiratory insufficiency, overt respiratory failure in these patients is unusual in childhood unless the scoliosis is severe (Cobb angle > 100 degrees) and associated problems such as muscle weakness, rigid spine syndrome or parenchymal lung disease are present. Scoliosis can also complicate inherited syndromes such as Marfan syndrome, neurofibromatosis and Ehlers–Danlos syndrome, but there are few serial data on respiratory decompensation in the paediatric age group in these disorders. A progressive, asphyxiating form of chest wall deformity (Jeune's syndrome) can cause respiratory failure in early childhood.

Rigid spine syndrome

The rigid spine syndrome is an interesting, but poorly defined clinical entity characterized by stiffness and marked reduction in flexion of the dorso-lumbar and cervical spine. The term was coined by Dubowitz.[40] It is plain that the features of the rigid spine syndrome accompany conditions such as congenital muscular dystropy, the Emery–Dreifuss syndrome and minimal change myopathy, but at present it seems sensible to keep these as separate diagnostic labels until further genetic studies establish the molecular basis of the disorders. The evidence available would suggest that an underlying myopathy is present as spinal electromyogram shows a myopathic pattern and creatinine phosphokinase (CPK) level is often elevated. Spinal rigidity seems to have a marked effect on the mechanical efficiency of the respiratory and accessory muscles, in addition to reducing chest wall compliance. It is possible that cervical spine immobility predisposes the individual to upper airway obstruction. This combination of factors means that respiratory failure can develop insidiously in the presence of a straight spine and relatively well-preserved vital capacity (e.g. > 1.5 litres).

In a study[41] of nine patients with rigid spine syndrome (aged 13–32 years), four patients who developed respiratory failure had a mean vital capacity of 40% predicted compared with a mean value of 68% predicted in individuals who remained normocapnic.

A fatal cardiomyopathy has been reported in one patient with the rigid spine syndrome.[42] Cardiac arrhythmias are a feature of the Emery–Dreifuss syndrome.[15]

CYSTIC FIBROSIS (CF) (see also Chapter 13)

Ventilatory failure is more common in adolescents and adults with CF, but may occur in childhood in severely affected patients. Chronic ventilatory decompensation is proceeded by a hypoxaemic normocapnic phase. NIPPV has been used successfully in acute hypercapnic exacerbations,[43] during physiotherapy to reduce falls in SaO_2 and respiratory muscle fatigue,[44] and as a bridge to transplantation. Nocturnal CPAP has been shown to improve overnight SaO_2 in CF patients with sleep-disordered breathing but did not reduce nocturnal CO_2 levels.[45] In a short term comparison[46] of O_2 therapy overnight and NIPPV, both therapies improved SaO_2, but only NIPPV reduced CO_2 levels. Long-term controlled studies are required to clarify this area.

OUTCOME OF PAEDIATRIC LONG-TERM MECHANICAL VENTILATION

Reports published over the last decade reflect the shift from invasive to non-invasive techniques, particularly in children with neuromuscular disease.[47,48] Although negative pressure ventilation has been used for many years in children, studies comparing different ventilatory techniques in this age range are lacking. Early work[24] suggesting that children below the age of 8 to 10 years were unable to cope with nasal

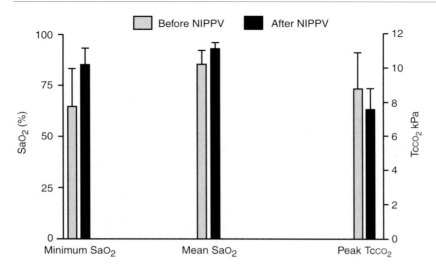

Figure 15.7 *Nocturnal arterial blood gas tensions before and after NIPPV in neuromusculoskletal disease (from Ref. 13).*

masks has been refuted.[14] Teague *et al.*[49] have demonstrated that bilevel NIPPV can be used effectively in children with alveolar hypoventilation due to chronic upper airway obstruction, craniofacial disorders and neuromuscular disease. Even children with developmental delay were able to tolerate the mask, and tracheostomy was avoided. We have reported the use of nocturnal mask ventilation[14] in 40 children with neuromusculoskeletal disease aged 9 months to 16 years. In these patients a significant improvement in nocturnal and diurnal arterial blood gas tensions was seen (Figures 15.7 and 15.8). The majority of children used pressure preset ventilators (e.g. BiPAP, Respironics Inc., Breas PV501 or the Nippy, B&D Electromedical). Around half were treated with full facemasks, with the older children preferring nasal masks. Growth velocity improved markedly in some patients. Three children (two SMA, one CMD) died over a mean of 30 months follow-up (range 1–105 months). Overall survival in another cohort of children requiring home ventilation was 85%. In most cases survival is related to the progression of the underlying condition, although it is clear that in some conditions (e.g. DMD), the natural history is the disorder is changed by the addition of ventilatory support. Other than in DMD, there are no firm data as yet on the quality of life in children and infants receiving NIPPV.

PRACTICAL POINTS

Establishing the diagnosis

A firm diagnosis is essential to provide prognostic information, plan future care and facilitate genetic counselling of the family. Advances in the interpretation of muscle biopsy histology have improved the diagnosis of many childhood neuro-

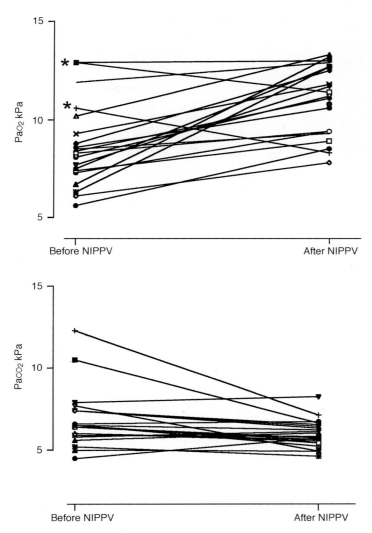

Figure 15.8 *Diurnal arterial blood gas tensions before and after NIPPV in neuro-musculoskeletal disease (from Ref. 13). *Values obtained on supplemental oxygen therapy.*

muscular conditions, but diagnostic uncertainty can be a problem when a child presents acutely in respiratory failure.

It is advisable to make every attempt to secure an unequivocal diagnosis in each case so that outcome can be properly assessed.

Identification of high risk cases and monitoring

Regular follow-up of children with a vital capacity of less than 50% predicted is recommended. In DMD patients a decline in lung function is often seen within

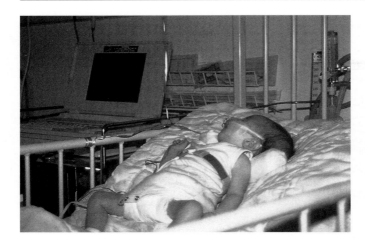

Figure 15.9
Paediatric sleep study using the Pneumograph 600 (Densa).

several years of the loss of ambulation. Symptoms of nocturnal hypoventilation such as headaches, poor sleep and fatigue are well-known, but in young children irritablilty, poor concentration and failure to thrive may be more prominent. In wheelchair bound patients cyanosis is frequently first observed when the child is eating or getting dressed. These features are an indication for nocturnal monitoring of respiration by oximetry and, where possible, measurement of transcutaneous/end-tidal CO_2, oronasal airflow and chest wall movement to establish the contribution of central hypoventilation and upper airway obstruction. Our practice in paediatric cases is to use nocturnal oximetry with transcutaneous CO_2 monitoring (Hewlett Packard model 47210A or Radiometer TINA system), and the Densa Pneumograph 600 or Edentrace to differentiate between obstructive and central respiratory disturbances (Figure 15.9). A number of screening systems can be applied in the home with relative ease, and some have the advantage of being suitable for monitoring patients of all sizes, from a neonate to 130 kg adult! Screening pulse oximetry is employed in some centres. If the child has slept well, a normal SaO_2 trace probably excludes significant sleep disordered breathing. Traces may be equivocal, however, in which case more detailed studies are indicated. Considerable experience is required in the interpretation of the results.[50]

An additional indication for nocturnal respiratory support support is recurrent respiratory infections associated with ventilatory insufficiency. For example, mask ventilation has been used in a 19-month-old child with intermediate SMA who had been hospitalized elsewhere for 6 months with recurrent right middle and lower lobe pneumonia, hypoxaemia and nocturnal hypercapnia. The introduction of nocturnal BiPAP delivered by a full facemask, facilitated discharge home and no further hospital admissions have been required during 12 months of follow-up. We have also used nocturnal CPAP via full facemask in a 3-year-old with SMA who presented with recurrent chest infections necessitating intubation and conventional ventilation on two occasions in the previous 3 months. In this child diurnal and nocturnal $PaCO_2$ were normal and so CPAP was used in preference to NIPPV. In 48 months of follow-up there have been no further chest infections, arterial blood gas tensions remain stable and growth velocity has markedly increased (see SMA discussion above).

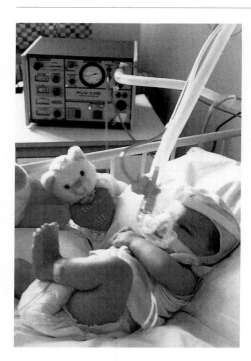

Figure 15.10 *Paediatric NIPPV in 9-month-old patient with congenital central hypoventilation syndrome.*

Choice and introduction of ventilatory system

T-IPPV will be needed for patients with either inadequate bulbar reflexes or extreme ventilator dependence. Previously it has been advocated that negative pressure ventilation is advisable in children under the age of 6 years who require nocturnal ventilatory support, and these techniques are used extensively in some centres. However, Barois[8] has cautioned that NPV in early childhood can create chest wall deformity, and it is now clear that nasal or facemask-IPPV can be used in children of less than 2 years (Figure 15.10). Consequently, it is no longer sensible to offer firm guidelines on the basis of age. As indicated above, CPAP may be suitable for children with recurrent chest infections and nocturnal hypoxaemia in the absence of marked CO_2 retention.

Masks

In very small children it may be necessary to use customized nasal or full facemasks (Figure 15.10), although commercially available masks are now produced in petite, paediatric and neonatal sizes (Respironics Inc., ResMed, Mallinkrodt) (Figure 15.11). The smallest size Adam circuit nasal pillows (to date) accommodate children of around 8–10 years of age or above. For children whose needs are not met by standard commercial masks, interfaces can be customized. Individualized interfaces are also often required in children with craniofacial disorders, or contractures of the jaw.

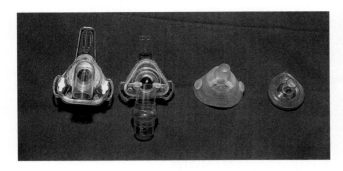

Figure 15.11
Paediatric interfaces. Left to right: Petite mask (Respironics, Inc.), SC mask (Respironics, Inc.), child mask (Hans Rudolf), Preemie-0 mask (Vital signs).

Ventilator

In the French series of paediatric cases[9] volume preset ventilators were used (Eole 1A/E, 2A/E, Monnal D, Lifecare PLV 100), but in other paediatric NIPPV studies bilevel pressure support ventilation predominates. In 40 Royal Brompton/ Hammersmith Hospital children started on NIPPV over half use the BiPAP S/T ventilator (Respironics Inc.) and most of the remainder use the Nippy (B&D Electromedical), VPAP (ResMed) or PV401 (Breas Co). In obese teenagers with DMD occasionally a more powerful volume preset ventilator e.g. BromptonPAC (Pneupac Ltd.) has been required to achieve satisfactory control of arterial blood gas tensions. Below the age of 18 months triggering of the BiPAP may be unreliable – we have found the PLV-100 (Lifecare), Breas PV401 or Harmony ventilator (Respironics, Inc.) can effective in this situation. Alternatively timed mode can be considered, but rates may not be sufficient in very small children.

ACUTE NIPPV IN CHILDREN

Other than the studies describing application in Type I SMA,[11,12] there are few reports of the use of NIPPV for acute respiratory failure in children. Fortenberry *et al.*[51] have described ICU-based experience with bilevel pressure support non-invasive ventilation in 28 children (mean age 8 years, range 4–204 months). Most children had pneumonia, and nine had underlying neurological, neuromuscular or immunocompromise disorders. NIPPV was used for a median of 72 hours with an average IPAP value of 12 cmH$_2$O and EPAP 6 cmH$_2$O. Within the first hour significant improvements in Paco$_2$, respiratory rate and Pao$_2$/Fio$_2$ ratio were achieved and radiological improvement was noted. Only three patients required intubation and no major complications occurred. In a further paediatric intensive care unit (PICU) study[52] of 34 severely ill children (pneumonia, asthma, post-operative respiratory failure, sleep disordered breathing), mean duration of NIPPV use was just over 6 days and significant improvements in Paco$_2$, Sao$_2$ and heart rate occurred. Three patients required intubation and the only notable complication was nasal bridge sores. NIPPV has also been employed in 26 children (median age 7.2 years) admitted to PICU with acute severe asthma.[53] Bilevel pressure support was used

(BiPAP, Respironics, Inc.) to complement maximal medical therapy, including inhaled beta-2 agonists and steroids. Intubation was not required in 19/26 patients, but 11 of the children tolerated NIPPV poorly.

No controlled studies have yet been performed, but these large case series do suggest that NIPPV is feasible and may help avoid intubation is some children with acute ventilatory failure. Bilevel pressure support devices have been used almost exclusively in these trials.

Starting NIPPV

Acclimatization to the ventilatory system is a highly individual affair and needs to be titrated to the child. If NIPPV is being started electively this is best achieved by an admission to hospital for a few days. Involvement of the parents or carers from the start of treatment is essential to build confidence and reduce anxiety. Young children and those with weakness of the small muscles of the hands or shoulder girdle will need help in securing the mask. Carers should be advised not to pull the straps securing the mask too tight as this distorts the contours of the mask and may lead to a nasal sore. Fortunately nasal bridge lesions seem less common in children. In those over around 8 years of age who are able to understand the rationale for treatment, NIPPV can be introduced at the child's pace during the day. Not surprisingly, boredom is a great enemy during intensive NIPPV use and can be alleviated using videos, story telling and games adapted to the situation. Encouragement and gentle persistence are necessary in the early stages. For younger children the chances of success are increased by introducing the mask at night after the child has dozed off. Full facemasks are often helpful, but inveterate thumbsuckers may be adequately ventilated with a nasal mask. Pacifiers can be helpful for younger children using nasal masks. Deadspace should be minimized where possible. The selection of masks is discussed in Chapter 3. Oximetry and transcutaneous CO_2 monitoring can be employed to establish appropriate ventilator settings, supplemented by arterialized ear lobe blood gas sampling which is well-tolerated by children. We perform overnight monitoring of oximetry and transcutaneous CO_2 to ensure control of nocturnal hypoventilation before discharge home. Average ventilator pressure settings in 40 consecutive children with neuromusculoskeletal disease treated with NIPPV at Royal Brompton Hospital, were IPAP 15 cmH_2O, EPAP 5 cmH_2O. If ventilation is required during the day in a child using a wheelchair, mask or mouthpiece ventilation can be continued using battery powered equipment (e.g. Lifecare PLV-100, Breas PV 401). Alternatively a pneumobelt can be used.

Problems with mask ventilation

There is evidence that the chronic use of tight fitting masks may affect facial growth, resulting in mid-facial hypoplasia in some children[54] (Figure 15.12). This seems more likely if the child starts NIPPV or CPAP below the age of 8 years and has weakness of the facial muscles. Regular evaluation of facial development is advisable[54]

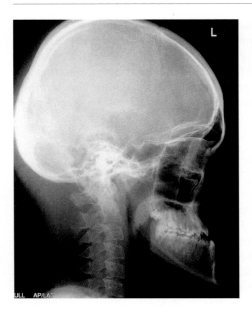

Figure 15.12 *Mid-facial hypoplasia in a 16-year-old patient with minimal change myopathy who started nocturnal nasal mask NIPPV aged 7 years.*

Alternation between facemasks, nasal masks, and nasal plugs, together with the use of customized masks, may distribute pressure more widely over the facial skeleton long-term, thereby reducing this problem. Ultimately better mask design, and further research on which children are more likely to be affected are required.

PAEDIATRIC CPAP (see also Chapter 16)

Indications for CPAP in children are more varied than those in adults (Box 15.5).

Box 15.5 *Paediatric indications for CPAP*

- Craniofacial syndromes (e.g. Pierre Robin, Crouzon, Treacher Collins, Apert)
- Persistent OSA post-tonsillectomy and adenoidectomy
- Down's syndrome
- Prader Willi syndrome
- Cerebral palsy
- Mucopolysaccharidoses
- Tracheobronchomalacia
- Laryngomalacia/bilateral vocal cord problems
- Bronchopulmonary dysplasia. Cystic fibrosis
- Neuromuscular conditions resulting in OSA

The commonest cause of obstructive apnoeas and hyponoeas during sleep in childhood is enlargement of the tonsils and adenoids. This problem may regress naturally with age or is dealt with by adenotonsillectomy. Surgery is discussed further in

Chapter 16. In a series of 413 children with OSA (mean age 5 years), Waters and colleagues[55] reported that 42% were treated with adenotonsillectomy and 19% with CPAP. OSA persists despite surgery in a small minority of children. Patients with congenital syndromes comprised 28% of those with OSA, and over 50% of those treated with CPAP. CPAP successfully reduced the respiratory disturbance index in 90% (72/80) of recipients. In those who received a formal CPAP titration study, 8/32 could not tolerate sufficient pressure to obviate all obstructive events because of the development of hypoventilation or central apnoeas. It is important to note that in all childhood forms of sleep disordered breathing, obstructive hypopnoeas are more common than overt apnoeas, and children have a greater tendency to develop nocturnal hypercapnia than adults. CPAP was poorly tolerated resulting in discontinuation of therapy in 18 patients, mainly due to parental non-acceptance of therapy or intolerance of the mask. In a further case series[56] of 18 children under the age of 2 years, the authors reported successful CPAP application in the majority. This study also demonstrates the dynamic nature of CPAP requirement in children, as growth in individuals with some syndromes e.g. Pierre Robin sequence may allow CPAP to be discontinued. It is our experience that children with learning disabilities can cope well with CPAP equipment, providing it is introduced at their pace. For individuals who fail CPAP therapy, but experience marked desaturation, oxygen therapy can be considered. Oxygen therapy appears to be more effective in children with OSA than adults, in whom apnoeic periods may be prolonged. Monitoring is required to ensure that SaO_2 is corrected and OSA is not exacerbated. Some children with learning disabilities may find nasal cannulae easier to cope with than a CPAP mask.

DISCHARGE HOME

The home care of a ventilator-dependent child poses particular problems, which are magnified if the condition is progressive. Although the child is more likely to thrive in the home environment, the family can experience high levels of stress[57,58] so that psychosocial support for caregivers is essential. Financial problems often add to the burden. Discharge planning and the impact of a ventilator-dependent child on the family are discussed in Chapter 18.

ADOLESCENT NEUROMUSCULAR CLINICS

In many patients with congenital neuromuscular disease e.g. DMD, ventilatory decompensation occurs in the late teenage years. This is just the time when patients transfer from paediatric to adult care, and a smooth transition does not always take place. As a result far too many teenagers present in acute respiratory failure, and have not been prepared for this possibility and potential treatment modes. The development of multidisciplinary Adolescent Neuromuscular Clinics (based on the Cystic Fibrosis model), run jointly by adult and paediatric clinicians should facilitate the hand over to adult care, and build confidence in the patient and his/her family.[30]

REFERENCES

1   Adams AB, Whitman J, Marcy T. Survey of long-term ventilatory support in Minnesota: 1986 and 1992. *Chest* 1993; **103**: 463–9.
2   Adams AB, Shapiro R, Marinii JJ. Changing prevalence of chronically ventilator-assisted individuals in Minnesota: increases, characteristics, and the use of non-invasive ventilation. *Respir Care* 1998; **43**: 635–6.
3   Fauroux B, Sardet A, Foret D. Home treatment for chronic respiratory failure in children: a prospective study. *Eur Respir J* 1995; **8**: 2062–6.
4   Robinson RO. Ventilator dependency in the United Kingdom. *Arch Dis Child* 1990; **65**: 1235–6.
5   Jardine E, O'Toole M, Paton JY, Wallis C. Current status of long term ventilation of children in the United Kingdom: a questionnaire survey. *BMJ* 1999; **318**: 295–9.
6   Melki J, Abdelhak S, Sheth P, *et al.* Gene for chronic proximal spinal muscular atrophies maps to chromosome 5 q. *Nature* 1990; **344**: 767–8.
7   Dubowitz V. Disorders of the lower motor neurone: the spinal muscular atrophies. In: Dubowitz V (ed.) *Muscle disorders in childhood*, 2nd edn. London: WB Saunders, 1995: 325–67.
8   Barois A, Estournet-Mathiaud B. Ventilatory support at home in children with spinal muscular atrophies (SMA). *Eur Respir Rev* 1992; **10**: 319–22.
9   Barois A, Estournet-Mathiaud B. Nasal ventilation in congenital myopathies and spinal muscular atrophies. *Eur Respir Rev* 1993; **3**: 275–8.
10 Thomas NH, Dubowitz V. The natural history of type I (severe) spinal muscular atrophy. *Neuromusc Disord* 1994; **4**: 497–502.
11 Birnkrant DJ, Pope JF, Martin JE, Repucci AH, Eiben RM. Treatment of type I spinal muscular atrophy with non-invasive ventilation and gastrostomy feeding. *Pediat Neurol* 1998; **18**: 407–10.
12 Bach JR, Niranjan V, Weaver B. Spinal Muscular Atrophy Type I. A noninvasive respiratory management approach. *Chest* 2000; **117**: 1100-1105.
13 Wang T-Y, Bach JR, Avilla C, Alba AS, Yang G-FW. Survival of individuals with spinal muscular atrophy on ventilatory support. *Am J Phys Med Rehabil* 1994; **71**: 207–11.
14 Simonds AK, Ward S, Heather S, Bush AB, Muntoni F. Outcome of domiciliary nocturnal mask ventilation in congenital neuromuscular-skeletal disorders. *Eur Respir J* 2000; **16**: 476–81.
15 Dubowitz V. The muscular dystrophies. In: Dubowitz V (ed.) *Muscle disorders in childhood*, 2nd edn. London: WB Saunders, 1995: 34–133.
16 Rideau Y, Gatin G, Bach J, Gines G. Prolongation of life in Duchenne's muscular dystrophy. *Acta Neurol* 1983; **5**: 118–24.
17 Baydur A, Gilgoff I, Prentice W, Carlson M, Fischer DA. Decline in respiratory function and experience with long term assisted ventilation in advanced Duchenne's muscular dystrophy. *Chest* 1990; **97**: 884–9.
18 Nigro G, Coni LI, Politano L, Bain RJI. The incidence and evolution of cardiomyopathy in Duchenne muscular dystrophy. *Int J Cardiol* 1990; **26**: 271–7.
19 Barbe F, Quera-Salva MA, McCann C, *et al.* Sleep-related respiratory disturbances in patients with Duchenne muscular dystrophy. *Eur Respir J* 1994; **7**: 1403-8.
20 Khan Y, Heckmatt JZ. Obstructive apnoeas in Duchenne muscular dystrophy. *Thorax* 1994; **49**: 157–61.

21 Alexander MA, Johnson EW, Petty J, Stauch D. Mechanical ventilation of patients with late stage Duchenne muscular dystrophy: management in the home. *Arch Phys Med Rehabil* 1979; **60**: 289–92.

22 Bach JR, O'Brien J, Krotenberg R, Alba AS. Management of end stage respiratory failure in Duchenne muscular dystrophy. *Muscle Nerve* 1987; **10**: 177–82.

23 Hill NS, Redline S, Carskadon M, Curran FJ, Millman RP. Sleep-disordered breathing in patients with Duchenne muscular dystrophy using negative pressure ventilators. *Chest* 1992; **102**: 1656–62.

24 Heckmatt JZ, Loh L, Dubowitz V. Night-time nasal ventilation in neuromuscular disease. *Lancet* 1990; **335**: 579–82.

25 Ellis ER, Bye PTB, Bruderer JW, Sullivan CE. Treatment of respiratory failure during sleep in patients with neuromuscular disease. *Am Rev Respir Dis* 1987; **135**: 148–52.

26 Raphael J-C, Chevret S, Chastang C, Bouvet F, The French Multicentric Group. A prospective multicentre study of home mechanical ventilation in Duchenne de Boulogne muscular dystrophy. *Eur Respir Rev* 1992; **2**: 312–16.

27 Leger P, Bedicam JM, Cornette A, *et al*. Nasal intermittent positive pressure ventilation. Long term follow-up in patients with severe chronic respiratory insufficiency. *Chest* 1994; **105**: 100–5.

28 Vianello A, Bevilacqua M, Salvador V, Cardaioli C, Vincenti E. Long-term nasal intermittent positive pressure ventilation in advanced Duchenne's muscular dystrophy. *Chest* 1994; **105**: 445–8.

29 Hill NS. Noninvasive positive pressure ventilation in neuromuscular disease. Enough is enough! *Chest* 1994; **105**: 337–8.

30 Simonds AK, Muntoni F, Heather S, Fielding S. Impact of nasal ventilation on survival in hypercapnic Duchenne muscular dystrophy. *Thorax* 1998; **53**: 949–52.

31 Bach JR. Standards of care in muscular dystrophy association clinics. *J Neuro Rehab* 1992; **6**: 67–73.

32 Bach JR, Campagnolo DI, Hoeman S. Life satisfaction of individuals with Duchenne muscular dystrophy using long-term mechanical ventilatory support. *Am J Phys Med Rehabil* 1991; **70**: 129–35.

33 Ahlstrom G, Gunnarsson L-G. Disability and quality of life in individuals with muscular dystrophy. *Scand J Rehab Med* 1996; **28**: 147–57.

34 Bach JR. Mechanical insufflation–exsufflation. Comparison of peak expiratory flows with manually assisted and unassisted coughing techniques. *Chest* 1993; **104**: 1553–62.

35 Barach AL, Beck GJ. Exsufflation with negative pressure: physiologic and clinical studies in poliomyelitis, bronchial asthma, pulmonary emphysema and bronchiectsis. *Arch Intern Med* 1954; **93**: 825–41.

36 Bach JR, Ishikawa Y, Kim H. Prevention of pulmonary morbidity for patients with Duchenne muscular dystrophy. *Chest* 1998; **112**: 1024–8.

37 Raphael J-C, Chevret S, Chastang C, Bouvet F. Randomised trial of preventive nasal ventilation in Duchenne muscular dystrophy. *Lancet* 1994; **343**: 1600–4.

38 Muntoni F, Hird M, Simonds AK. Preventative nasal ventilation in Duchenne muscular dystrophy. *Lancet* 1994; **344**: 340 (letter).

39 American Thoracic Society. Idiopathic congenital central hypoventilation syndrome. Diagnosis and management. *Am J Respir Crit Care Med* 1999; **160**: 368–73.

40 Dubowitz V. *A colour atlas of muscle disorders in childhood*. London: Wolfe Medical Publications, 1989.

41 Ras GJ, Van Staden M, Schultz C, Stubgen J-P, Lotz BP, Van der Merwe C. Respiratory manifestations of rigid spine syndrome. *Am J Respir Crit Care Med* 1994; **150**: 540–6.

42 Colver AF, Steer CR, Godman MJ, Uttley WS. Rigid spine syndrome and fatal cardiomyopathy. *Arch Dis Child* 1981; **56**: 148–51.

43 Padman R, Lawless S, Von Nessen S. Use of BiPAP by nasal mask in the treatment of respiratory insufficiency in pediatric patients: preliminary investigation. *Pediat Pulmonol* 1994; **17**: 119–23.

44 Fauroux B, Boule M, Lofaso F, *et al*. Chest physiotherapy in cystic fibrosis: improved tolerance with nasal pressure support ventilation. *Pediatrics* 1999; **103**: E32.

45 Regnis JA, Piper AJ, Henke KG, Parker S, Bye PT, Sullivan CE. Benefits of nocturnal nasal CPAP in patients with cystic fibrosis. *Chest* 1994; **106**: 1717–24.

46 Gozal D. Nocturnal ventilatory support in patients with cystic fibrosis: comparison with supplemental oxygen. *Eur Respir J* 1997; **10**: 1999–2003.

47 Nelson VS, Carroll JC, Hurvitz EA, Dean JM. Home mechanical ventilation of children. *Dev Med Child Neurol* 1996; **38**: 704–15.

48 Ellis ER, McCauley VB, Mellis C, Sullivan CE. Treatment of alveolar hypoventilation in a six-year-old girl with intermittent positive pressure ventilation through a nose mask. *Am Rev Respir Dis* 1987; **136**: 188–91.

49 Teague WG, Fortenberry JD. Noninvasive ventilatory support in paediatric respiratory failure. *Respir Care* 1995; **40**: 86–96.

50 Poets CF. Polysomnographic sleep studies in infants and children. In: Zach M, Carlsen K-H, Warner JO, Sennhauser FH (eds). *New diagnostic techniques in paediatric respiratory medicine: European respiratory monograph*. Sheffield: European Respiratory Society Journals, 1997: 179–213.

51 Fortenberry JD, Del Torro J, Jefferson LS, *et al*. Management of paediatric acute hypoxaemic respiratory insufficiency with bilevel positive pressure (BiPAP) nasal mask ventilation. *Chest* 1995; **108**: 1059–64.

52 Padman R, Lawless ST, Kettrick RG. Noninvasive ventilation via bilevel positive airway pressure support in pediatric practice. *Crit Care Med* 1998; **26**: 169–73.

53 Teague WG, Lowe E, Dominick J. Non-invasive pressure support ventilation (NIPPV) in critically ill children with status asthmaticus. *Am J Respir Crit Care Med* 1998; **157**: A542.

54 Li KK, Riley RW, Guilleminault C. An unreported risk in the use of home nasal continuous postive airway pressure and home nasal ventilation in children. *Chest* 2000; **117**: 916–18.

55 Waters KA, Everett FM, Bruderer JW, Sullivan CE. Obstructive sleep apnea: the use of nasal CPAP in 80 children. *Am J Respir Crit Care Med* 1995; **152**: 780–5.

56 Downey III R, Perkin RM, MacQuarrie J. Nasal continuous positive airway pressure use in children with obstructive sleep apnea younger than 2 years of age. *Chest* 2000; **117**: 1608–12.

57 Aday LH, Wegener DH, Anderson RM, Aitken MJ. Home care for ventilator-assisted children. *Health Affairs* 1989; **Summer**: 137–47.

58 Lantos JD, Kohrman AF. Ethical aspects of pediatric home care. *Pediatrics* 1992; **89**: 920–4.

16

Continuous positive airway pressure (CPAP) therapy

A K SIMONDS

INTRODUCTION

Continuous positive airway pressure (CPAP) therapy was introduced as a treatment for obstructive sleep apnoea (OSA) by Sullivan and colleagues[1] in 1981. It has revolutionized the approach to this condition, virtually abolishing the need for tracheostomy which was previously recommended for severe OSA. However, major controversy remains regarding the effectiveness of CPAP in mild OSA[2,3] and the association between OSA and cardiovascular/cerebrovascular disease. CPAP also has a role in patients with acute hyoxaemia due to conditions such as pneumonia, pulmonary oedema, and exacerbations of COPD; and may be effective in some adults and infants with central sleep apnoea. As the major application is in OSA, this use will be covered in detail. Alternative approaches including weight loss strategies, the mandibular advancement splint/oral devices, upper airway surgery and pharmacological measures will be compared and contrasted with CPAP.

SLEEP APNOEA SYNDROMES

An apnoeic episode is defined as 10 seconds or more of cessation of airflow at the nose and mouth. The apnoea is obstructive in origin if respiratory effort occurs throughout the apnoea, and central if there is no accompanying respiratory effort. Episodes of reduction in airflow (> 10 seconds) are called hypopnoeas; exact definitions vary from laboratory to laboratory (Box 16.1). The syndrome of obstructive sleep apnoea can be described as multiple episodes of apnoea or hyponoea associated with clinical impairment e.g. increased somnolence or altered cardio-

---

Box 16.1 *Definitions*

- Obstructive sleep apnoea/hypopnoea syndrome: a condition characterized by repetitive obstruction of the upper airway often leading to desaturation and arousals from sleep
- Obstructive apnoea: cessation of airflow for 10 seconds or more associated with continued respiratory effort
- Central apnoea: cessation of airflow for 10 seconds or more unaccompanied by respiratory effort
- Hypopnoea (varying definition): reduction in airflow or respiratory effort by 50% for 10 seconds or more
- Upper airways resistance syndrome: condition characterized by flow limitation leading to arousals from sleep

---

Box 16.2 *Diagnostic criteria*

Individuals must fulfill criterion A or B, plus C.
A. Excessive daytime sleepiness that is not better explained by other factors
B. Two or more of the following that are not better explained by other factors:
  - Choking or gasping during sleep
  - Recurrent awakenings from sleep
  - Unrefreshing sleep
  - Daytime fatigue
  - Impaired concentration
C. Overnight monitoring demonstrates five or more obstructed breathing events per hour during sleep. These events may include any combination of obstructive apnoeas/hypopneas or respiratory effort related arousals

pulmonary function. Diagnostic criteria suggested by the taskforce of the American Academy of Sleep Medicine[4] are given in Box 16.2. Somnolence arises as apnoeic/hypopnoeic episodes are terminated by arousal, and in the presence of multiple arousals sleep becomes fragmented and unrefreshing. Most workers in the field would agree that a spectrum exists which extends from simple snoring, through symptomatic snoring to the obstructive sleep apnoea syndrome. The presence of more than 15 apnoeas and hyponoeas per hour (apnoea/hypopnoea index, AHI) during sleep is usually regarded as abnormal, but some clinicians and epidemiologists regard the upper limit of normal for AHI as a score of 5. Of greater importance than AHI is the physiological impact on sleep quality, arterial oxygen desaturation and cardiovascular function, and this should always be assessed on an individual basis. Snoring causing airflow limitation, in the absence of apnoeas or desaturation, can fragment sleep and cause somnolence – this condition is known as the upper airways resistance syndrome. It is important to note that the criteria used to diagnose and quantify OSA in children differ from those used for adults.[5,6] This is partly because significant desaturation can occur in children with episodes lasting less than 10 seconds, and few normative data exist.

A prevalence study[7] of adults aged 30–60 years in the USA showed that OSA was present in 9% of males and 4% of females; symptoms related to sleep disorder were reported in 4% of males and 2% of females. Other epidemiological studies have produced comparable results.[8] In a UK study[9] of sleep disordered breathing 1% of men had more than 10 dips in arterial oxygen saturation/hour. OSA is therefore a common condition and a brisk growth in patients requiring treatment is likely to be seen. In females an increasing incidence of OSA is seen after the menopause. A report from the Royal College of Physicians (UK)[10] estimates that symptomatic OSA affects around 1.5% of middle-aged men, with a prevalence in women of 0.75%. This translates to a figure of 180,000 affected individuals in the UK. Only around 4% of these are currently receiving CPAP therapy.[10]

OSA has been shown to cause nocturnal swings in blood pressure and prelimi-nary results from the American Sleep Heart Health and Wisconsin Cohort studies suggest that diurnal hypertension may ensue. Prospectively there is a dose depen-dent association between sleep disordered breathing at baseline and the presence of hypertension at later follow-up.[11] From a mechanistic point of view, sympathetic overactivity occurs during apnoeic episodes and is correlated with the severity of AHI. In population studies a causal relationship between OSA and cardiac/cerebrovascular morbidity has not been demonstrated, although case control studies have suggested a significant association. In a Swedish cohort Mooe et al.[12,13] found that men and women with an AHI of greater than 14 or 15 respectively were more likely to have angiographically proven coronary artery disease (odds ratio 4.5 for men and 4.1 for women) than those without sleep disordered breathing. Odds ratios were corrected for BMI, smoking, hypertension and diabetes. In the Wisconsin Sleep cohort study[14] multiple logistic regression analysis has shown that individuals with an AHI > 30 compared with those with an AHI < 2 were three times as likely to have coronary artery disease. Partinen et al.[15] found an associa-tion between regular snoring and cerebral infarction (risk ratio 2.8), moreover the risk ratio rose to 10.3 when habitual snorers and non-snorers were compared. However, this work suffers from potential recall bias and the fact that strokes can cause sleep disordered breathing as well be a result of it. Further population based prospective studies such as the ongoing Sleep Heart Health Study should clarify matters.

ASSESSMENT AND INVESTIGATION

Common presenting features of OSA include snoring, apnoeas witnessed by partner, hypersomnolence, and nocturnal choking (Box 16.3). Cardiorespiratory examination should be carried out and attention directed to the upper airway (e.g. large tonsils and adenoids, nasal septal deviation or polyps). The clinician should be alert to the presence of underlying predisposing conditions such as neurological disorders (e.g. previous CVA, myotonic dystrophy), or endocrine disease such as hypothyroidism and acromegaly.

Box 16.3 *Presenting features of obstructive sleep apnoea*

Daytime somnolence
Concentration problems at work and home
Nocturnal choking
Poor sleep quality
Partner concerned by snoring and/or apnoeas witnessed during sleep
Morning headaches
Fallen asleep/concentration problems while driving
Impotence
Nocturnal polyuria

The investigation of patients with suspected OSA has been reviewed recently. Snoring, obstructive sleep apnoea and central sleep apnoea can be distinguished by overnight monitoring of respiration (sleep study – see Box 16.4). The American Academy of Sleep Medicine[4] has summarized evidence supporting various monitoring components, including respiratory impedance plethysmography,

---

Box 16.4 *Types of sleep monitoring studies*

- Oximetry (+/- spirometry)
- Limited multichannel respiratory monitoring: oronasal airflow, respiratory effort, body position, oximetry, snoring
- Polysomnography: Respiratory vaiables – oronasal airflow, respiratory effort, oximetry, snoring plus electroencephalogram (EEG), electro-oculogram (EOG), electromyogram (EMG) to stage sleep, and may include monitoring of intrathoracic pressure (using oesophageal balloon)
- CPAP titration: intelligent 'autoset' machines or polysomnography with manual titration
- Oximetry (+/- multichannel respiratory variables) plus transcutaneous or end-tidal CO_2 monitoring: nocturnal hypoventilation suspected or used for ventilator setting titration

---

pneumotachometer, oesophageal pressure, oronasal airflow etc. However, although rigorous, this assessment does not take into account the diagnostic accuracy of a number of such techniques when used in combination.

Oximetry alone lacks sufficient sensitivity and specificity to be adequate as a screening investigation for OSA. However, it has been argued that nocturnal oximetry combined with the measurement of FEV_1 and FVC provides sufficient predictive power to institute therapeutic measures.[16] Spirometry allow patients with chronic lung disease to be identified in whom nocturnal desaturation may be due to hypoventilation alone. By contrast another study[17] comparing home oximetry with polysomnography showed relatively poor correlation between assessment measures. However, it can be concluded that oximetry may help recognize severe OSA patients. Polysomnography is viewed by many as the gold standard investigation, but it is demanding in technician time and cost and has never been independently validated. Early data suggest that limited multichannel monitoring which includes assessment of snoring, airflow respiratory effort and oxygenation may be a practical substitute for conventional polysomnography for clinical purposes.[18] Suitable alternatives are video/oximetry/snoring detection systems or monitoring of nasal flow profile/snoring and oximetry. It should be noted that few of these multichannel systems have been subject to detailed comparison with full polysomnography, although validation has been carried out in some such as the Edentrace (Figure 16.1) and Sullivan Autoset system (ResMed). Operator skills, a firm understanding of the algorithm used to distingiush respiratory events, use of an appropriate oximetry sampling frequency, visual inspection of raw data to eliminate artifacts and training in sleep study interpretation are important, but frequently underestimated determinants of diagnostic accuracy. A highly symptomatic patient should not have the diagnosis of OSA rejected on the basis of a negative multichannel screening study alone. Polysomnography should be available for such cases where limited multichannel screening produces equivocal results, or when sleep–wake disorders other than OSA are suspected e.g. narcolepsy, benign idiopathic hypersomnolence. For patients with suspected alveolar hypoventilation due to chest wall disease, neuromuscular disorders or COPD, CO_2 monitoring is advisable (Chapter 10). A suggested approach to investigation is given in Box 16.5.

Box 16.5 *An approach to the investigation of sleep disordered breathing*

Category	Monitoring
High probability of OSA	Limited multichannel respiratory study If negative proceed to polysomnography
Low probability of OSA	Limited multichannel respiratory study
Possibility of non-respiratory sleep/wake disorder e.g. narcolepsy	Polysomnography
Parasomnia	Polysomnography plus video system
Patient at risk of nocturnal hypoventilation	Multichannel respiratory variables or oximetry plus CO_2 monitoring
Titration of CPAP	Autoset CPAP titration, or polysomnography with manual titration
Titration of assisted ventilation and/or O_2 therapy	Oximetry and CO_2 monitoring

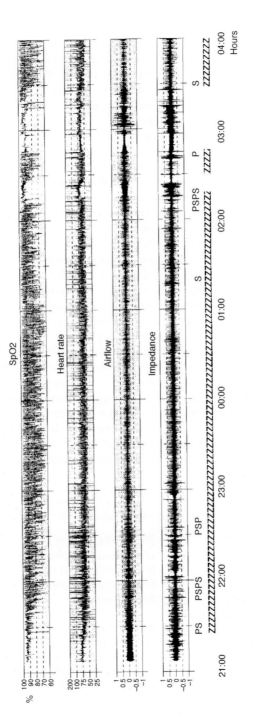

Figure 16.1 *Multichannel limited sleep study (Edentrace) showing severe obstructive sleep apnoea. Respiratory disturbance index in this patient was 79 and his Epworth sleepiness score 19. Spo_2: arterial oxygen saturation; Z: snoring; P: prone position; S: supine position.*

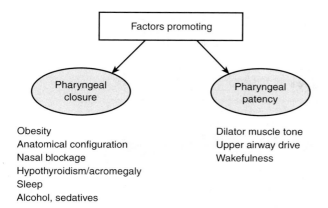

Figure 16.2 *Balance of forces acting on the upper airway.*

PATHOPHYSIOLOGY AND MECHANISM OF ACTION OF CPAP IN OSA

During sleep the patency of the upper airway is preserved by a balance between forces predisposing to airway collapse and those responsible for actively dilating the airway (Figure 16.2).

Dynamic viewing of the airway during sleep using fluroscopy[19] has shown that airway collapse commonly begins in the oropharyngeal region, progressing to the hypopharynx or laryngopharynx. The soft palate was pulled down as a plug into the oropharynx in many patients. Endoscopic visualization during sleep[20] has confirmed that airway collapse occurs in a number of regions either simultaneously or progressively. In this study of 45 patients the following patterns were seen: primary narrowing at the level of the nasopharynx plus other sites of secondary narrowing in 40%, primary site of narrowing nasopharynx plus other sites of primary narrowing 22% and primary narrowing only in the nasopharynx in 18%. Other combinations of collapse were seen in the remaining patients. It is suggested that upper airway collapse occurs due to the effect of negative pressure during inspiration acting on hypotonic pharyngeal walls. However, it has been demonstrated that airway collapse can occur during central apnoeas or at end expiration, indicating that negative intraluminal pressure is not a prerequisite. Passive collapse or positive extraluminal pressure may contribute.

CPAP exerts its effect by splinting the upper airway open throughout its length. Additional benefits include an increase in functional residual capacity and a reduction in the inspiratory work of breathing. In each case the level of continuous positive pressure needs to be titrated to the individual, to achieve maximum benefit (Figure 16.3).

INDICATIONS FOR CPAP

Obstructive sleep apnoea/upper airway resistance syndrome

CPAP can be effective therapy for all forms of OSA and the upper airway resistance syndrome (UARS). The decision to start CPAP is dependent on the severity of the

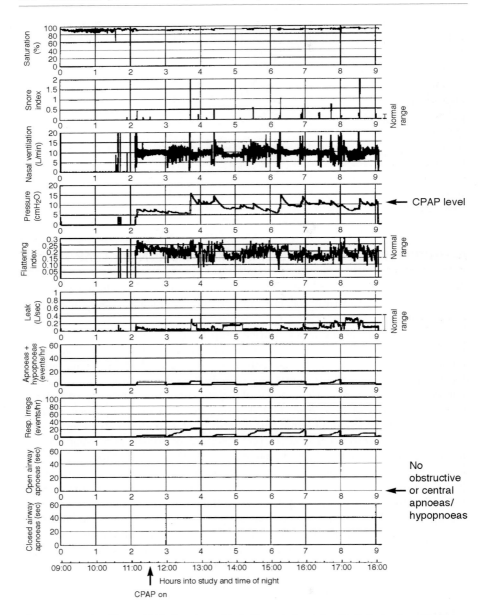

Figure 16.3 *Intelligent CPAP titration with Sullivan Autoset (ResMed) device in patient with baseline study shown in Figure 16.1. Note improvement in arterial oxygen saturation and abolition of apnoea and hypopnoeas. Median CPAP requirement is 7.8 cmH₂O with a 90th centile requirement of 11 cmH₂O.*

effects of the sleep disordered breathing and the feasilbility of suitable alternative measures. The diagnosis of OSA should be established by monitoring of breathing during sleep as described above. In particular daytime hypersomnolence is a key indication for intervention. Hypersomnolence can be quantitated subjectively using self-completed questionnaires such as the Epworth Sleepiness Scale (ESS)[21] (Box 16.6) or Stanford Sleepiness Scale. The ESS offers a validated, comprehensive approach to sleepiness in various everyday conditions, but as with all patient completed questionnaires it is dependent on user accuracy in answering the questions. The median sleep latency time (MSLT) can be established using polysomnography and offers a more objective measure, although not all UK sleep laboratories offer this facility routinely, and the MSLT may not be a reliable indicator of the impact of hypersomolence at an individual level. In practice, hypersomnolence can be described as falling asleep inappropriately during the day in spite of a normal duration of nocturnal sleep. Sleepiness when driving is a particular concern, in view of the increased incidence of road traffic accidents in OSA patients.[22] The presence of significant desaturation or cardiovascular complications such as nocturnal arrhythmias and angina, and uncontrolled hypertension should lower the threshold for instituting CPAP. Several studies comparing CPAP either to sham CPAP[23] or a placebo control tablet[24,25] have now confirmed the efficacy of CPAP in decreasing sleep disordered breathing, reducing daytime somnolence both subjectively and objectively, and improving the patient's quality of life.

Box 16.6 The *Epworth Sleepiness Scale (from Johns)*[21]

This scale assesses your level of sleepiness during the day.

How likely are you to doze off or fall asleep in the following situations, in contrast to feeling just tired? This refers to your usual way of life in recent times. Even if you have not done some of these things recently try to work out how they would have affected you. Use the following scale to choose *the most appropriate number* for each situation.

| 0 = would **never** doze | 1 = **slight** chance of dozing |
| 2 = **moderate** chance of dozing | 3 = **high** chance of dozing |

Situation	Chance of dozing
Sitting and reading	....
Watching TV	....
Sitting inactive in a public place (e.g. theatre or a meeting)	....
As a passenger in a car for an hour without a break	....
Lying down for a rest in the afternoon when circumstances permit	....
Sitting and talking to someone	....
Sitting quietly after lunch without alcohol	....
In a car, while stopped for a few minutes in the traffic	....

A score of 10 or above is abnormal.

Reversible causes of OSA include obesity, and endocrine disorders such as hypothyroidism and acromegaly. If OSA is severe, CPAP can be used while the patient loses weight or until endocrine treatment has taken effect. Hormone replacement therapy may have a role in post-menopausal female patients, but is unlikely to effect a cure.[26]

Standards for the use of CPAP in sleep apnoea syndromes have been set recently by the American Thoracic Society[27] and a Consensus conference.[28]

BODY POSITION MODIFICATION

Adopting the supine position when awake decreases supraglottic airflow and this effect is magnified in OSA patients. While body position during sleep is likely to play a role in the tendency to pharyngeal airway collapse, intra-pharyngeal pressure studies suggest that the level and extent of collapse does not differ in supine and lateral positions. Positional OSA is regarded as present if AHI in the supine position is twice or more that in the lateral position. An interplay between body position, sleep stage and body mass index is inevitable. Positional OSA is more commonly seen in thin patients with mild to moderate OSA. Although AHI tends to be higher in REM than non-REM sleep, in some patients with positional OSA in NREM sleep, positional dependence is lost in REM sleep. Numerous ploys have been used to try to reduce sleep in the supine position, including the time-honoured cotton reel or tennis ball sewn into the back of the pyjamas. Electrical positional alarm devices have also been used, and some degree of training effect may take place. A short randomized trial[29] of CPAP versus a backpack used to maintain the lateral position in patients with mild to moderate positional OSA showed both treatments to have similar efficacy, therefore this area warrants further attention. However, it has been noted that most studies to date take no account of neck position which may be a more important determinant of upper airway compromise than total body position. Positional manipulation is unlikely to be effective in patients with an AHI of more than 10 in the lateral position.

WEIGHT REDUCTION

At least 50% of OSA patients are obese. In some patients loss of weight may be curative and in others it is likely to reduce the severity of the condition, and so weight reduction should always be encouraged where appropriate. Sleep physicians have been castigated for not paying sufficient attention to weight loss in their patients.[2] Unfortunately most patients fail to lose sufficient weight, or any weight lost is quickly regained. No major study has yet assessed the role of the anti-obesity drug Orlistat (Xenical, Roche) in OSA. Surgery for morbid obesity carries a significant morbidity, but may be appropriate in a minority of grossly obese patients. Ballester et al.[30] have recently compared the efficacy of a weight loss and sleep hygiene programme (conservative therapy) compared with conservative therapy plus CPAP in patients with an average AHI of around 50 and BMI of 32–34. In the group with conservative therapy alone weight loss was 3.1 kg over 3 months compared with 1.1 kg in the CPAP group. A greater improvement in daytime sleepiness and quality of life was seen in the CPAP users. The authors estimated that the odds of deriving a treatment response to CPAP compared with conservative therapy alone, was 6.52 (odds ratio 2.51–17.6, 95% CI).

ORAL DEVICES

Dental appliances have been an important breakthrough in the treatment of snoring and mild OSA over the last decade. The mandibular advancement splint (MAS) (Figure 16.4) fits over the upper and lower teeth promoting the mandible to a more prognathic position. This increases the cross-sectional area of the pharynx particularly in the velopharyngeal region,[31] and may stimulate increased activation of muscles which enhance airway patency. Several crossover studies have shown the MAS to be as effective as CPAP in mild to moderate OSA.[32–34] It can also control socially disruptive snoring in some patients. However, assessment is problematical as studies have used devices of different design, and compliance is hard to document accurately. In one crossover trial of the MAS versus CPAP in patients with an AHI of less than 40, the fall in Epworth sleepiness score and AHI compared with baseline study was comparable in MAS and CPAP treatment limbs, although there was a tendency to better control of the AHI in the CPAP arm. The majority of patients preferred the MAS. Amalgamating the results of these studies, it is clear that the MAS is a useful alternative to CPAP in patients with UARS and mild to moderate OSA, but dental appliances are unlikely to provide sufficient control in severe OSA. The MAS may however prove better than nothing in severe OSA patients who cannot tolerate CPAP.[35] Potential complications with the MAS include temporo-mandibular joint discomfort, but in practice this seems uncommon. It is important that the MAS is carefully fitted to the individual's dentition and the position of the lower component slowly advanced over time. Devices on the market include the Silensor (Erkodent GmbH, Tuttlingen, Germany) and 'Negus' models. They cannot be used in edentulate patients and should be avoided in children with growing dentition. Patients with habitual teeth grinding at night may prove difficult subjects and usually need more rigid devices.

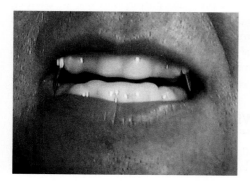

Figure 16.4 *The mandibular advancement splint (courtesy of Dr P L'Estrange).*

DEVICES TO PROMOTE NASAL PATENCY

The Nozovent™ is a nasal dilator which has been advocated to reduce snoring. It is a plastic spring device which is placed within the nares. Hoffstein et al.[36] have shown that its effect on snoring is trivial, although some individuals claim benefit. There is no evidence that it is effective in OSA. Nasal strips (3M) are available over the counter and consist of wire enforced bands which are placed over the nose. The stated aim is to improve nasal airflow and occasional patients report benefit. However, the strips have not been systematically evaluated and are expensive. Many patients have already tried the nasal strips before seeking further help.

UPPER AIRWAY SURGERY

Nasal surgery

Optimizing the nasal airway by correcting a deviated septum, removal of polyps or treating rhinitis will decrease upstream resistance, thereby reducing the tendency to pharyngeal collapse. These measures should be considered in individuals with symptomatic nasal blockage. However, as the main level of airway obstruction is usually in the pharynx, nasal surgery may reduce snoring and modify OSA, but rarely abolishes the condition. In individuals with structural nasal airway obstruction surgical attention may faciliate the use of CPAP.

Tonsillectomy and adenoidectomy

Enlargement of the tonsils and/or adenoidal tissue is the commonest cause of upper airway obstruction in children with sleep apnoea and can be visualized easily on examination. Lymphoid growth is maximum at the age of around five years, but occasionally tonsils remain hypertrophied in adolescence and young adulthood rather than regressing. Tonsillectomy in this situation is usually helpful regardless of age. Individuals with OSA undergoing tonsillectomy and adenoidectomy have a higher incidence of post-operative complications than those operated on for other indications. Post-operative worsening of OSA may occur due to oedema and the respiratory depressant effect of anaesthetic drugs and analagesics. Indeed, in severe OSA sedative pre-medication can provoke acute upper airway obstruction. Adults and children in this situation should be very closely monitored, pre- and post-operatively. In children important risk factors for post-operative complications are age less than three years, a respiratory distress index (RDI) of > 10, minimum SaO_2 during apnoeas or hypopnoeas $< 70\%$, and the presence of craniofacial syndrome or chromosomal disorder. Not surprisingly, pre-operative failure to thrive, cor pulmonale, obesity and a recent respiratory tract infection are also associated with higher morbidity.

Uvulopalatopharyngoplasty (UVPP)

This procedure was pioneered by Fujita in 1981 and usually includes resection of the uvula, part of the soft palate and pharnyx (Figure 16.5). The aim is to improve

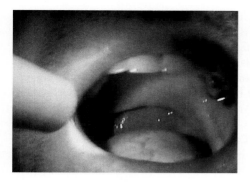

Figure 16.5 *Airway appearance following uvulopalatopharyngoplasty (UVPP).*

the airway and stiffen it so that collapse during sleep is resisted. Many patients are attracted by the possibility of a once and for all cure to the problem of OSA, rather than a lifetime of CPAP. However, the outcome of UVPP is difficult to interpret as surgical technique can vary from surgeon to surgeon, and not all subjects have undergone long term polysomnographic follow-up. Although some centres have reported early benefit, evidence suggests that in a proportion of patients subjective reduction in snoring hypersomnolence is not accompanied by a marked decrease in apnoea/hypopnoea index. Indeed the decrease in snoring may mask continued severe obstructive episodes. In addition, UVPP may be complicated by palatal incompetence and pharyngeal stenosis. Late results can also be disappointing, although a study[37] which compared UVPP and CPAP in patients with mild or moderate OSA showed no difference in long-term survival between the two treatments. This finding contrasts with results from an earlier study[38] which showed increased mortality in UVPP patients.

In view of these problems attempts have been made to select the patients most likely to respond to UVPP.[39,40] Launois *et al.*[41] suggest that individuals with airway collapse at nasopharyngeal level, without secondary areas of collapse elsewhere are the best candidates for UVPP. Airway compromise at hypopharyngeal level is unlikely to respond to UVPP, as surgery is carried out rostral to this site.

Myatt and colleagues[42] carried out a multicentre prospective study of modified UVPP in 21 selected patients with snoring and mild OSA. Subjects with velopharyngeal level obstruction were identified by nasendoscopy during midazolam induced sleep. All had a BMI of less than 30 and had an Epworth sleepiness score of 8 or more, and AHI between 5 and 30. Following surgery Epworth sleepiness scores fell from 10.9 to 5.6 ($p < 0.0.004$) and mean AHI showed a downward trend from 18 to 10. Partners reported a reduction in snoring. At 12 weeks post-operatively none of the patients had nasal regurgitation, loss of taste or alteration of voice. However, it is vital that long-term results from UVPP are obtained and these compared systematically with the MAS and CPAP.

Laser-assisted uvulopalatoplasty (LAUP)

This procedure differs from conventional UVPP in that laser application to the soft palate is used to shorten the palate and uvula with the aim of reducing vibration of these structures and hence, snoring. The lateral pharyngeal wall and tonsils are not involved in the procedure. Therapy is often given over several sessions. Kamami has reported that snoring was eliminated or reduced in 77% of 34 patients who underwent laser assisted uvulopalatoplasty. However, it should be stressed that there are no peer-reviewed outcome data on the results of LAUP for snoring and no evidence whatsover that it has a role in the management of OSA. In view of the controversy surrounding LAUP, the American Sleep Disorders Association has produced a series of recommendations on the topic.[43] These suggest that LAUP should not be recommended in OSA. Candidates with snoring and symptoms of sleep disordered breathing should be evaluated with monitoring of respiration during sleep to excude OSA. Patients should be informed that the benefits, risks and side effects of LAUP have not yet been established. When used in snorers, LAUP may delay the subsequent diagnosis of OSA, by removing the warning feature of snoring. As with conventional UVPP, care should be taken when prescribing sedatives or sedative analgesia to individuals undergoing upper airway surgery.

Radiofrequency volumetric tissue reduction of the soft palate has also been attempted. In a pilot study[44] this form of tissue ablation was found to be safe in snorers with an AHI of < 15 when performed in an outpatient setting. However, the study size was small and follow-up only short-term.

UVPP VERSUS CPAP

There is persuasive evidence showing that CPAP is preferable to UVPP in severe OSA. The situation in less severe cases is not as clear. While it is important not to be prescriptive, our practice is to use CPAP as the treatment of choice in moderate or severe OSA, especially when somnolence is marked (Epworth sleepiness score > 12, AHI exceeds 30 and/or episodes are associated with hypoxaemia and cardivascular stress. Individuals with severe snoring alone, or snoring and mild OSA undergo full airway assessment including sleep nasendoscopy. If this indicates nasopharygeal airway compromise the advantages and disadvantages of surgery are discussed with the patient. Patients treated with surgery for OSA undergo a sleep study after the procedure and continue long-term follow-up. As indicated above, further studies comparing CPAP with UVPP and the MAS in patients with mild OSA are urgently needed.

It has been suggested that CPAP treatment cannot be used effectively in patients who have undergone UVPP. We have *not* found this to be the case, although the extent of the surgery is clearly an important factor.

Maxillofacial surgery

A complex staged surgical approach to OSA has been developed at Stanford, USA. Here, maxillo-mandibular advancement is used to enlarge the pharynx. Results from this centre are encouraging,[45] but have not been duplicated widely. At present this type of radical surgery is advisable only in those with severe cranio-facial disproportion.

Tracheostomy

Bypassing the upper airway by tracheostomy abolishes obstructive episodes, but is associated with considerable morbidity in its own right and imposes significant social limitations on the patient. Any additional central apnoea component may not be adequately treated with a tracheostomy alone. Since the advent of CPAP, a formal tracheostomy for OSA is rarely needed. Minitracheostomy has been used as a temporizing measure,[46] but the stoma is probably too small for effective ventilation.

Pharmacological treatment

Although a number of drug treatments have been recommended for OSA, including medroxyprogesterone and strychnine, the only agent that produces a significant improvement in nocturnal oxygenation and AHI is protriptyline. This non-sedative tricyclic drug appears to act by reducing REM-sleep related sleep disordered breathing,[47] and may have an independent action on upper airway tone.[48] A mild beneficial effect in snoring has also been demonstrated.[49] However, anticholinergic side effects including constipation, urinary hesitancy and impotence are common, doses above 10 mg at night are poorly tolerated, and the drug is due to be withdrawn from the market by the manufacturer. It is not clear whether nortriptyline has similar effects. The 5HT antagonist fluoxetine has REM suppressant properties and may aid weight loss. It has been shown to be of some value in OSA,[50] and further studies with newer drugs are likely.

EFFECTS OF CPAP IN OBSTRUCTIVE SLEEP APNOEA

When established correctly, CPAP immediately controls sleep disordered breathing and rapidly reduces daytime somnolence.[23] Retrospective analysis suggests that long term CPAP lessens morbidity and mortality due to OSA,[38] however this conclusion is not supported by prospective epidemiological trials. It is now probably unethical to withhold CPAP therapy from individuals with moderate or severe OSA, as these subjects at the very least will be denied relief of daytime somnolence. Long-term studies of the impact of CPAP on morbidity and mortality in mild OSA are needed.

INDICATION FOR CPAP THERAPY IN CENTRAL SLEEP APNOEA

Central sleep apnoea can be divided into two categories: patients with alveolar hypoventilation due to impaired chemosensitivity, and those with increased respiratory drive. The latter group includes individuals with periodic (Cheyne–Stokes) respiration due to cardiac failure. In some of these patients symptoms of sleep fragmentation *and* cardiac function may improve with the introduction of CPAP therapy.[51] However, CPAP may worsen symptoms in occasional patients with severe left ventricular dysfunction[52] and so should only be used with careful monitoring and follow-up. Recently the Autoset CS device (ResMed) has been developed for use in patients with Cheyne–Stokes respiration due to cardiac failure. This attempts to capture respiratory cycling and then reduce overall ventilation, thereby increasing CO_2 level. Initial studies suggest it may be more effective than CPAP and O_2 therapy in Cheyne–Stokes patients. CPAP may also have a role in neonates with apnoea syndromes. This work is at an early stage and there are few controlled data available.

CPAP THERAPY IN ACUTE HYPOXAEMIC LUNG DISEASE

CPAP has an established role in treating refractory hypoxaemia in patients with acute pulmonary oedema[53] and severe pneumonia.[54] The treatment works by increasing alveolar recruitment and functional residual capacity, decreasing anatomical shunting, and reducing the work of breathing. In these acute situations CPAP therapy is generally provided in an ICU or on high dependency ward using demand flow generator systems supplied with a piped oxygen/air blender. CPAP in acute COPD is discussed elsewhere (Chapter 3).

CHOICE OF CPAP EQUIPMENT FOR DOMICILIARY USE (Figure 16.6)

A wide range of portable CPAP systems is available. As described above, the CPAP unit is a flow generator which should be capable of delivering a constant pressure throughout the respiratory cycle. Ideally, it should be reliable, portable, inexpensive and function as noiselessly as possible. Systems cost between £200 and £400 (328 and 656 Euros respectively). Many can provide compliance data. More expen-

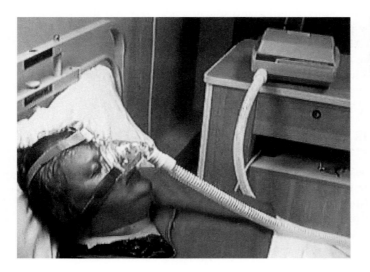

Figure 16.6 *Nasal continuous positive airway pressure therapy (CPAP).*

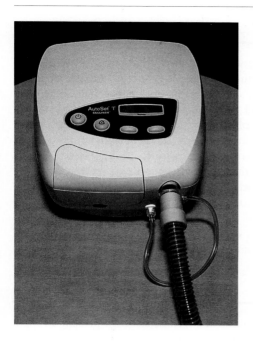

Figure 16.7 *Autoset T variable CPAP device (ResMed).*

sive models (e.g. Sullivan Autoset T (Figure 16.7), Horizon, De Vilbiss) deliver variable CPAP and patients can download information on pressure requirements overnight. Several studies comparing different CPAP devices show that there is little to choose between them in performance characteristics.[55] There is also no evidence that variable CPAP offers advantages over conventional fixed level CPAP,[56] although it is possible that some selected cases (e.g. those with tolerance problems) may benefit. Cost is often the main determinant in purchasing the equipment.

Many machines provide a gradual ramped increase in CPAP to the preset level in the first 5–20 minutes of use. Some individuals, particularly those beginning treatment or those who require high CPAP levels find this helpful. Others find the ramp unnecessary and prefer to 'get on with' the pre-determined pressure as soon as the mask is in place. We do not routinely provide humidification, but this may be indicated in some patients with side effects as described below.

MASK SELECTION

This is discussed in Chapters 3 and 6. Nasal pillows or plugs (Adam circuit, Puritan Bennett) are as efficient at delivering CPAP as a nasal mask.[57] If the patient is severely hypersomnolent or confused mouth leaks will reduce the efficiency of treatment. Here a full facemask is recommended. These masks have a quick release mechanism to reduce the risk of aspiration in an obtunded patient, although clearly such a patient would require close observation. Individualized masks or nosepieces can be constructed for patients who cannot be adequately fitted with an 'off the peg' mask.

STARTING CPAP

As with any new treatment the aim and principles of CPAP therapy should be explained to the patient. Starting pressures of between 5 and 10 cmH$_2$O are usual, although some individuals require higher values. Several centres have developed algorithms to predict the pressure level required, but these have not always been validated prospectively. Engelman and colleagues[58] have shown that the most important factors determining CPAP pressure are collar size and apnoea/hypopnoea index, which together explained 53% of the variance in prescribed CPAP levels.

It is often helpful to first try CPAP during an afternoon nap, so that any early problems can be identified and solved before nocturnal monitoring. Acclimatization rates are very variable. The more somnolent the patient the more likely he/she is to tolerate the treatment and therefore a CPAP titration study may be feasible on the first night of treatment. Others find they sleep poorly using CPAP at first and so an early titration study may be unrepresentative.

CPAP TITRATION

Conventional CPAP titration studies require the technician to be present all night to carry out polysomnography and adjust CPAP level until obstructive episodes and their consequences are abolished. As the degree of sleep fragmentation and number of arousals determines the degree of daytime somnolence, ideally CPAP should reduce arousals to a minimum. This requires EEG, EOG and EMG monitoring which adds to the cost of the study, and is not available in all centres. However, autonomic phenomena such as change in heart rate and blood pressure seem to accurately reflect arousals and can be more easily monitored.[59]

'INTELLIGENT' (AUTOSETTING) CPAP

It is likely that 'intelligent' CPAP machines (e.g. Autoset T, Resmed; Horizon, DeVilbiss; Morphee Plus, Laboratoire Pierre Medical Verrieres Le Buisson) will become used increasingly to establish patients on CPAP. These machines detect flow in the mask and automatically adjust CPAP until normal flow is restored (Figure 16.3). Safeguards are incorporated so that the CPAP level is not increased in response to central apnoeas. These autoset systems obviate the need for a technician to be in attendance overnight and make it easier for titration studies to be carried out at home. The long-term benefits of autoset systems compared with conventional CPAP titration are being examined, but they do not appear to offer major advantages. The Sullivan Autoset Clinical system (ResMed) can be use in diagnostic and CPAP titration mode.

CPAP OR BILEVEL PRESSURE SUPPORT VENTILATION?

The majority of patients with OSA are normocapnic by day and show no evidence of marked nocturnal CO$_2$ retention. CPAP is usually sufficient to control desaturation in these individuals. It has been postulated that the availability of two levels of pressure with the BiPAP machine (Respironics Inc.) may increase patient comfort and improve compliance over CPAP alone. However, in practice similar levels of compliance are seen (CPAP 74%, BiPAP 77% in a 6-month follow-up study.[60] BiPAP does have a role however in hypercapnic patients. These usually present with a combination of OSA plus COPD, massive obesity or respiratory muscle weakness. By improving minute ventilation BiPAP enhances CO_2 clearance, and reduces the work of breathing more effectively than CPAP.[61] In some individuals with severe end-stage OSA complicated by respiratory failure and cor pulmonale, BiPAP may be used in hospital intensively to rapidly correct arterial blood tensions. Once stability has been achieved it may be possible to switch to CPAP for maintenance therapy at home.

COMPLIANCE

Compliance with CPAP therapy is determined by a number of features the most important being the trade-off between symptom improvement and side effects as experienced by the patient. Compliance has been assessed subjectively and objectively.

Hoffstein and colleagues[62] used a questionnaire to assess the pattern of CPAP use and side effects in 148 subjects. Response rate was 65%. Seventy per cent of subjects prescribed CPAP continued to use it, with 81% believing it to be an effective treatment. Around 60% felt more awake during the day, and snoring was reported to be improved or eradicated by 76 patients. Seventeen patients were unable to persist with treatment. Interestingly, the side effects in these patients did not differ from those who continued CPAP – the chief problems being claustrophobia, nasal discomfort and the nuisance of having to use the equipment every night. In the most failed users, a marked improvement in AHI was obtained, so compliance did not clearly correspond to the efficiency of treatment. An ANTADIR survey of 3225 CPAP users found that 89% of respondents reported they used CPAP every night. A total of 76% said they used CPAP throughout the night, and overall 73% reported use all night, every night. There was good agreement between the patients' reported compliance and figures obtained from internal time clocks. Satisfaction with CPAP therapy was correlated with objective and subjective compliance. The two most frequent complaints were dry mouth and throat (52%) and noise of the machine (42%). A dry mouth and nasal symptoms were more common in patients with a pressure setting of more than 12 cmH$_2$O.

In other work reported, use by patients has been found to overestimate compliance. Kribbs et al.[63] have examined this issue objectively using hidden microprocessor time clocks. In this study although 60% of patients claimed to use CPAP every night, monitoring showed that only 46% used the treatment for at least 4 hours per night for 70% of the days studied. Those using CPAP regularly tended to be more hypersomnolent at the start of treatment and experience greater benefit with use. The commonest complaints in this study were inconvenience and nasal stuffiness.

Confirmatory data from the Edinburgh group[58] suggest that despite encouragement their patients used CPAP for only 4.7 hours at night on average. There was no correlation between CPAP use and improvement in multiple sleep latency or apnoea/hypopnoea index, but longer CPAP duration was related to a greater improvement in Epworth sleepiness scale, quality of life and depression.[64] Reeves-Hoche et al.[65] have shown a similar level of use (mean 4.2 hours/night), and found no factors that would predict the likelihood of good or poor compliance, although there is a tendency for poor compliers to have an increased number of CPAP side effects.

A European prospective study[66] has attempted to examine CPAP compliance in more detail. A total of 121 consecutive patients newly diagnosed with OSA (mean AHI 62, SD 29) were randomly allocated to groups with or without an inbuilt compliance monitor which measured the time spent at effective CPAP level. Regular CPAP use was defined as use for at least 4 hours per day for more than 70% of days. At 1, 2 and 3 months after starting therapy, 77%, 82% and 79% of patients were regular users. These results are encouraging and suggest that patient support and education play an important role in increasing compliance. This study showed no difference in clinical, polysomnographic or side effect profile between good and poor compliers, although clinical impression suggests that compliance may be poor in individuals with few symptoms who have been prompted to seek help because of the concerns of their bed partner.

Overall, there is still a need for CPAP therapy to become more user-friendly. Hoy et al.[67] have explored whether intensive educational input and support at the start of therapy improves use. CPAP use did improve in those receiving intensive compared to routine support (5.4 ± 0.3 v 3.9 ± 0.4 hours/night), and there were greater beneficial effects on symptom control, reaction time and mood – indicating that time invested at the start of therapy is worthwhile. Prompt attention to side effects and practical problems, improved mask design, education of the patient and family about the consequences of untreated OSA, and accurate titration of CPAP setting are all likely to improve the acceptability of treatment.

PRACTICAL PROBLEMS

Nasal stuffiness/rhinitis

It is suggested that nasal congestion or streaming may be most marked in patients with hyper-responsiveness to cold air, but this has not been confirmed. In individuals with occasional nasal obstruction at the time of an upper respiratory tract infection, ephedrine 0.5% nasal drops or dexarhinaspray for a short period are usually effective. Frequent use of ephedrine should be discouraged as this may lead to rebound nasal congestion. Patients with a history of perennial or seasonal rhinitis should undergo a trial of nasal corticosteroid. Nasal streaming may respond to ipratroprium nasal spray or a combination of ipratropium and nasal corticosteroid.

An alternative or additional approach is to add humidification. A low level of humidification can be provided by heat and moisture exchangers (HMEs). These can be helpful to tide an individual through an upper airway infection, but should be changed regularly. Cold or heated water bath humdifiers provide an increasing level of humidification, but add to the bulk of the equipment and are not necessary on a routine basis.

Mask discomfort

See Chapter 6.

Claustrophobia

This is often an early problem and usually responds to encouragement and support. The nasal plugs cover less of the face and may be helpful in this situation. A continued sensation of claustrophia and a feeling of suffocation should prompt a check on the CPAP setting as this may be inadequate or too high.

Mouth leaks

See Chapter 6.

Noise

Sound levels are similar in most systems[55] and most bed partners find the sound of the CPAP machine preferable to snoring. Some patients place the machines outside the bedroom door to reduce noise levels. This is acceptable providing CPAP levels at the mask are maintained.

Persistent sleepiness in the CPAP patient

Causes of persistent somnolence in OSA patients using CPAP are shown in Box 16.7. The problem needs to be addressed systematically. Initially CPAP compliance and sleep hygiene should be checked. Sleep hygiene includes such issues as ensuring

Box 16.7 *Causes of persistent somnolence in the CPAP patient*

Cause	Action
CPAP setting too low or too high	Titration study
Poor compliance with CPAP	Tackle compliance problems. Consider other therapy e.g. MAS
Poor sleep hygiene (e.g. insufficient time in bed)	Sleep hygiene advice
Additional sleep disorder e.g. periodic leg movement syndrome, or narcolepsy	Investigate by polysomnography
Co-morbidity (e.g. hypothyroidism)	Clinical assessment

sufficient time in bed, reducing caffeine intake, avoiding sedative medication etc. A further autoset titration study may be required to ensure that the optimal level of CPAP is being applied. Additional causes should also be considered. Full polysomnography may show co-morbidity such as periodic leg movement syndrome. We have recently seen two patients with OSA *and* narcolepsy. Finally, if no remediable factor can be found, judicious use of stimulant medication or modafinil may be considered if somnolence proves intractable This role for modafinil is currently experimental. It should be remembered that most studies show that sleepiness scores are improved, but not returned to normal by CPAP.

Cost/funding of CPAP equipment and cost-effectiveness

In some areas in the UK and elsewhere there are long waiting lists for CPAP machines. This has caused severe problems in some regions where patients are deprived of an effective treatment, and may resort to paying for their machine. This is inequitable. Problems with provision were exacerbated by the meta-analysis of Wright *et al.*[2] which suggested that widespead use of CPAP was unjustified. Subsequent trials have confirmed that CPAP therapy is evidence-based medicine (see above) which has helped, but not resolved the problem. The Royal College of Physicians Report on Sleep Apnoea and Related Conditions[10] strongly advises that purchasers should make adequate provision for funding of equipment, and also ensure that sufficient facilities for sleep studies are available in their region. It is clear that NHS patients should not have to buy a CPAP machine, if full investigation proves confirms symptomatic moderate or severe OSA. Recently it has been shown that health care utilization (hospital admission days) is reduced in OSA patients receiving CPAP therapy,[68] and the cost per stay is lower than for control (untreated) patients.[69,70] Such healthcare economic analyses do not even begin to take into account the cost of road traffic accidents related to untreated OSA, although clearly this is difficult to quantify.

Problems also exist in funding private sleep studies, as some insurance companies will cover this investigation and others do not. This is anomalous, and in view of the health risk that untreated OSA poses, does not make economic sense.

COMMON QUESTIONS ABOUT CPAP FROM PATIENTS

1   Should CPAP be used every night?

Many patients experiment with CPAP use to answer this question themselves. During the first night off CPAP after a period of effective use, symptoms are usually improved compared with pre-treatment levels, probably due to the reduction in sleep deprivation. Reduction in pharyngeal oedema will also enhance airway calibre. After several nights, symptoms commonly return.

In patients who lose a significant amount of weight, or who receive effective treatment for endocrine disorders, or upper airway surgery, a repeat sleep study should be carried out to determine whether CPAP therapy is still required.

2   What arrangements should be made for service and maintenance of equipment?

CPAP machines should be serviced once a year. Manufacturer's instructions should be observed. The service is a simple procedure and may be carried out locally or the machine sent away to the dealer, although the latter is less acceptable. Filters should be changed regularly according to the manufacturer's guide. Silicone nasal masks should last for 6 to 12 months if they are well cared for.

3   What arrangements should be made for taking CPAP equipment abroad?

During airflights CPAP equipment should be transported by hand as cabin luggage. Carry holdalls are available for most CPAP models or these can be bought off the peg. Patients should take with them a report stating CPAP requirements. In addition to health insurance cover, arrangements should be made regarding insurance of the equipment depending on whether the machine is on loan or belongs to the patient. It is important to ensure that there will be no problems with voltage incompatiblity in the country to be visited. Many CPAP machines operate with dual voltage (220/110) and are convenient for patients visiting the USA. For travellers in Europe, centres participating in the Eurolung Assistance Scheme[71] may be able to help in the event of equipment problems.

4   Driving and OSA – what are the facts?

As indicated above, individuals with OSA are at risk of being involved in road traffic accidents as a result of lapses in concentration and falling asleep at the wheel. This risk may be as much as seven times that of the normal population. The Medical Advisory Branch of the Driver and Vehicle Licensing Agency (DVLA) recommend that driving should cease if excessive sleepiness is present. Driving is permitted once satisfactory control of symptoms is achieved. It is the duty of the licence holder to inform the DVLA if his/her condition poses a risk to driving. Vocational drivers (Schedule 2) of large goods vehicles or passenger carrying vehicles (LGV/PCV) formally known as HGV/PSV drivers, who have a confirmed diagnosis of OSA should cease driving. Driving may be resumed subject to review when it is confirmed by a specialist that the condition has been adequately controlled for at least 12 months (DVLA, Update 1993). It is the duty of the doctor to warn his/her patients of the dangers of somnolescence and driving and ensure that treatment is optimal.

5   Use of CPAP in orthodox Jewish patients on the Sabbath

Some patients opt to use a timer to start their CPAP machine on the Sabbath night. Many will wish to discuss the issue with their rabbi. If a night without CPAP is felt to pose a significant health risk, use is usually sanctioned.

REFERENCES

1   Sullivan CE, Issa FG, Berthon-Jones M, Eves L. Reversal of obstructive sleep apnoea by continuous positive pressure applied through the nares. *Lancet* 1981; **1**: 862–5.

2   Wright J, Johns R, Melville A, Sheldon T. Health effects of obstructive sleep apnoea and the effectiveness of continuous positive airways pressure: a systematic review of the research evidence. *BMJ* 1997; **314**: 851–60.

3   Stradling J. Sleep apnoea and the misuse of evidence-based medicine. *Lancet* 1997; **349**: 201–202.

4   American Academy of Sleep Medicine Task Force. Sleep-related breathing disorders in adults: recommendations for syndrome definition and measurement techniques in clinical research. *Sleep* 1999; **22**: 667–89.

5   Marcus CL, Omlin KJ, Basinski DJ, *et al*. Normal polysomnographic values for children and adolescents. *Am Rev Respir Dis* 1992; **146**: 1235–9.

6   American Thoracic Society. Cardiorespiratory sleep studies in children. Establishment of normative data and polysomnographic predictors of morbidity. *Am J Respir Crit Care Med* 1999; **160**: 1381–7.

7   Young T, Palta M, Dempsey J, Skatrud J, Weber S, Badr S. The occurrence of sleep-disordered breathing among middle-aged adults. *N Engl J Med* 1993; **328**: 1230–5.

8   Bearpark H, Elliott L, Cullen S, *et al*. Home monitoring demonstrates high prevalence of sleep disordered breathing in men in the Busselton population. *Sleep Res* 1991; **20A**: 411.

9   Stradling JR, Crosby JH. Predictors and prevalence of obstructive sleep apnoea and snoring in 1001 middle aged men. *Thorax* 1991; **46**: 85–90.

10 Gibson GJ, Douglas NJ, Stradling JR, London DR, Semple SJG. Sleep apnoea: clinical importance and facilities for investigation and treatment in the UK. Addendum to the 1993 Royal College of Physicians Sleep Apnoea Report. *J Royal Coll Phys* 1998; **32**: 540–4.

11 Peppard P, Young T, Palta M, Skatrud J. Prospective study of the association between sleep-disordered breathing and hypertension. N *Engl J Med* 2000; **342**: 1378–84.

12 Mooe T, Rabben T, Wiklund U, Franklin KA, Eriksson P. Sleep-disordered breathing in men with coronary artery disease. *Chest* 1996; **109**: 659–63.

13 Mooe T, Wiklund U, Franklin KA, Eriksson.P. Sleep-disordered breathing in women: occurrence and association with coronary artery disease. *Am J Med* 1996; **101**: 251–6.

14 Young T, Peppard P. Sleep-disordered breathing and cardiovascular disease. Epidemiological evidence for a relationship. *Sleep* 2000; **23**: S122–S126.

15 Partinen M, Palomaki H. Snoring and cerebral infarction. *Lancet* 1985; **2**: 1325–6.

16 Chiner E, Signes-Costa J, Arriero JM, Marco J, Fuentes I, Sergado A. Nocturnal oximetry for the diagnosis of the sleep apnoea hypopnoea syndrome: a method to reduce the number of polysomnographies? *Thorax* 1999; **54**: 968–71.

17 Golpe R, Jimenez A, Carpizo R, Cifrian JM. Utility of home oximetry as a screening test for patients with moderate to severe symptoms of obstructive sleep apnea. *Sleep* 1999; **22**: 932.

18 Douglas NJ, Thomas S, Jan MA. Clinical value of polysomnography. *Lancet* 1992; **339**: 347–50.

19 Pepin JL, Ferretti G, Veale D, *et al*. Somnofluoroscopy, computed tomography, and cephalometry in the assessment of the airway in obstructive sleep apnoea. *Thorax* 1992; **47**: 150–6.

20 Morrison DL, Launios SH, Isono S, Feroah TR, Whitelaw WA, Remmers JE. Pharyngeal narrowing and closing pressures in patients with obstructive sleep apnea. *Am Rev Respir Dis* 1993; **148**: 606–11.

21 Johns MW. A new method for measuring daytime sleepiness: the Epworth sleepiness scale. *Sleep* 1991; **14** (6): 540–5.

22 Young T, Blustein J, Finn L. Sleep disordered breathing and motor vehicle accidents in a population-based sample of employed adults. *Sleep* 1997; **20**: 608–13.

23 Jenkinson C, Davies RJO, Mullins R, Stradling JR. Comparison of therapeutic and subtherapeutic nasal continuous positive pressure airway pressure for obstructive sleep apnoea: a randomised prospective parallel trial. *Lancet* 1999; **353**: 2100-5.

24 Engleman HM, Martin SE, Deary IJ, Douglas NJ. Effect of continuous positive airway pressure treatment on daytime function in sleep apnoea/hypopnoea syndrome. *Lancet* 1994; **343**: 572–5.

25 Engelman HM, Martin SE, Kingshott RN, MacKay TW, Deary IJ, Douglas NJ. Randomised placebo controlled trial of daytime function after continuous positive airway pressure (CPAP) therapy for sleep apnoea/hypopnoea syndrome. *Thorax* 1998; **53**: 341–5.

26 Cistulli PA, Barnes DJ, Grunstein RR, Sullivan CE. Effect of short term hormone replacement therapy in postmenopausal women with obstructive sleep apnea. *Am Rev Respir Dis* 1993; **147**: A686.

27 American Thoracic Society. Indications and standards for use of nasal continuous positive airway pressure (CPAP) in sleep apnea syndromes. *Am J Respir Crit Care Med* 1994; **150**: 1738–45.

28 Loube DI, Gay PC, Strohl KP, Pack AI, White DP, Collop NA. Indications for positive airway pressure treatment of adult obstructive sleep apnea patients. A consensus statement. *Chest* 1999; **115**: 863–6.

29 Jokic R, Klimaszewski A, Crossley M, Sridhar G, Fitzpatrick MF. Positional treatment vs continuous positive airway pressure in patients with positional obstructive sleep apnea syndrome. *Chest* 1999; **115**: 771–81.

30 Ballester E, Badia JR, Hernandez L, *et al*. Evidence of the effectiveness of continuous positive airway pressure in the treatment of sleep apnea/hypopnea syndrome. *Am J Respir Crit Care Med* 1999; **159**: 495–501.

31 Ryan CF, Love LL, Peat D, Fleetham JALAA. Mandibular advancement oral appliance therapy for obstructive sleep apnoea: effect on awake calibre of the velopharynx. *Thorax* 1999; **54**: 972–7.

32 Clark GT, Blumenfield I, Yoffe Nea. A crossover study comparing the efficacy of continuous positive airway pressure with anterior mandibular positioning devices on patients with obstructive sleep apnea. *Chest* 1996; **109**: 1477–83.

33 Ferguson KA, Ono T, Lowe AA, *et al*. A randomized study of an oral appliance vs nasal continuous positive airway pressure in the treatment of mild-moderate obstructive sleep apnea. *Chest* 1996; **109**: 1269–75.

34 Ferguson KA, Ono T, Lowe AA, *et al*. A short-term controlled trial of an adjustable oral appliance for the treatment of mild to moderate obstructive sleep apnoea. *Thorax* 1997; **52**: 362–8.

35 Pancer J, Al-Faifi S, Al-Faifi M, Hoffstein V. Evaluation of a variable mandibular advancement appliance for treatment of snoring and sleep apnea. *Chest* 1999; **116**: 1511–18.

36 Hoffstein V, Mateika S, Metes A. Effect of nasal dilation on snoring and apneas during different stages of sleep. *Sleep* 1993; **16**: 360–5.

37 Keenan SP, Burt H, Ryan F, Fleetham JA. Long-term survival of patients with obstructive sleep apnoea treated by uvulopalatopharyngoplasty or nasal CPAP. *Chest* 1994; **105**: 155–9.

38 He J, Krygen M, Zorich F, Conway W, Roth T. Mortality and apnea index in obstructive sleep apnea. *Chest* 1988; **94**: 9–14.

39 Sher AE, Thorpy MJ, Shprintzen RJ, Spielman AJ, Burack B, McGregor PA. Predictive value of the Mueller maneuver in selection of patients for uvulopalatopharygoplasty. *Laryngoscope* 1985; **95**: 1483–7.

40 Katsantonis GP, Maas CS, Walsh JK. The predictive efficacy of the Mueller maneuver in uvulopalatopharyngoplasty. *Laryngoscope* 1989; **99**: 677–80.

41 Launois SH, Feroah TH, Campbell WN, Issa FG, Morrison D, Whitelaw WA. Site of pharyngeal narrowing predicts outcome of surgery for obstructive sleep apnea. *Am Rev Respir Dis* 1993; **147**: 182–9.

42 Myatt HM, Croft CB, Kotecha BT, Ruddock J, Mackay IS, Simonds AK. A three-centre prospective pilot study to elucidate the effect of uvulopalatopharyngoplasty on patients with mild obstructive sleep apnoea due to velopharyngeal obstruction. *Clin Otolaryngol* 1999; **24**: 95–103.

43 American Sleep Disorders Association. Practice parameters for the use of laser-assisted uvulopalatoplasty. *Sleep* 1994; **17**: 744–8.

44 Powell NB, Riley RW, Troell RJ, Li K, Blumen MB, Guilleminault C. Radiofrequency volumetric tissue reduction of the palate in subjects with sleep-disordered breathing. *Chest* 1998; **113**: 1163–74.

45 Riley RW, Powell NB, Guilleminault C. Maxillary, mandibular and hyoid advancement for treatment of obstructive sleep apnea: a review of 40 patients. *J Oral Maxillofac Surg* 1990; **48**: 20–6.

46 Hasan A, McGuigan J, Morgan MDL, Matthews H. Minitracheotomy: a simple alternative to tracheostomy in obstructive sleep apnoea. *Thorax* 1989; **44**: 224–5.

47 Brownell LG, West P, Sweatman P, Acres JC, Kryger MH. Protriptyline on obstructive sleep apnea. A double-blind trial. *N Engl J Med* 1982; **307**: 1037–42.

48 Bonora M, St John WM, Bledsoe TA. Differential elevation by protriptyline and depression by diazepam of upper airway respiratory motor activity. *Am Rev Respir Dis* 1985; **131**: 41–5.

49 Series F, Marc I. Effects of protriptyline on snoring characteristics. *Chest* 1993; **104**: 14–18.

50 Kopelman PG, Elliott MW, Simonds AS, Cramer D, Ward S, Wedzicha JA. Short term use of fluoxetine in asymptomatic obese subjects with sleep related hypoventilation. *Int J Obes* 1992; **16**: 825–30.

51 Takasaki Y, Orr D, Popkin J, Rutherford R, Liu P, Bradley TD. Effect of nasal continuous positive airway pressure on sleep apnea in congestive heart failure. *Am Rev Respir Dis* 1989; **140**: 1578–84.

52 Davies RJO, Harrington KJ, Ormerod OJM, *et al*. Nasal continuous positive airway pressure in chronic heart failure with sleep disordered breathing. *Am Rev Respir Dis* 1993; **147**: 630–4.

53 Rasanen J, Vaisanen IT, Hikkila J, Nikki P. Acute myocardial infarction complicated by left ventricular dysfunction and respiratory failure: the effects of continuous airway pressure. *Chest* 1985; **87**: 158–62.

54 Brett A, Sinclair DG. Use of continuous positive airway pressure in the management of community acquired pneumonia. *Thorax* 1993; **48**: 1280–81.

55 Wiltshire N, Kendrick AH, Catterall JR. Comparison of nine different nasal CPAP systems. *Thorax* 1994 (in press).

56 Boudewyns A, Grillier-Lanoir V, Willemen MJ, De Cock WA, Van de Heyning PH. Two months follow up of auto-CPAP treatment in patients with obstructive sleep apnoea. *Thorax* 1999; **54**: 147–9.

57 Simonds AK, Cramer D, Wedzicha J. Nasal plugs (Adams circuit) for the delivery of CPAP and non-invasive intermittent positive pressure ventilation. *Thorax* 1991; **46**: 291P (abstract).

58 Engelman HM, Martin SE, Douglas NJ. Compliance with CPAP therapy in patients with the sleep apnoea/hypopnoea syndrome. *Thorax* 1994; **149**: 263–6.

59 Davies RJO, Vardi-Visy K, Clarke M, Stradling JR. Identification of sleep disruption and sleep disordered breathing profile from systolic blood pressure profile. *Thorax* 1993; **48**: 1242–7.

60 Reeves-Hoche MK, Hudgel D, Meck R, Zwillich CW. BiPAP vs CPAP: patient compliance in the treatment of obstructive sleep apnea, six month data in a two year study. *Am Rev Respir Dis* 1993; **147**: A251.

61 Elliott MW, Aquilina R, Green M, Moxham J, Simonds AK. A comparison of different modes of non-invasive ventilatory support: effects on ventilation and inspiratory muscle effort. *Anaesthesia* 1994; **49**: 279–83.

62 Hoffstein V, Viner S, Mateika S, Conway J. Treatment of obstructive sleep apnea with nasal continuous positive airway pressure. Patient compliance, perception of benefits, and side effects. *Am Rev Respir Dis* 1992; **145**: 841–5.

63 Kribbs NB, Pack AI, Kline LR, Smith PL. Objective measurement of patterns of nasal CPAP use by patients with obstructive sleep apnea. *Am Rev Respir Dis* 1993; **147**: 887–95.

64 Douglas NJ, Engelman HM. CPAP therapy: outcomes and patient use. *Thorax* 1998; **53**: S47–S48.

65 Reeves-Hoche MK, Meck R, Zwillich CW. Nasal CPAP: an objective evaluation of patient compliance. *Am Rev Respir Dis* 1994; **149**: 149–54.

66 Pepin J-L, Krieger J, Rodenstein D, *et al.* Effective compliance during the first 3 months of continuous positive airway pressure. A European prospective study of 121 patients. *Am J Respir Crit Care Med* 1999; **160**: 1124–9.

67 Hoy CJ, Vennelle M, Kingshott RN, Engelman HM, Douglas NJ. Can intensive support improve continuous positive airway pressure use in patients with sleep apnea/hypopnea syndrome? *Am J Respir Crit Care Med* 1999; **159**: 1096–110.

68 Bahammam A, Delaive K, Ronald J, Manfreda J, Roos L, Kryger MH. Health care utilization in males with obstructive sleep apnea syndrome two years after diagnosis and treatment. *Sleep* 1999; **22**: 740–7.

69 Kryger MH, *et al.* Utilization of health care services in patients with severe obstructive sleep apnoea. *Sleep* 1996; **19**: S111–S116.

70 Kapur V, *et al.* The medical cost of undiagnosed sleep apnea. *Sleep* 1999; **22**: 749–55.

71 Smeets F. Travel for technology-dependent patients with respiratory disease. *Thorax* 1994; **49**: 77–81.

17

Physiotherapy and nursing during non-invasive positive pressure ventilation

JULIA BOTT, PENNY AGENT AND SUSAN CALLAGHAN

PHYSIOTHERAPY (Julia Bott and Penny Agent)

INTRODUCTION

Physiotherapists need to work closely alongside other members of the multi-disciplinary team to promote best care for the patient on non-invasive positive pressure ventilation (NIPPV). The role the physiotherapist plays will vary from centre to centre, but understanding the core skills and aims of the profession may facilitate decisions as to the best use of these team members.

Physiotherapy is a healthcare profession which emphasises the use of physical and emotional approaches in the promotion, maintenance and restoration of an individual's physical, psychological and social well-being, encompassing variations in health status. The core skills used by chartered physiotherapists include manual therapy, therapeutic exercise and electrophysical modalities.[1]

Physiotherapy treatment is achieved through a combination of assessment, advice and education, and hands-on intervention. The aims of respiratory physio-therapy[2] are to:

- Reduce fear and anxiety
- Reduce breathlessness and the work of breathing
- Improve efficiency of ventilation
- Mobilize and aid expectoration of secretions
- Improve knowledge and understanding
- Reduce (thoracic) pain
- Maintain or improve exercise tolerance and functional ability.

As NIPPV both improves ventilation and is an electrophysical modality, it seems logical that physiotherapists will be participants in its administration. Indeed, physiotherapists have been involved with NIPPV since its inception[3] and have contributed to the growing wealth of knowledge in the area.[3–10] Debate continues as to which is the most suitable healthcare professional group to administer this treatment. However, a key factor in forming a team in any insti-tution is that it is composed of individuals possessing the appropriate skills, with the interest and availability, to administer NIPPV competently and effectively. These skills are:

- Patient handling and communication
- Respiratory physiology
- Knowledge of ventilators
- Familiarity with interfaces e.g. masks
- Knowledge of pressure area care
- Time to spend with the patient
- Patience!

Respiratory physiotherapists are likely to have all the prerequisite skills, with a distinct core skill being patient handling, a vital ingredient in the success of non-invasive techniques,[5] particularly in acute respiratory failure. The techniques of applying NIPPV are covered in other sections of this book. For the purposes of this chapter we will identify standard physiotherapy treatments, with reference to the aims that they fulfil, and explore their modifications and adaptations for the patient receiving NIPPV.

As is the case with physician and nurse care, a detailed assessment of a patient is standard physiotherapy practice today and it should accurately define the patient's problems allowing a treatment plan to be developed. Initially this assess-ment must be made at each visit. A first general premiss is that physiotherapy treat-ment must be realistic, effective and, above all, acceptable to the patient in all but extreme circumstances.

An account of the patient's problems and relevant physiotherapy action will follow.

FEAR AND ANXIETY

Individuals who require ventilatory support may have an abnormal respiratory pattern and be breathless, anxious or confused. Anxiety can be greatly increased if patients do not understand their condition or the ventilatory equipment around them, or if their breathing feels 'out of control'. Therefore, a very important aspect of any physiotherapeutic intervention, as with the management of NIPPV, is psychosocial skills, in particular managing a patient's anxiety and fear. Good communication, counselling and health education all play their part in alleviating a patient's stress.[11] However, as these topics are covered in detail in the section on nursing in the second part of this chapter, and in Chapters 6 and 18, they will be omitted here.

Relaxation

Although the teaching of formal relaxation techniques would not be appropriate in an acutely ill patient, helping a breathless patient to relax will assist in reducing his or her anxiety level. Relaxation is better achieved if the patient's anxieties can be alleviated, so is facilitated by the techniques mentioned above. Moreover, relaxation, combined with other techniques (see below) may help reduce the work of breathing and will improve synchronization of respiration with the ventilator.

BREATHLESSNESS, INCREASED WORK OF BREATHING, AND INEFFICIENT VENTILATION

Physiotherapy has much to offer the patient who is breathless. The use of simple positioning and breathing techniques can assist in a reduction in breathlessness and the work of breathing, and enhance ventilation.

Positioning

The positioning of patients for the following reasons is the first step in any physiotherapy treatment:[12]

- comfort
- improvement in the mechanics of breathing and
- optimization of the ventilation/perfusion ratio.

Correct positioning will help alleviate breathlessness and will vary depending on the individual and underlying pathology. High sitting, forward lean sitting (FLS) and high side lying are comfortable positions, provided the patient is well supported. All patients ventilated with NIPPV should be encouraged to adopt a comfortable and relaxed posture.

In breathless patients with severe hyperinflation and low flat diaphragms, FLS may be used for the delivery of NIPPV. The key features of this position are that

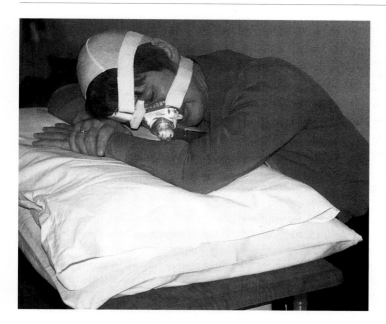

Figure 17.1
Forward lean sitting (FLS) position.

the patient should be comfortable with the arms fully supported on a table with appropriate numbers of pillows to support the head and allow the patient to relax (Figure 17.1). This can be achieved in a chair or sitting over the edge of the bed. FLS relies on the incompressibility of the abdominal contents to load the diaphragm, forcing it into a more domed and lengthened position, thereby improving its length/tension ratio[13] and consequently its force of contraction. This position has been shown to bring about a decrease in the work of breathing,[14] a reduction in the sensation of breathlessness,[13–15] reversal of the paradoxical abdominal wall motion[14] and a decrease in expiratory reserve volume and minute ventilation, without detriment to arterial blood gas tensions,[15] in patients with severe chronic obstructive pulmonary disease (COPD) and asthma.

Passive fixing of the shoulder girdle, by supporting the elbows, assists with relaxation and accessory muscle action. It is possible that, in addition to improving diaphragm function, the pressure exerted by the abdominal contents may passively assist by reducing hyperinflation. FLS may not be the most comfortable position for every patient and some will find supported upright sitting preferable. Modification to FLS may be required in patients with severe ankle oedema, or severe neuromuscular disease. In this situation high side lying may be appropriate. Good positioning of the patient should not affect the position of the NIPPV interface on the face.

Breathing control

In conjunction with positioning, breathing control should be taught both while breathing spontaneously and during NIPPV use. Breathing control is defined as 'gentle breathing using the lower chest with relaxation of the upper chest and shoulders. It is breathing at normal tidal volume and at a natural rate. Expiration is unforced'.[16] Care must be taken in the situation when an individual's chest is chronically hyperinflated with shortened diaphragm length, not to enforce an apparent pattern of 'diaphragmatic breathing'. In this case, encouraging abdominal movement inappropriately may increase, rather than decrease, work of breathing as the patient attempts to produce a movement they are no longer capable of achieving.[17] Optimal ventilation with NIPPV attempts to mimic breathing control and patients should be encouraged to relax during ventilation. The aim should be for the patient to master breathing control in everyday life and adapt it for use when breathless or during activity.

Intermittent positive pressure breathing

Intermittent positive pressure breathing (IPPB) is a longstanding, indeed the first, form of NIPPV and has long been established as a means of correcting ventilatory failure,[18] having the same effect as voluntary hyperventilation but without the increased work.[19] As with newer modes,[20,21] reduction in the work of breathing is a key feature of this mode of ventilation.[22,23] Physiotherapy has incorporated use of intermittent positive pressure breathing (IPPB) devices (e.g. 'The Bird') in treatment for decades,[24] as passive thoracic expansion is helpful during physiotherapy treatments.[25] However, it has been shown that synchrony with the equipment is vital or the patient will experience an increase in the work of breathing, usually as a result of operator inexperience[23] – a useful reminder of the importance of familiarity with equipment.

EXCESS BRONCHIAL SECRETIONS

Patients requiring the use of NIPPV may have excess bronchial secretions. These may simply be due to an acquired respiratory tract infection, or pre-existing respiratory disease. Initially, NIPPV was predominantly used in patients with chronic

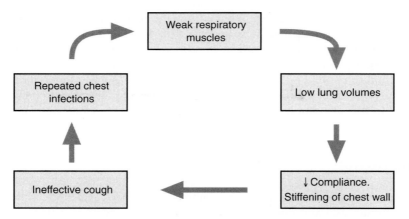

Figure 17.2 *Problems associated with advancing neuromuscular weakness and the rationale behind the need for physiotherapy.*

disorders, including COPD. However with its increased application in acute respiratory failure (ARF) in patients with cystic fibrosis or neuromuscular conditions suffering from severe chest infections, airway clearance techniques either in conjunction with NIPPV or alone, are essential. Figure 17.2 highlights the problems associated with advancing neuromuscular weakness and the rationale for physiotherapy.

Historically, non-invasive ventilation (NIV) has been used to assist ventilation only. More recently, it has been adapted to assist airway clearance as well as improve ventilation. Many specific airway clearance techniques exist, but none, as yet, has been evaluated in conjunction with NIPPV to date.

Hydration and humidification

Mucociliary clearance mechanisms damaged by disease may be further impaired when using NIPPV due to dehydration, caused by reduced fluid intake and the increased flow of cold air through the upper airways. This can result in increased viscosity of bronchopulmonary secretions, impaired cilial action and subsequent secretion retention. Adequate humidification for patients with secretions is vital and may be achieved when using NIPPV through:

1 Drinking. Patients should be encouraged to increase fluid intake, if allowed. Drinking whilst using NIPPV can be taught; the patient is instructed to sip small amounts carefully through a straw, swallowing on expiration.
2 Heated water bath humidifier, e.g. MR290 (Fischer & Paykel), Sullivan® HC100 and Sullivan® Humidaire™ (ResMed, UK).
3 Heat and moisture exchanger (HME). This method is less efficient via nasal mask ventilation as exhaled water vapour may be expired through the mouth.

Airway clearance techniques: no equipment required

ACTIVE CYCLE OF BREATHING TECHNIQUES

The active cycle of breathing techniques (ACBT) is defined as 'a cycle of breathing control, thoracic expansion exercises and the forced expiration technique (FET)'.[16] In patients with cystic fibrosis, it has been demonstrated to be an effective method of aiding removal of secretions, in combination with postural drainage (PD)[26–29] and chest clapping (percussion) and shaking or vibrations[26,28,29] with no detriment to arterial oxygen saturation (SaO_2)[28] and some improvement in pulmonary function.[29] Little work has been done on this method in other conditions. It must be borne in mind that the majority of the studies have used this technique in combination with PD and/or chest clapping and shaking or vibrations. In addition, to compound the confusion, the technique in the early studies was called FET and was used in combination with breathing control and thoracic expansion and would be called ACBT today.

Although the effects of ACBT have not been assessed in patients on NIPPV it is easy to replicate by adapting the patient's machine settings (Figure 17.3). As previously discussed, the equivalent of breathing control is achieved by using the patient's normal tidal volume (V_T) settings on the ventilator. Increasing V_T, inspiratory

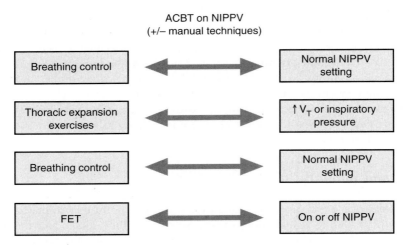

Figure 17.3 *Replication of ACBT on NIPPV.*

pressure (IPAP), or inspiratory time (Ti) can simulate thoracic expansion exercises. To perform a forced expiratory manoeuvre, the circuit may be disconnected at the expiratory valve. Adaptation of the circuit so that it can be used with a mouthpiece is often beneficial to the patient. ACBT when using NIPPV, as in the spontaneously breathing patient, can be performed in any position.

AUTOGENIC DRAINAGE

Autogenic drainage (AD) originated in Belgium in the late 1960s. It is a method of controlled breathing in which the patient adjusts the rate, location and depth of respiration.[30] Traditionally it involves three phases of breathing at different lung volumes, starting with very low, to 'unstick', moving higher, to 'collect' and ending with the highest volume to 'evacuate'.[31] It is usually performed in sitting and studies on this technique do not include chest clapping and shaking or vibrations. In patients with cystic fibrosis it has been shown to be equally effective and acceptable as ACBT.[32] The effects of AD have not been investigated in non-cystic fibrosis patients or those using NIPPV. Theoretically though, as with ACBT, it may be simulated with adjustment of settings as appropriate. It is primarily recommended for patients already familiar with this technique as it is lengthy to teach and requires good co-operation and concentration. However, in those patients already using AD, the combination with NIPPV can be beneficial.[33]

POSTURAL DRAINAGE

Positioning has been traditionally used successfully by physiotherapists to assist with the removal of secretions that are viscous enough to flow with gravity assistance,[34] with,[26–29, 35] or without[34,35] the addition of FET and/or chest clapping and shaking or vibrations.[26,28,29] The positions used are specific to the drainage of individual lung segments. Breathless patients, however, are commonly unable to achieve those that require the head-down position. This is likely to be due to the possible excessive load induced in moving the abdominal contents against gravity. These positions may then need to be modified, but can still be used in conjunction with other airway clearance techniques with or without the application of NIPPV/IPPB. The use of assisted ventilation may allow some offloading of this work and enable them to adopt gravity assisted positions or allow for extension of the treatment time in these positions to allow effective drainage and clearance.

MANUAL TECHNIQUES

Combined with PD, these techniques are considered 'conventional' chest physio-therapy. However, they are also the least uniformly applied of all chest physio-therapy techniques[36] and remain controversial. These techniques have been subject to a great deal of bad press, with some authorities advocating their omission. We should not forget, however, that much of the research reportedly evaluating other modalities has, in fact, included these techniques[26,28,29] along with the approach under test. It is equally possible to add chest clapping and shaking or vibrations to a secretion clearance treatment on NIPPV, as it is without. Chest clapping is customarily performed during periods of increased tidal volume, as in patients with cystic fibrosis this was shown to avoid arterial oxygen desaturation.[28] Research is variable on this technique, both in quality and published outcome, but in patients with copious secretions, rapid two-handed chest clapping has been found to assist more rapid removal of secretions compared to PD and ACBT alone or the combi-nation of PD, ACBT and slow, single-handed clapping.[37] This is in agreement with van der Schans,[36] who in a recent review of chest physiotherapy techniques, concluded that the efficacy of mucus clearance by manual techniques appears to be frequency dependent.

Chest shaking and/or vibration is performed on expiration only and care should be taken to ensure that the direction of the compression is in line with the expira-tory chest wall movement, i.e. down and in, not up towards the mouth, as is sometimes taught. For the patient receiving NIPPV, performing these manouevres with alternate breaths may be more comfortable.

ASSISTED COUGH TECHNIQUES

In any patient with reduced thoracic expansion and abnormal breathing pattern, or severe neuromusculoskeletal disease e.g. paralytic kyphoscoliosis or muscular dystrophy, the ability to cough effectively may be impaired. There are a number of techniques available to assist with spontaneous cough:

- Supine
  - Costophrenic angles of ribs
  - Heimlich-type assist
  - Anterior chest compression
- Side lying
  - Heimlich-type assist
  - Lateral chest compressions with Heimlich-type assist

- Sitting
  - Self-assisted.

Each requires careful placement of the patient, and the therapist's hands, to ensure the forces are correctly applied (Figure 17.4). As with chest shaking/vibration, it is essential that the force is applied on expiration only and care should be taken to ensure that the direction of the compression is in line with the expiratory chest wall movement, i.e. down and in, with the exception of the techniques incorporating the Heimlich-type assist, when the abdominal pressure is up and in. The specific components are beyond the scope of this chapter. However, for further details, the reader is referred to the work of Massery.[38]

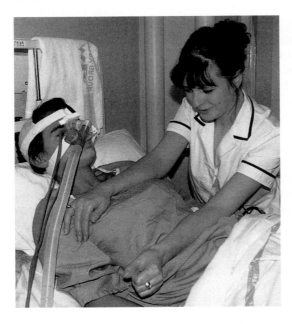

Figure 17.4 *Assisted cough – anterior chest compression with Heimlich-type assist.*

COUGH STIMULATION

If all other techniques fail to induce a cough in a person for whom it is essential, and in whom muscle strength is sufficient to produce an effective cough, stimulation of the trachea may be necessary. This is done by means of gently rubbing the throat in the region of the cricoid cartilage. Strong stimulation is unnecessary. This is relatively ineffective and it should be remembered that the technique is unpleasant and is a last resort.

Airway clearance techniques: requiring equipment

POSITIVE EXPIRATORY PRESSURE (PEP)

The positive expiratory pressure (PEP) mask is widely used for airway clearance throughout Europe. The patient breathes in and out 5–20 times through a flow resistor, which creates a positive pressure in the airways during exhalation.[39] A manometer is used in the circuit to ensure the pressure is at 10–20 cm H_2O during expiration. This technique is performed in sitting. Research on this device is conflicting; Kaminska et al.[40] found, in a 6-week study comparing and alternating PEP with conventional treatment in the home, that patients with chronic bronchial sepsis did not produce as much sputum when using the PEP as when performing conventional treatment. In contrast, McIlwaine and coworkers[41] found in a year long study that PEP was superior to conventional treatment in patients with cystic fibrosis. Hofmeyr et al.[42] compared three treatment packages in patients with cystic fibrosis and demonstrated an advantage of the package that consisted of ACBT and PD alone, compared with PEP added to ACBT and PD or to ACBT and PEP combined in sitting. This study merely added to the evidence that PD is effective and suggests, perhaps, that ACBT and PEP should not be combined. Van der Schans[43] concluded that PEP may temporarily increase lung volume but does not enhance mucus transport. This technique is suitable when NIPPV is being used simultaneously, but only with a mouthpiece.

FLUTTER

The Flutter is a pipe-shaped device, which generates a controlled oscillating positive pressure and interruptions of the expiratory flow when exhaling through it. It can be used in sitting or supine lying. A number of studies have been conducted comparing the Flutter with various airway clearance techniques.[44–46] Pike et al.[46] found no differences in sputum weight, pulmonary function or SaO_2 when Flutter with forced expirations was compared with ACBT in patients with cystic fibrosis. As with PEP, it is possible to use the Flutter in conjunction with NIPPV to good effect,[33] but this combination has not been formally studied.

IPPB

Physiotherapy has incorporated use of IPPB in treatments for chest clearance for many years.[24,25] It is used as a means of providing passive inflation during relaxed breathing and deep breathing sections of physiotherapy treatments, as in ACBT (Figure 17.3). The ease with which the operator can adjust the breath size and speed makes it well suited to this. Moreover, the pattern of airflow is such that it better replicates a deep, sharp intake of breath than many of the newer models on the market, due to their increasing sophistication in triggering and smoothness of action. For these reasons, many patients who use longer term NIPPV choose to switch to this mode for their physiotherapy.

HAYEK HIGH FREQUENCY OSCILLATOR

The Hayek oscillator is a negative pressure ventilator (see Chapter 2). There are 12 sizes of cuirass available making this a suitable technique for children and adults alike. It can provide external high frequency oscillation (EHFO) in its 'secretion mode', when it is used as an airway clearance technique. The Hayek EHFO was compared with the ACBT for clearance of secretions in children with cystic fibrosis,[47] but when using it the patients had lower sputum weight and pulmonary function than when using ACBT. However, in the authors' experience, the Hayek in EHFO mode has been successfully used in assisting the clearance of secretions in patients with Duchenne muscular dystrophy (DMD), as an alternative to ACBT with manual techniques and assisted cough. Some patients may experience discomfort with the cuirass, and the machine itself is not portable.

EMERSON IN–EXSUFFLATOR

The In–Exsufflator (cough machine) assists patients in clearance of retained bronchopulmonary secretions by exsufflation with negative pressure. The machine gradually applies a positive pressure to the airway, then rapidly shifts to a negative pressure. It can be used with a mouthpiece or facemask and the rapid change in pressure simulates a cough by producing a high expiratory flow rate from the lungs.

The benefits of the In–Exsufflator have been studied in a variety of neuromuscular conditions e.g. poliomyelitis,[48] amyotrophic lateral sclerosis,[49] muscular dystrophy,[50] and may be particularly suitable for patients on NIPPV when suctioning or a tracheostomy are not appropriate (see Chapter 15).

SUCTIONING

In extreme instances, naso- or oropharyngeal suctioning may be required, with or without an artificial airway inserted. In this situation the patient will often be drowsy, have sputum retention, and despite the physiotherapist's best efforts to induce a spontaneous or assisted cough, will be unable to cough effectively. All the standard precautions should be adhered to[51] and the NIPPV mask will need to be temporarily, and as briefly as possible, removed. It is imperative that the patient is adequately oxygenated throughout this procedure.

Individuals in the terminal stage of respiratory failure may become distressed by secretions in the upper airways. In this situation, oropharyngeal suction with the Yankauer sucker may be most appropriate. Alternatively, preparations to dry the secretions may be preferred, e.g. hyoscine hydrobromide. During this final phase of the patient's life, it is vital that the patient's own wishes are considered a priority in treatment decisions.[52]

PAIN

Many patients with chest disease suffer from pain whether it is post-operative, or due to musculoskeletal dysfunction, or of unknown cause. Physiotherapists are skilled at the assessment and treatment of pain with a number of modalities available. These include:

- Manual therapy with, for example, joint mobilizations, muscle-lengthening techniques, neural tissue release
- Postural correction

- TENS
- Acupuncture/pressure
- Heat therapy.

These techniques may be applied successfully to patients on or off NIPPV. Further discussion of these techniques is beyond the scope of this chapter, but a more detailed description of these techniques with reference to respiratory disease is available.[16]

OXYGEN THERAPY

Supplemental oxygen (O_2) may be required and can either be entrained via a porthole in the mask or more commonly via a small connector further down the circuit and hence away from the patients' face. With most NIPPV machines, it is not possible to measure accurately the fraction of inspired O_2 (FiO_2). This may need to be increased during active physiotherapy and a pulse oximeter can be used to ensure the patient is adequately oxygenated during treatment. Although caution still needs to be exercised, in practice increasing the concentration is unlikely to produce further hypercapnia or drowsiness. This was confirmed by Starke et al.[53] in their study using IPPB with two different O_2 concentrations of 24% and approximately 45%. Flow rate adjustments must be returned to the resting setting at the end of treatment.

In addition the physiotherapist should consider that the patient on NIPPV may need several bedside oxygen outlets available, for example, for:

- Venturi mask
- Entrainment into NIPPV mask or tubing
- Nasal cannulae
- IPPB.

Tubing for each of the above uses should be labelled clearly, particularly if the flow rates differ.

NEBULIZER THERAPY

When the patient is not totally ventilator dependent, bronchodilators or other nebulizers (inhaled steroids, antibiotics, mucolytics) may be administered conventionally by the prescribed method. However, in those patients who are unable to discontinue NIPPV even briefly, there are a number of methods available:

1 Administered concurrently via a mouthpiece run from a compressor (Figure 17.5 (a)). However, with the advent of active venturi nebulizer systems, some patients may experience difficulty with this method.
2 Administered within NIPPV circuit in a T-piece system, (Figure 17.5 (b)) via a facemask. A large percentage of the drug may be deposited in the nasal passages with this method.

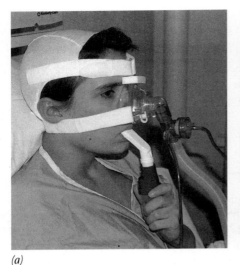

(a)

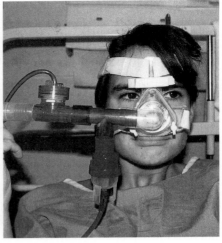

(b)

Figure 17.5
Methods of administering nebulizer therapy in conjunction with NIPPV. (a) administered concurrently via a mouthpiece; (b) within NIPPV circuit in a T-piece system; (c) via a T-piece with a mouthpiece attachment.

(c)

3 Administered via a T-piece in the circuit with a mouthpiece attachment (Figure 17.5 (c)). This method may be the most effective and most comfortable for the patient.
4 Administered via IPPB.

REHABILITATION

A comprehensive rehabilitation programme is an important component of the physiotherapy treatment in most patients' long-term care. The benefits of pulmonary rehabilitation are well documented, predominantly for patients with COPD[54–56] and in cystic fibrosis there is evidence that exercise also assists with secretion clearance.[57] These studies are in spontaneously ventilating patients. With the rise in use of NIPPV in both the acute and the chronic settings, there is an increasing need to continue individualized rehabilitation in these patients. This should be commenced as early as possible, even when the patient may be acutely ill.[12] The ventilator circuit should be long enough to allow the patient to perform simple activities beside the bed; and this should be encouraged. Increased mobility is confidence-boosting, reduces the risk of venous thromboembolism and pressure sores, and will also assist with nursing care as the patient may be able to get out of bed for activities such as using a commode.

Ambulatory NIPPV

With the technological advances of portable ventilatory machinery, e.g. Hippy ventilator (B&D Electromedical, UK) and battery packs available for a wider variety of NIPPV equipment, ambulatory NIPPV is now a realistic possibility for many patients.

A number of studies have confirmed the benefits of its use in exercise.[58–61] To date the studies have concentrated on patients with COPD. Typically these patients have an increased ventilatory load at rest which is exacerbated during exercise.[59]

In summary, the benefits of respiratory pressure support during exercise are thought to be:

- Reduction in breathlessness/dyspnoea[59–61]
- Improved exercise tolerance[59]
- Reduction in muscle fibre fatigue.[61]

The amount of IPAP required to achieve these benefits varies with individuals. Interestingly, Highcock et al.[62] found no benefit in the use of the Hippy ventilator (B&D Electromedical, UK) for patients with COPD performing a shuttle walk test because there was an inadequate flow generation at higher levels of demand. With the development of advanced technology these problems may be overcome, and further evidence is needed in a wider variety of patient groups. However, ambulatory NIPPV has the potential to play a key role in enhancing patients' exercise capacity and increasing the benefit derived from pulmonary rehabilitation programmes. It may also lead to greater independence while using NIPPV thereby facilitating a better quality of life.

In conclusion, the physiotherapists' role in caring for the patient on NIPPV and their family can be complex and far-reaching. It can range from traditional interventions for chest clearance, rehabilitation, and reduction in the work of breathing, through anxiety reduction by education and relaxation, to setting up and revising ventilator parameters and supervising oxygen and nebulizer delivery.

REFERENCES

1   Chartered Society of Physiotherapy (London). *The curriculum framework*. 1996.
2   Bott J, Moran F. Physiotherapy and NIPPV. In: Simonds A (ed.) *Non-invasive respiratory support*. London: Chapman and Hall, 1995: 133–42.

3   Ellis ER, Bye PTP, Bruderer JW, Sullivan CE. Treatment of respiratory failure during sleep in patients with neuromuscular disease. *Am Rev Respir Dis* 1987; **135**: 148–52.

4   Ellis ER, Grunstein RR, Chan S, Bye PTP, Sullivan CE. Non-invasive ventilatory support during sleep improves respiratory failure in kyphoscoliosis. *Chest* 1988; **94**: 811–15.

5   Bott J, Keilty SEJ, Brown AM, Ward EM. Nasal intermittent positive pressure ventilation. *Physiotherapy* 1992; **78**: 93–6.

6   Bott J, Bauduoin SV, Moxham J. Nasal intermittent positive pressure ventilation in the treatment of respiratory failure in obstructive sleep apnoea, *Thorax* 1991; **45**: 457–8.

7   Piper AJ, Parker S, Torzillo PJ, Sullivan CE, Bye PJP. Nocturnal nasal IPPV stabilizes patients with cystic fibrosis and hypercapnic respiratory failure. *Chest* 1992; **102**: 846–50.

8   Bott J, Carroll MP, Conway JH, *et al*. Randomised controlled trial of nasal ventilation in acute ventilatory failure due to chronic obstructive airways disease. *Lancet* 1993; **341**: 1555–7.

9   Piper AJ and Wilson G. Nocturnal nasal ventilatory support in the management of daytime hypercapnic respiratory failure. *Austral Physiother* 1996; **42**, I: 17–29.

10 Piper AJ, Ellis ER. Non-invasive ventilation. In: Pryor JA, Webber BA (eds). *Physiotherapy for respiratory and cardiac problems.* London: Churchill Livingstone,1998: 101–20.

11 Sim J. Interpersonal aspects of care: communication, counselling and health education. In: Pryor JA, Webber BA (eds). *Physiotherapy for respiratory and cardiac problems.* Edinburgh: Churchill Livingstone, 1998: 211–26.

12 Dean E. The effects of positioning and mobilization on oxygen transport. In: Webber BA, Pryor JA (eds). *Physiotherapy for respiratory and cardiac problems,* 2nd edn. London: Churchill Livingstone, 1998.

13 Sharp JT, Drutz WS, Moisan T. Postural relief of dyspnoea in severe chronic obstructive pulmonary disease. *Am Rev Respir Dis* 1980; **122**: 201–11.

14 O'Neill S, McCarthy DS. Postural relief of dyspnoea in severe chronic airflow limitation. *Thorax* 1983; **38**: 595–600.

15 Barach AL. Chronic lung disease: Postural relief of dyspnoea. *Arch Phys Med Rehab* 1974; **55**: 494–504.

16 Webber BA, Pryor JA, Bethune DD, Potter HM, McKenzie D. Physiotherapy techniques. In: Webber BA, Pryor JA (eds). *Physiotherapy for respiratory and cardiac problems.* Edinburgh: Churchill Livingstone, 1998: 137–211.

17 Gosselink RAAM, Wagenaar RC, Rijswijk H, Sargeant AJ, Decramer MLA. Diaphragmatic breathing reduces efficiency of breathing in patients with chronic obstructive pulmonary disease. *Am J Respir Crit Care Med* 1995; **151**: 1136–42.

18 Sukumalchantra Y, Park SS, Williams MH. The effect of intermittent positive pressure breathing (IPPB) in acute ventilatory failure. *Am Rev Respir Dis* 1965; **92**: 85.

19 Emmanuel GE, Smith WM, Brisco WA. The effect of IPPB and voluntary hyper-ventilation upon the distribution of ventilation and pulmonary blood flow to the lung in COPD. *J Clin Invest* 1966; **45**: 1221–32.

20 Elliott MW, Aquilina R, Green M, *et al*. A comparison of different modes of non-invasive ventilatory support: effects on ventilation and inspiratory muscle effort. *Anaesthesia* 1994; **49**: 270–83.

21 Carrey Z, Gottfried SB, Levy RD. Ventilatory muscle support in respiratory failure with nasal positive pressure ventilation. *Chest* 1990; **97**: 150–8.

22 Torres G, Lyons HA, Emerson P. The effects of IPPB on the interpulmonary distribution of inspired air. *Am J Med* 1960; **29**: 946.

23 Ayres SM, Kozam RL, Lukas DS. The effects of intermittent positive pressure breathing on intrathoracic pressure, pulmonary mechanics and the work of breathing. *Am Rev Respir Dis* 1963; **87**: 370–9.

24 Gaskell DV, Webber BA. *The Brompton Hospital guide to chest physiotherapy*, 3rd edn. Oxford: Blackwell, 1977: 78–83.

25 Bott J, Keilty SEJ, Noone L. Intermittent positive pressure breathing – a dying art? *Physiotherapy*, 1992; **78**: 656–60.

26 Pryor JA, Webber BA, Hodson ME, Batten JC. Evaluation of the forced expiration techniques as an adjunct to postural drainage in the treatment of cystic fibrosis. *BMJ* 1979; **2**: 417–18.

27 Sutton PP, Parker RA, Webber BA, *et al*. Assessment of the forced expiration technique, postural drainage and directed coughing in chest physiotherapy. *Eur J Respir Dis* 1983; **64**: 62–8.

28 Pryor JA, Webber BA, Hodson ME. Effect of chest physiotherapy on oxygen saturation in patients with cystic fibrosis. *Thorax* 1990; **45**: 77.

29 Webber BA., Hofmeyr JL., Morgan MDL., Hodson ME. Effects of postural drainage, incorporating the forced expiration technique on pulmonary function in cystic fibrosis. *Br J Dis Chest* 1986; **80**: 353–9.

30 David A. Autogenic drainage – the German approach. In: Pryor JA (ed.) *Respiratory care*. Edinburgh: Churchill Livingstone, 1991: 65–78.

31 Schoni MH. Autogenic drainage: a modern approach to physiotherapy in cystic fibrosis. *J Roy Soc Med* 1989; **82** (Suppl 16): 32–7.

32 Miller S, Hall DO, Clayton CB, Nelson R. Autogenic Drainage and the Active Cycle of Breathing techniques. *Thorax* 1995; **50**: 165–9.

33 Gummery L. Personal communication, 2000.

34 Wong JW, Keens TG, Wannamaker EM. Effects of gravity on tracheal mucus transport rates in normal patients and in patients with cystic fibrosis. *Pediatrics* 1977; **60**: 146–52.

35 Verboon JM, Bakker W, Sterk PJ. The value of the forced expiration technique with and without postural drainage in adults with cystic fibrosis. *Eur J Respir Dis* 1986; **69**: 169–74.

36 Van Der Schans CP, Postma DS, Koeter GH, Rubin BK. Physiotherapy and bronchial mucus transport. *Eur Respir J* 1999; **13**: 1477–86.

37 Gallon A. Evaluation of chest percussion in the treatment of patients with copious sputum production. *Respir Med* 1991; **85**: 45–51.

38 Massery M. Respiratory rehabilitation secondary to neurological deficits: treatment techniques. In: Frownfelter DL (ed.) *Chest physical therapy and pulmonary rehabilitation – an interdisciplinary approach*, (2nd edn). Chicago: Year Book Medical Publishers, 1987: 529–62.

39 Hardy KA. A review of airway clearance: new techniques, indications, and recommendations. *Respir Care* 1994; **39**: 87–105.

40 Kaminska TM, Pearson SB. A comparison of postural drainage and positive expiratory pressure in the domiciliary management of patients with chronic bronchial sepsis. *Physiotherapy* 1988; **74**,5: 251–4.

41 McIlwaine PM, Wong LT, Peacock D, Davidson AG. Long-term comparative trial of conventional postural drainage and percussion versus positive expiratory pressure physiotherapy in the treatment of cystic fibrosis. *J Pediatr* 1997; **131**,4: 570–4.

42 Hofmeyr JL, Webber BA, Hodson ME. Evaluation of positive expiratory pressure as an adjunct to chest physiotherapy in the treatment of cystic fibrosis. *Thorax* 1986; **41**: 951–4.

43 Van der Schans CP, van der Mark TW, de Vries G. Effect of positive expiratory pressure breathing in patients with cystic fibrosis. *Thorax* 1991; **46**: 252–6.

44 Lindemann H. The value of physical therapy with VRP1 Desitin ('Flutter'). *Pneumonologie* 1992; **46**(12): 626–30.

45 Pryor JA, Webber BA, Hodson ME, Warner JD. The flutter VRP1 as an adjunct to chest physiotherapy in cystic fibrosis. *Respir Med* 1994; **88**: 677–81.

46 Pike SE, Machin AC, Dix KJ, Pryor JA, Hodson ME. Comparison of flutter VRP1 and forced expirations (FE) with active cycle of breathing techniques (ACBT) in subjects with cystic fibrosis. *Netherlands J Med* 1999; **54**: 555 (abstract).

47 Phillips GE, Pike SE, Jaffe A, Bush A. Comparison of the active cycle of breathing techniques and external high frequency oscillation with a cuirass for clearance of secretions in children with cystic fibrosis. *Respir Crit Care Med* 1999; **159**; 3: A687.

48 Bach JR, Smith WH, Michaels J, *et al.* Airway secretion clearance by mechanical exsufflation for post poliomyelitis ventilator-assisted individuals. *Arch Phys Med Rehab* 1993; **74**: 170–7.

49 Hanayama K, Ishikawa Y, Bach JR. Amyotrophic lateral sclerosis – successful treatment of mucus plugging by mechanical insufflation–exsufflation. *Am J Phys Med Rehab* 1997; **76**: 338–9.

50 Bach JR, Isahikaura Y, Healeyung K. Prevention of pulmonary morbidity for patients with Duchenne muscular dystrophy. *Chest* 1997; **112**: 1024–8.

51 Hough A. *Physiotherapy in respiratory care. A problem solving approach*. London: Chapman and Hall, 1991.

52 Latimer, T. Caring for seriously ill and dying patients: the philosophy and physics. *Can Med Assoc J* 1991; **1**: 859–64.

53 Starke ID, Webber BA, Branthwaite MA. IPPB and hypercapnia in respiratory failure: the effect of different concentrations of inspired oxygen on arterial blood gas tensions. *Anaesthesia* 1979; **34** (3): 283–7.

54 Ries AL, Kaplan RM, Limberg TM, Prewitt LM. Effects of pulmonary rehabilitation on physiologic and psychosocial outcomes in patients with chronic obstructive pulmonary disease. *Ann Intern Med* 1995; **122**: 823–32.

55 Goldstein RS, Gort EH, Stubbling D, Arendano MA, Guyatt GH. Randomised controlled trial of respiratory rehabilitation. *Lancet* 1994; **334**: 1394–7.

56 Lacasse Y, Wong, Guyatt GH, Goldstein RS. Meta-analysis of respiratory rehabilitation in chronic obstructive pulmonary disease. *Lancet* 1996; **348**: 1115–19.

57 Dodd ME. Exercise in cystic fibrosis adults. In: Pryor JA (ed.) *Respiratory Care*. Edinburgh: Churchill Livingstone, 1991: 27–50.

58 Dolmage TW, Godstein RE. Proportional assist ventilation and exercise tolerance in subjects with COPD. *Chest* **111**: 948–54.

59 Keilty SEJ, Ponte J, Fleming TA, Moxham J. Effect of inspiratory pressure support on exercise tolerance and breathlessness in patients with severe stable chronic obstructive pulmonary disease. *Thorax* 1994; **49**: 990–4.

60   Maltais F, Reissmann H, Gottfried SB. Pressure support reduces inspiratory effort and dyspnoea during exercise in chronic airflow obstructions. *Am J Respir Crit Care Med* 1995; **155**: 1027–33.

61   Polkey MJ, Kryoussis D, Mills GH, *et al*. Inspiratory pressure support reduces slowing of inspirational muscle relaxation rate during exhaustive treadmill walking in severe COPD. *Am J Respir Crit Care Med* 1996; **154**: 1146–50.

62   Highcock MP, Smith IE, Shneerson JM. The Hippy ventilator: effects of a portable ventilator on exercise tolerance in COPD. *Thorax* 1997; **52** (Suppl 6): 28.

NURSING (Susan Callaghan)

INTRODUCTION

Nurses are central to the care and management of patients using NIPPV. They provide 24-hour direct patient care and support within the hospital setting, and their contribution is essential to the multiprofessional team. Nursing management of patients using NIPPV is a complex and challenging task and it is important that knowledge, skills and abilities are identified to develop advanced nursing practice in caring for this group of patients.[1] Advising and supporting families and carers is an increasingly important part of the professional role.[2] The quality of the nurse's relationship with the patient and their carers may contribute to the success of NIPPV. Advanced treatment techniques and a faster throughput of patients means that effective ways of communicating with patients are more important than ever. Nurses are able to reassure patients by explaining what is happening to them during new types of treatment and how to cope following discharge from hospital. Nurses are at the interface between hospital care and the community.

THE ROLE OF THE NURSE IN INPATIENT RESPIRATORY CARE

The goals of respiratory care are to reduce illness, optimize well-being, and provide comprehensive and continuing care.[3]

All patients admitted for NIPPV will have a respiratory assessment from the nurse which involves assessment (identifying problems), planning (setting goals and identifying how to achieve them), implementation (putting the plan into action) and evaluation (assessing the overall results). The respiratory assessment can also be used to explore the full impact of the disease and treatment on the patient in physical, psychological and psychosocial terms. The rehabilitative aspects of care also need to be addressed as most patients using NIPPV will have chronic health-care problems. Good communication and establishing a firm patient–nurse partnership is an essential step in helping patients to live and learn to manage their respiratory illness and NIPPV. Nursing intervention should assist patients to manage their own care and treatment.[4] Involving their families and carers in a supporting role is beneficial for them. Increasingly this group of patients will be cared for on respiratory and general medical wards where NIPPV is having a growing influence on the management of lung and neuromuscular diseases.[5]

Knowledge of the different types of ventilatory equipment and their performance is essential if the nurse is to advise, monitor and care for patients using NIPPV.

NURSING SKILLS WHEN CARING FOR PATIENTS USING NIPPV

These can be identified by setting standards of care and monitoring learning outcomes. A comprehensive knowledge and understanding of cardiorespiratory physiology and pathophysiology is necessary if nurses are to make informed respiratory assessments.[6]

A respiratory nurse should also have knowledge of oxygen, humidification and suction therapy, as well as other breathing techniques described in this chapter.

It is important that the nurse respects the patient's individuality at all times and helps him/her to achieve their own level of independence and adapt to meet their daily needs.

The nurse will be faced with a variety of patient problems, some will be common to all respiratory diseases and others will be specific to NIPPV treatment.

Implications of NIPPV

Many patients receiving NIPPV treatment will have a chronic incurable illness in which symptoms may be palliated, but not eradicated. The way the patient lives with their disease and manages the medical and nursing intervention will have an effect on the use of NIPPV, and the course of their disease.[7]

Dependence on ventilatory support may be accompanied by loss of mobility and independence as well as social isolation.[8] Even those only using NIPPV at night may experience problems such as a sense of loss of autonomy, relationship difficulties and psychological distress.

Nurses and the multiprofessional team need to develop appropriate counselling skills[9] and an understanding of the psychosocial and psychological needs of the patient using NIPPV so as to foster a positive outlook towards treatment.

Coping with anxiety

Many patients are anxious when they are told they will need NIPPV. Lack of knowledge increases anxiety which can be alleviated by clear explanation of the procedure.[10] To promote successful adaptation and coping, patient education is crucial.[11] Time taken to explain and familiarize the patient and family with the equipment will help them relax, making it easier to begin treatment. Reassurance is particularly important in patients undergoing NIPPV as they may feel extremely vulnerable. Reassurance offered by high-visibility nursing care and positive reinforcement of explanations will reduce anxiety, stress and help with coping strategies.[12] Problem-focused coping strategies help chronically ill individuals deal with their illness and the treatments that confront them.[13]

Patients should be encouraged to ask questions and discuss with the nurses any concerns or discomforts about their treatment. Introductions to other patients using NIPPV may also be beneficial to those patients who are anxious about the equipment as talking to other users may alleviate these fears.

In the acute application of NIPPV, calming and relaxing the patient may be very difficult and the nurse may have to sit with the patient holding the mask on their face. Nurses, particularly those present during the night, play a crucial role in helping the patient adjust to using the ventilator. It is therefore crucial that night staff are involved in regular training and educational sessions on NIPPV.

Giving psychological support

As well as the physical needs, assessment should also focus on the psychological needs of the patient so that a partnership is developed and an holistic approach to patient care can be employed.[14] Anxiety and loss of independence can exacerbate the patient's feeling of helplessness and decrease in self-esteem. The nurse's role is to recognize this vicious cycle and to prevent situations that lead to despair and hopelessness.[15] Hope is the key to motivation, and motivation will encourage the patient to use the ventilator and adapt to a new lifestyle. Not surprisingly it has been shown that NIPPV is embraced positively because of beneficial effects on patient's quality of life.[16] Additionally the key to the success of long term ventilation is physiological stability.[17]

Respiratory disease has major social implications. Patients' social needs often become evident when discussing physical symptoms. Restricted mobility can bring isolation and loneliness, and the nurse will need good interpersonal skills to listen to the patient's problems. Listening, clarifying and offering advice and information are major aspects of the nurse's role.[18]

As using the ventilator can make patients feel inadequate and low in self-esteem, it is important for a nurse to avoid letting the patient become over-dependent. Continued independence is vital for self-esteem and dignity; therefore as far as possible the nurse should allow the patient to do things him/herself, and then provide positive feedback.

Patient/carer education and compliance

Education and learning are extremely important determinants of patient compliance. Learning is a form of adaptation in that a person will seek knowledge to meet a specific need.[19] If the long-term NIPPV patient is to accept ventilation as part of their daily routine, they will need a complete understanding of their disease and the practicalities of treatment.

Many centres provide competency plans which are completed by both trainer and patient to facilitate the acquistion of practical skills. These include use of non-invasive ventilation; and areas such as suctioning, tracheostomy care, and changing a tracheostomy in patients receiving invasive ventilation. This written confirmation of training forms part of a general risk management strategy in the patient discharged home on ventilatory support (see Chapter 18). An example is shown in Table 18.3.

An accurate record of the length of time the patient uses NIPPV is important to assess initial compliance problems. After establishing the ideal duration of ventilator use, a care plan can be agreed that will incorporate treatment with independent activities.

The nurse needs to pay close attention to early difficulties when using NIPPV, and have a good understanding of how to solve these (see Chapters 5 and 6). Time should be devoted to problems which affect patient comfort, as well as those which limit the efficiency of ventilation,[20] although these aspects are inevitably linked. It is important to encourage patients to report the problems with tolerance and also symptoms of underventilation which include: dyspnoea, fatigue, morning headaches, and poor sleep quality. Overventilation may occasionally occur, particularly in patients with neuromuscular disease: symptoms include profound fatigue, dizziness and parasthesiae. Such experiences should prompt urgent monitoring of diurnal and nocturnal arterial blood gas tensions and adjustment of ventilator settings as necessary.

Individuals will often feel much better after using NIPPV for a few days. Paradoxically, those requiring long-term use may then become reluctant to continue with NIPPV and will need reinforcement and persuasion to use their ventilator, and a further explanation of why this is necessary. Some NIPPV users have fears about their body image during treatment causing them to feel self-conscious in front of family, other patients and visitors. Body image is a key element of many healthcare interventions, and its disturbance is potentially damaging to patients.[21] Our practice is to manage NIPPV patients within a general respiratory ward area, so that NIPPV is seen as another form of respiratory therapy like LTOT or nebulizer use. Other experienced ventilator users on the ward are often extremely supportive towards new users and can provide a valuable non-medical perspective.

Pressure area care

One of the most commonest problems with NIPPV is pressure sores on the bridge of the nose and around the mask. A variety of preventative measures including polystyrene spacer wedges, adhesive towelling tape on the mask and protective skin dressings can be used to protect the bridge of the nose. A recent nursing research project in this Unit has evaluated two commonly used pressure-relieving dressings

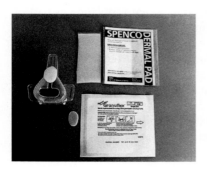

Figure 17.6 *Strategies for reducing nasal pressure sores.*

for the prevention of nasal bridge pressure sores. Patients using Granuflex (ConvaTec Ltd.) had less deterioration in the nasal bridge pressure area over time compared with a comparison group and patients using Spenco Dermal[22] (Figure 17.6). The risk of sacral and other pressure sores is high in some patients, especially those with weaning problems, because of impaired physical mobility related to muscle weakness or paralysis. An individual assessment of disability and equipment needs is required.[23] Special adjustable beds, mattresses and lifting aids should be available. Adjustable beds are almost always necessary for patients with Duchenne muscular dystrophy and other disorders associated with profound neuromuscular weakness.

Health promotion

Health education is also essential to help people with chronic illness maximize their potential.[24] The nurse's role as a health educator is crucial in enabling patients with chronic illness to function at their optimum level in hospital and at home. Health promotion should include basic knowledge about common lung conditions, smoking cessation and compliance with treatment and medication.[25] These activities are traditionally directed to medical information, but it is important to raise awareness to the responsibilities of the patient during treatment with NIPPV. Information can be given verbally, and reinforced through educational literature and the use of videos, many of which are provided by support groups, such as the British Lung Foundation's 'Breathe Easy' groups. These groups have a very valuable role to play in allaying anxiety in both patients and carers.

Nutrition

A nutritional assessment by the nurse on admission is essential and this should include, weight history, oral intake changes and symptoms that affect nutrition such as dysphagia and breathlessness.[26] As eating is generally contraindicated during acute NIPPV because of the risk of aspiration, it is important to monitor the patient's nutritional intake. Optimal nutrition is very important to patients using NIPPV especially those with neuromuscular disorders, who often have profound weight loss, muscle atrophy and weakness. This loss of muscle bulk involves the respiratory muscles, which therefore also become weak. Adequate nutrition can minimize wasting and help to maintain muscle bulk. The nurse needs to identify problems so that early referral to the dietician or for assessment of swallowing problems may be carried out. Nasogastric feeding can be carried out while using NIPPV, but care is needed to prevent mask pressure over the nasogastric tube causing a pressure sore. Some patients with swallowing problems or severe nutritional problems benefit from the introduction of a percutanous gastrostomy.

Terminal care

The management of patients using NIPPV in the terminal phase of their disease is difficult. At this stage one is aiming for symptom palliation and the best possible quality of life for the patient and their family. Quality of life will mean different things to different people and these views may change with the evolution of the disease.[27] Retaining autonomy and being able to participate in management decisions are vital for the patient. While most patients continue ventilatory support in the terminal phase for symptom relief some may request discontinuation of the ventilator. This needs sensitive handling,[28] but the patient's wishes are paramount. The use of opiates should be considered and a high level of nursing presence is needed to monitor, assess and adjust treatment to symptoms[29] at this stage. Terminal care of ventilator dependent patients is discussed further in Chapter 14.

Discharge planning for the ventilator dependent patient

It is essential that the transition from hospital to home is as smooth as possible. This requires good communication and a multidisciplinary approach.[20] The nurse is in a central position to coordinate other health professionals and support services. Discharge planning should start as soon as the patient is admitted. Full assessment of the home situation should be carried out, followed by a care needs assessment as soon as the clinical situation is stabilized.

Before discharge competency training in aspects of ventilatory care should be completed. Medical and nursing advice should be available on a 24-hour basis and the patient and carers given instructions on how to access this. Technical support, information about replacement supplies, care of equipment and provision for emergency breakdown and repair service must be provided. Information regarding ventilator settings should be given to the patient and family.

Discharging a ventilator dependent patient can be difficult and time consuming. Establishing community funding for home care is often problematical.[31] A partnership between the community and hospital in planning, teaching and training is essential.

CONCLUSION

The use of NIPPV has increased significantly over the last few years. As the main care providers respiratory nurses are in a key position to coordinate other health professionals in a collaborative cost-effective approach in patients using ventilatory support. Nurses must ensure that the delivery of care is evidenced based, and that health care needs are met through effective education and training in the use of NIPPV.

REFERENCES

1   Jones S. Applying nasal intermittent positive pressure ventilation. *Nursing Times* 1995; **91**: 32–3.
2   Department of Health. *Making a difference – strengthening the nursing, midwifery and*

health visiting contribution to health and healthcare, the new NHS. London: Department of Health, 1999.

3   Dance FH. The future of the respiratory care profession. In: Burton G, Hodgkin J, Ward J. (eds). *Respiratory care. A guide to clinical practice,* 4th edn. Philadelphia: Lippincott, 1997: 101–9.

4   Litchfield, M. Practice wisdom. *Adv Nurs Sci* 1999; **22**: 62–73.

5   Callaghan S. Neuromuscular lung disorders. In: Shuldham C. (ed.) *Cardiorespiratory nursing.* Cheltenham: Stanley Thornes, 1998: 211–29.

6   Fields D. Every breath you take. *Nurs Times* 1997; **93**(26): 28–30.

7   Molema J, Rameckers EM, Rolle T. Empowerment of patients: a threat or a help? *Monaldi Arch Chest Dis* 1995; **50**: 337–9.

8   Heslop A. A study to evaluate the intervention of a nurse visiting patients with disabling chest diseases in the community. *J Adv Nurs*1988; **13**: 71–7.

9   Hill MC, Johnson J. Professional practice. An exploratory study of nurses' perceptions of their role in neurological rehabilitation. *Rehab Nurs* 1999; **24**(: 152–7.

10   McGrath J, Adams L. Patient-centered goal planning: a systemic psychological therapy? *Top Stroke Rehab* 1999; **6**: 43–50.

11   Howard JE, Davis J, Roghman K. Respiratory teaching of patients: how effective is it? *J Adv Nurs* 987; **12**: 207–14.

12   Lazarus RS. The psychology of stress and coping. *Issues Ment Nurs* 1985; **7**(1–4): 399–418.

13   Parson EJ. Coping and well-being strategies in individuals with COPD. *Health Values* 1990; **14**(3): 17–23.

14   Trnobranski PH. Nurse patient negotiation: assumption or reality? *J Adv Nurs* 1994; **19**: 733–7.

15   Bain L. Neurodegenerative diseases: sustaining hope. *Profess Nurse* 1996; **11**: 515–16.

16   Ledger P, Bedicam JM, Cornette A. Nasal intermittent positive pressure ventilation: long term follow up of patients with severe chronic respiratory insufficiency. *Chest* 1994; **105**: 100–5.

17   Baydur A, Layne E, Aral H, *et al.* Long term non-invasive ventilation in the community for patients with musculoskeletal disorders: 46 years experience and review. *Thorax* 2000; **55**: 4–11.

18   Robinson J. *Focus on care. A practical guide to planning and delivery of community care.* London: King's Fund, 1991.

19   Rankin SH, Duffy KL. *Patient education issues, principles and guidelines.* Pennsylvania: Lippincott, 1983.

20   Thomas S. Motor neurone disease, a progressive disease requiring a co-ordinated approach. *Profess Nurse* 1993 **8**): 583–5.

21   Price R. *Body image: nursing concepts and care.* New York: Prentice Hall, 1990.

22   Callaghan S, Trapp M. Evaluating two dressings for the prevention of nasal bridge pressure sores. *Profess Nurse* 1998; **13**: 361–4.

23   Doyle DL, Stern NP. Negotiating self-care in rehabilitation nursing. *Rehab Nurs* 1992; **17**: 319–26.

24   Brown S, Mann R. Breaking the cycle. Control of breathlessness in chronic lung disease. *Profess Nurse* 1990; **3**: 325–8.

25   Cortis JD, Lacey AE. Measuring the quality and quantity of information-giving to in-patients. *J Adv Nurs* 1996; **24**: 674–81.

26 Blackburn GL, Bistrian BR, Maini BS. Nutritional and metabolic assessment of hospitalised patient. *J Parent Enteral Nutr* 1977; **1**: 11–22.
27 Robert D, Willig TN, Leger P. Patient experiences of nasal ventilation in neuromuscular disorders. *Eur Respir Soc J* 1994; **6**: 599–606.
28 Polkey MI, Lyall RA, Davidson AC, Leigh PN, Moxham J. Ethical and clinical issues in the use of home non-invasive mechanical ventilation for palliation of breathlessness in motor neurone disease. *Thorax* 1999; **54**: 367–71.
29 Skilbeck J, Mott L, Smith D, Page H, Clark D. Nursing care for people dying from chronic obstructive airways disease. *Internat J Palliat Nurs* 1997; **13**: 100–106.
30 Simonds AK. Discharging the ventilator-dependent patient. *B J Intens Care* 1998; March/April: 47–51.

Discharging the ventilator dependent patient and the home ventilatory care network

A K SIMONDS

GOALS OF HOME VENTILATION

Discharging a ventilator-dependent patient home is a challenging process that needs to be achieved as seamlessly as possible. The complexity of arrangements will clearly differ in a patient receiving 24-hour tracheostomy ventilation for a progressive neuromuscular disease, compared to a stable scoliotic patient using nocturnal nasal ventilation. For the purposes of this chapter ventilator dependency is defined as the requirement for ventilatory support at least six hours a day for more than 30 days. The goals of long-term home ventilation are shown in Box 18.1.

Box 18.1 *Goals of home ventilation*

- To extend life
- To enhance the quality of life
- To reduce morbidity
- To improve physical and physiological function
- To deliver treatment safely and cost effectively

It is self-evident that patients should be medically stable at the time of discharge with no imminent change predicted in their clinical state or ventilatory needs. From a paediatric perspective it has been suggested that a child becomes a candidate for long term home ventilatory support after 'one month of clinical and physiologic stability requiring no major diagnostic intervention or changes in respiratory support that result from ventilation or oxygenation abnormalities'.[1] This recommendation holds for adults too of course, but in practice suitability for home ventilation may be obvious sooner. Motivation of the patient and their family is hugely important. No discharge will be successful unless the individual is committed to ventilatory support and believes it will benefit him/her.

CHANGING DEMOGRAPHICS

The last two decades has seen a substantial rise in the number of ventilator dependent patients due an increase in number of patients surviving critical illness (e.g. cervical cord trauma), technological developments, and the impact of non-invasive ventilation. Adams et al.[2] found that non-invasive ventilation was responsible for 47% of the growth in chronic ventilator-assisted individuals in Minnesota between 1992 and 1997. An awareness that NIPPV may alter the natural history of a condition and palliate symptoms has also lead to the appplication of ventilatory support in situations where hitherto it was felt inappropriate to provide such assistance (e.g. amyotrophic lateral sclerosis (ALS)/motor neurone disease). This is in line with a shift in societal expectations for patients with chronic disorders.[3]

In the Minnesota series[2] there was a 110% increase in ventilator dependent patients between 1986 and 1992 and 42% increase from 1992 to 1997. The 1998 report from the Antadir Observatory (the French national database) shows that the uptake of NIPPV increased almost exponentially from 1988, with 500 persons receiving NIPPV in 1990, 3000 by 1996 and 4500 in 1998 (Figure 1.3). By contrast, 2000 individuals were using tracheostomy ventilation in 1988, this figure had increased to 2500 in 1996, but subsequently shows a falling trend to 2000 patients using T-IPPV in 1998. The US survey found that 35% of patients were receiving ventilatory support for less than 24 hours a day i.e. the majority were highly ventilator-dependent. This differs from results elsewhere which suggest that the greater proportion of patients receiving home ventilation use only nocturnal, or nocturnal and part-time diurnal NIPPV. The discrepancy can be explained by the fact that the US study included only patients using ventilators with a back-up respiratory rate, so that those using bilevel machines without back-up rate (spontaneous mode) at night were excluded.

The USA study,[2] demonstrated that the age groups showing most increase in ventilatory dependence were those under 11 years and over 70 years. Obstructive lung disease was the main indication for ventilatory support in the older patients, and the French data also show that the rate of uptake of home ventilation is increasing more rapidly in obstructive rather than restrictive conditions. Not surprisingly, in view on the younger age of recipients and chronicity of the conditions, the neuromuscular group were ventilated for longer periods (> 5 years) in the home.

DECISION-MAKING

As described in Chapters 10–15, consensus recommendations regarding the use of domiciliary ventilation tend to be based on long-term uncontrolled series, rather than randomized controlled studies. However, in restrictive chest wall disorders and neuromuscular conditions involving the respiratory muscles, the alternative to ventilatory support once hypercapnic respiratory failure has developed is almost certainly death, therefore randomized controlled studies are unlikely and almost certainly unethical. In COPD, the situation is quite different, and currently domiciliary NIPPV is only recommended in certain circumstances (Chapter 12).

NON-INVASIVE OR TRACHEOSTOMY VENTILATION?

Tracheostomy ventilation (T-IPPV)

The need for a long-term tracheostomy is determined by bulbar function, upper airway patency, and the ability to clear bronchial secretions effectively. Previously, T-IPPV was automatically used in patients with a high level of ventilator dependency i.e. those requiring respiratory support for more than 16 hours a day. However, non-invasive modes (often in combination) can be used for some 24-hour ventilator-dependent patients, although this is not usually practical in babies and very small children. Some patients can be taught glossopharyngeal ('frog') breathing in which successive breaths are gulped and stacked, to increase ventilator free time.

A comprehensive assessment of swallowing function is important to determine bulbar competence. When carrying out these tests with a tracheostomy tube *in situ*, it should be remembered that the tracheostomy tube itself can impair swallowing function as it reduces anterior movement of the larynx, may change pressures above and below the epiglottis, decreases pharyngeal sensation and can compress the oesophagus and pharynx. Cuff inflation exaggerates this effect. Where possible swallowing function should be tested with the tracheotomy cuff deflated, and if compromise of pharyngeal and oesphageal function is suspected, a reduction in the size of the tube should be considered.

The volume of secretions, and frequency of suctioning in the absence of an acute chest infection is also a useful guide. A patient who cannot swallow his own saliva will require T-IPPV. A methylene blue dye (or Ribena) test is commonly used as bedside evaluation, but this is not highly sensitive. If aspiration is suspected, but not confirmed on bedside testing, video-fluoroscopy can be performed. However, it should be noted that a minor degree of swallowing dysfunction does not necessarily mean that decannulation and NIPPV is contraindicated, indeed this is relatively common in Duchennne muscular dystrophy (DMD) and ALS patients. In this situation, modification of the diet to increase consistency of the food, and attention to body position when eating is important.

The advantages and disadvantages of different tracheostomy tubes are shown in Table 18.1. In individuals with chronic severe aspiration who are unable to speak e.g. following a brainstem CVA, a low pressure cuffed, non-fenestrated

Table 18.1 *Advantages and disadvantages of types of tracheostomy*

Type	Advantages	Limitations
Uncuffed	Lowest risk of tracheal trauma Insertion easier than cuffed tube. Best vocalization	Leaks Cannot increase diameter e.g. for night ventilation Risk of aspiration
Low pressure cuff	Option to seal leak Can vary external diameter by cuff inflation Helps prevent aspiration	May cause tracheal trauma Insertion may be more difficult than uncuffed tube
Fenestrated low pressure cuffed	Useful for patients able to breathe spontaneously during the day, but who need nocturnal ventilation Helps prevent aspiration	Reduced frequency of tube changes as can clean inner cannula. May cause granuloma formation
Fome cuff (Bivona)	Good for long-term placement Least potential for tracheal damage Helps prevent aspiration	Can be difficult to place and remove Cuff may reflate spontaneously
Talking tracheostomy	Opportunity for speech in patients who require permanent cuff inflation Helps prevent aspiration	Needs separate air source which is noisy and limits mobility. Air can dry secretions Requires tracheostomy port occlusion by switch or finger
Customized tracheostomy	Very helpful in patients with abnormal anatomy e.g. severe scoliosis	Costs more than standard tubes

tracheostomy tube is indicated for safety. Cuff pressure should not exceed 20 cmH$_2$O. For patients who are able to speak, but have major aspiration problems, a speaking tracheostomy tube with separate port to direct low flow air upward through the larynx can be tried. In those with minimal or no aspiration difficulties, trial cuff deflations should be attempted while monitoring tube aspirate, oximetry and arterial blood gas tensions. A major leak around the tracheostomy may limit the efficiency of ventilation, but this can usually be redressed by altering ventilatory settings or changing from a volume to pressure preset ventilator.

In adults who can be satisfactorily managed with the tracheostomy cuff deflated, and are able to breathe spontaneously for short periods, a fenestrated tracheostomy is useful to facilitate speech. Indeed, every step possible should be taken to allow patients to speak, or if this is not possible to communicate with assistive aids as this is crucial to morale and allows patients to take part in decision-making more easily.

Great difficulty in creating a tracheostomy is sometimes be experienced in patients with cervical and chest wall deformity due to a high scoliosis, kyphosis, ankylosing spondylitis or contractures etc. For these individuals standard tracheostomy tubes are often inadequate. Some manufacturers (e.g. Portex Ltd.) will customize tracheostomy tubes for the individual. We have found that computerized tomography scans of the tracheal region are very helpful in obtaining accurate measurements of the depth and length of tube required (Figure 18.1).

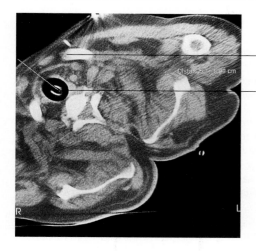

— Distance from stain to trachea

— Tracheostomy tube

Figure 18.1 *Computerized tomogram of neck region to determine the dimensions of trachesotomy tube required in spina bifida patient.*

Non-invasive ventilation

In patients with preserved bulbar function and a < 24-hour ventilator dependence, non-invasive ventilation is usually the approach of choice. NIPPV modes are preferred by both patients and their carers if this is feasible.[4] NIPPV has also been used successfully in totally ventilator-dependent patients (Chapter 14). The selection of patients for non-invasive ventilation and choice of equipment is discussed in Chapters 2 and 10. A step down in ventilatory support from T-IPPV to NIPPV can be achieved in weaning patients and those recovering from spinal cord injury or a brainstem CVA. A step up from NIPPV to T-IPPV may be needed in patients with progressive conditions such as DMD and motor neurone disease/ALS.

HOME CARE NETWORK

The success of any home care programme depends on a support network which inspires confidence in all parties. The components of this are shown in Box 18.2.

Access to medical advice

Patients and their families will inevitably need medical guidance from time to time e.g. whether to start a course of antibiotics, queries about ventilator settings, or the side effects of treatment such as nasal bridge sores and gastric distension. These may be simply dealt with by telephone, or require a home visit, outpatient assessment or admission. A team member with adequate experience of ventilatory support should be available on a 24-hour basis to triage the calls and arrange suitable follow-up. All patients should have access to a telephone. Individuals should be able to self-refer for admission if their condition rapidly deteriorates.

Box 18.2 *Home care network plan*

1 • Ready access to medical advice, home visits, hospital admission and respite care
  • Regular monitoring of medical progress
  • Risk management assessment (see Figure 18.4)
2 Technical support
  • replacement of disposables and hardware
  • emergency equipment breakdown repair service
  • regular maintenance of equipment in the patient's home
3 Patient and family education. Training of caregivers. Competency agreements. Reassessment and retraining as necessary
4 Close liaison with the general practitioner and other medical and ancillary teams involved with care
5 Social services support
6 Advice regarding practical arrangements for work, school (including statementing of children), holidays, transportation of equipment, and fitness for airline travel
7 Information on patient support schemes (International Ventilator Users Network, Breathe Easy clubs, Muscular Dystrophy Association, Duchenne Family Support Group, Motor Neurone Disease Association, Scoliosis Association UK, Brompton Breathers etc.)

*No individual should be discharged without a support network in place, although the level of back-up required will necessarily vary from patient to patient.

Other hospital departments such as the Accident and Emergency Unit/Emergency Room should be aware of these procedures. An open access 'walk-in' clinic for patients receiving non-invasive ventilation and CPAP, staffed by a respiratory support technician/nurse is very helpful for sorting out minor technical difficulties, before these develop into major problems. During home visits the clinical state of the patient, and ventilator performance can be assessed. A portable oximeter and vitalograph are useful for these visits.

The frequency of routine follow-up assessments will vary from patient to patient. Shared care is particularly helpful for patients who live long distances from the ventilation centre and often serves an as impetus for the development of local home ventilation programmes.

Risk minimization assessment

It is impossible to totally eliminate hazards for the home ventilator user, as equipment can fail and tracheotomies can and do block, whether at home or in hospital. However, every step should be taken to anticipate risks and minimize these as far as possible. In the author's experience the commonest cause of ventilator-related problems in the UK is mains power failure,[5] followed by accidental disconnection of ventilator tubing, and blockage/failure to replace the tracheostomy.

Most ventilators contain mains power failure, high pressure and low pressure alarms, but some bilevel models, do not (e.g. BiPAP S, S/T, Respironics Inc). In patients with a moderate degree of ventilatory dependency and marked nocturnal hypoventilation, alarms are advisable. However, some ventilator-dependent patients will sleep through alarms, or may be unable to summon help themselves. Carer arrangements in these patients need to be closely reviewed. For patients highly dependent on mask or tracheostomy ventilation it is sensible to put a battery pack in circuit with the ventilator and mains power, so that if there is a power cut, the ventilator will automatically switch to battery power. Connections between the tracheostomy/mask, circuit tubing and ventilator should be as secure as possible (bayonet type preferable to push-in), and the circuit tubing supported to prevent dragging. Tracheostomy patients should be provided with a smaller size tracheostomy tube in case there are problems changing the tube caused by granulation tissue, stenosis etc. Training of carers with written instructions of how to manage problems will help improve the proficiency of the home team, decrease anxiety and build confidence. Regular reappraisal of skills and retraining where necessary, is required. All concerned should understand that ventilation at home is never going to be 100% safe, and there is inevitably a less developed emergency back-up system than in hospital. For medico-legal reasons, all the measures taken to minimize risk in each individual should be recorded in the hospital notes. These recommendations are summarized in Table 18.2. Central reporting of adverse events would help disseminate the lessons learned more widely.

Technical support

Patients need to have an action plan to put into practice if their ventilatory equipment malfunctions. Many using nocturnal non-invasive ventilation will cope for several days without ventilatory support; highly ventilator-dependent patients will need an immediate solution to the mechanical problem. For patients who cannot breathe independently for more than a few hours a 'back-up' ventilator is essential. Similarly a battery option should be available to cope with power cuts and travel outside the home. (The authorities can be notified in the UK so that power reconnection after a power cut will occur as a priority in ventilator users).

In the UK there are several nationwide service and maintenance schemes which are coordinated by the large hospital units and carried out by engineers from the commercial sector (see Appendix I). Patients from other hospitals can be entered in these schemes. It is helpful to categorize patients as to their degree of ventilatory dependency. This allows engineers to give precedence to those who require urgent attention. A simple way to do this is on the basis of one night, two night and three night need i.e. a 'one night' patient cannot function for more than one disturbed night without a ventilator, a 'two night' patient can not cope for more than two nights etc. Patients are asked to notify the equipment problem by telephone to the coordinating centre. This call should be screened to ensure that there is no simple remedy to the problem (e.g. change of fuse). The engineer is then contacted. Ideally, the technical problem is dealt with in the patient's home, but if a repair cannot be effected a substitute ventilator of the same make is provided. An alternative is for service and maintenance to be carried out by the local hospital. This may work well, but it should be remembered that ventilators break down at weekends and on bank holidays when many in-hospital biomedical

Table 18.2 *Risk minimization in the home ventilator patient*

Potential problem	Risk management
Ventilator breakdown	Regular service and maintenance. Emergency contact line to report problems. Emergency technician call out to patient's home available. Back-up ventilator in patients who cannot breathe for 1 night without ventilatory support.
Mains power failure	Battery pack. Mains power alarm. Battery paced in circuit with mains power and ventilator in ventilator-dependent patient at night. Ambu bag available for ventilator-dependent patients
Accidental disconnection from ventilator	Low pressure and low volume alarms. Firm attachment of ventilator/circuitry connections. Support of ventilator tubing to prevent dragging on tracheostomy or mask.
Tracheostomy blocked	Efficient suction with battery power or manual operation. Carers trained to change tracheostomy. Optimize humidification. High pressure alarm.
Tracheostomy falls out	Improve tube fixation. Carers trained to change tracheostomy. Smaller size tracheostomy tube available.
Medical problems	Immediate access to hospital care available. Patient and carers trained to recognize early signs of chest infection and ventilatory decompensation. Carers trained in resuscitation skills.
General	Training of carers in skills necessary for the care of the individual, with written competency agreements Access to telephone hotline to discuss problems and most suitable course of action. Written plan of action for predictable problems e.g. equipment failure.

engineering departments are closed. Patients often have great difficulty in transporting their equipment to the hospital.

Finally, some manufacturers and dealers offer service and maintenance deals for their own brand of ventilator or CPAP machine. Not all of these schemes include a 24-hour breakdown service and so would be inappropriate in a highly ventilator-dependent individual.

Home ventilators need servicing once or twice a year depending on the model. This will include a check on electrical safety. CPAP machines should be serviced once a year. Oxygen concentrators are independently serviced in the home by the providing company.

Disposables such as masks, headgear, tubing etc. can be supplied by the hospital or direct from the manufacturers. On average NIPPV users will need one to two commercial masks a year. Customized facepieces have a variable lifespan. New ventilator tubing and headgear is needed once a year. Occasionally patients benefit from a disposable heat and moisture exchanger (e.g. Portex thermovent) when secretions or rhinitis are a problem. These should be discarded after 24 to 48 hours.

T-IPPV patients have a far greater requirement for technical support in the home and a full description of their needs is beyond the scope of this text. However, support equipment should include suction machine and suction tubes, spare tracheostomy tube (including smaller sized tube in case of difficulties with placement), stoma dressings, saline, syringes and humidifier.

Patient and family education

Before home discharge each ventilator user, their family and carers need to understand:

- The nature of the patient's underlying respiratory condition and its consequences
- The basic principles of the ventilator and how to connect the power supply, circuit, exhalation valve and mask correctly
- The ventilator settings required by the user. How to attach oxygen from concentrator and humidification, if required
- The function of the alarms
- How to change the filter and carry out simple cleaning and maintenance
- A simple problem-solving approach to medical or technical problems in the home
- What to do and who to contact if the ventilator or other equipment malfunctions.

It is helpful to provide a patient-orientated handbook to reinforce these practical aspects and a record of the patient's ventilatory settings, mask type, and oxygen flow rate (if applicable). Written competency agreements can be signed off by both trainer and patient carer to confirm these educational areas have been covered (see below).

Patients/carers are also responsible for the routine maintenance of their ventilatory equipment which will include changing or washing the filters on positive pressure ventilators, and rinsing the mask and tubing. The mask and ventilator tubing should be washed in soapy water every week and dried thoroughly. Sterilization is not required and may damage the mask. Individuals using negative pressure equipment will need to wash pneumojackets regularly.

The training of patients and carers regarding T-IPPV is necessarily more detailed. Carers need to be competent in suction, changing the tapes and dressings round the stoma site, and replacing the tracheostomy tube. They need to be able to recognize signs of respiratory distress and be familiar with resuscitation procedures. It is our practice to complete competency training agreements with all patients and their carers requiring home T-IPPV. An example of a training plan is given in Table 18.3.

Ideally, for the patient and carer home ventilation should form part of a comprehensive pulmonary/neuromuscular rehabilitation programme.

Table 18.3 *Training plan to establish competency in carers*

(a) Example of a training plan for carers responsible for patient with a tracheostomy

Name of patient:.................   **Carers to be included**:..... **Consultant** ....

Named nurse ....

Physiotherapist ....

Topics   **Trainer** .... **Dates of teaching sessions**

Respiratory assessment

Suctioning

Skin care of tracheostomy site

Tape change

Tracheostomy tube change

Resuscitation (CPR) training

(b) Example of competency training agreement for suctioning a tracheostomy

Patient's name...   Carer's name...

Knowledge

Simple anatomy of trachea, bronchi and lungs

Reason for tracheostomy, type, and airway problems of patient

Explanation of why and how often suction likely to be needed

Evidence of chest infection, need for humidification

Signature of carer ....   Date ....

Signature of trainer ....   Date ....

Practical skills

Assessment of the need for suctioning

Understanding of size of suction catheter, suction pressure required and operation of suction pump

Demonstration of correct suction technique (pre-measured)

Recognition of problems related to suctioning

Signature of carer..   Date ....

Signature of trainer..   Date ....

Liaison with other team members

Clear information on the patient's medical and ventilatory requirements needs to be available to all involved parties, and they should be involved in decision-making at every opportunity. It is helpful for other team members to have a copy of the ventilator handbook and record of ventilator settings.

Advice regarding travelling with the ventilator/benefits

As indicated in Chapter 11, many patients receiving nocturnal non-invasive ventilation return to a near normal quality of life and understandably want to take part in normal activities, including foreign travel. This is usually feasible in nocturnal non-invasive ventilator users and, with planning, more handicapped individuals with well-controlled respiratory failure can also travel extensively. NIPPV ventilators are easier to transport than portable negative pressure systems which tend to be excessively bulky. Independent arrangements regarding oxygen requirements and transportation of ventilatory equipment should be made well in advance. The fitness of any individual to fly depends on their general health, baseline PaO_2 and $PaCO_2$, ventilatory dependency, the altitude (cabin pressurization), duration of flight and level of physical activity during the flight. Uncontrolled hypercapnia, severe hypercapnia in response to oxygen therapy and bullous lung disease are all contraindications to air travel. 'Fitness to fly' tests where the arterial blood gas tensions are measured before and during a simulated flight are very helpful for calculating oxygen requirements and ensuring that hypercapnia is not precipitated. As ventilation will inevitably deteriorate during sleep in those who require nocturnal ventilatory support and obstructive sleep apnoea will become manifest without CPAP, patients are advised not to sleep during the flight, or use their ventilator with a battery pack. Short haul fights or stop-overs are therefore preferable to long haul flights. The ventilator should always travel as cabin luggage. Patients should be provided with a letter from their medical attendant to authorize this requirement. The BiPAP range (Respironics Inc), VPAP II (ResMed) and many other models are dual voltage and useful for trips to North America. The standard voltage in other destinations should be checked and a suitable adapter plug obtained. All heavily ventilator-dependent patients should travel with a fully charged battery pack. Wet acid batteries are not allowed on airflights, but the batteries listed in Chapter 8 are acceptable. A summary of recommendations for air travel in ventilator dependent patients is given in Box 18.3. These are in keeping with British Thoracic Society Guidelines on managing passengers with lung disease planning air travel.[6]

A Eurolung Assistance scheme has been set up for ventilator and oxygen-dependent travellers.[7] This is an association of health professionals, medical technology services, tourism agencies and insurance companies which promotes travel in such patients. The Eurolung Assistance Directory published by the group provides useful information on the availability of support services, including oxygen suppliers throughout Europe, and also gives details of specific airline requirements for technology-dependent individuals.

Support groups

Many patients and families find it valuable to share their experiences. Addresses of relevant agencies are given in Appendix II. Some hospitals provide newsletters and research updates on ventilatory equipment.

Box 18.3 *Recommendations for air travel in the ventilator-dependent patient*

- Inform airline in advance
- Take short haul flights, where possible
- Travel with a record of diagnosis, ventilator settings, recent blood gas results and contact number of ventilator centre
- Take ventilator as cabin luggage
- Sleep before travelling, so as to keep awake as much as possible during flight
- Avoid alcohol, keep hydrated, and eat light meals
- Ensure voltage compatibility of ventilator with country of destination
- Consider supplemental oxygen if Sao_2 < 93% on air (use with ventilator if hypercapnia likely)

Additional requirements for 24-hour tracheostomy ventilator-dependent patients:
- Back-up ventilator required
- Battery pack (dry battery) and charger required
- Battery or foot operated suction machine
- Spare tracheostomy tube
- Tracheostomy cuff filled with saline not air
- Carer competent to change tracheostomy tube and operate ventilator
- Ambu bag available for resuscitation

DISCHARGE OF THE VENTILATOR DEPENDENT CHILD: A MODEL OF CARE

Following the disturbing finding that many ventilator dependent children were spending excessive periods of time in intensive care units because of delays in discharge,[8] a UK Working Party on Paediatric Long-term Ventilation has developed core guidelines to facilitate the discharge of ventilator dependent children.[3] In outline, once the requirement for home ventilation has been established, it is recommended that a multidisciplinary discharge team is formed, and a needs assessment carried out. The needs assessment will include:

- Identification of funding source for the home care package (in the UK this will usually be the health authority for the child's home area. Social services fund any non-professional carers)
- Equipment requirements
- Equipment maintenance
- Housing review
- Home carers
- Training of carers.

The guidelines make it clear that each home care team should be led by a qualified paediatric nurse, but other carers do not need a nursing qualification. A comprehensive training programme should be provided for all carers. The parents and other family members will usually form part of the care team, but they should not be overburdened. The level of care/support in the home will be determined by a number of factors including:

- Non-invasive or invasive ventilation
- Level of ventilator dependency
- Child ambulant or paralysed/has limited mobility
- Other family demands and work pressures.

Families with ambulant children using nocturnal mask ventilation may require very little care assistance in the home, whereas a child with a high cervical cord injury who is 24-hour T-IPPV dependent may require a team of 4–6 carers. Similar principles apply to adult patients.

ALTERNATIVES TO HOME CARE

It should be recognized that not all families can cope with a ventilator dependent member, and some patients do not have families. Some excellent community care facilities do exist, but these are limited. For adults, independent living in the home with a team of carers is also possible and should be encouraged. Planning this type of care package is inevitably more complex than a set-up where family members provide the majority of care, but is very worthwhile. An acute care unit or ICU is *not* the place to care for a long-term ventilator dependent patient from a practical, humanitarian, or economic point of view.

WORLD PERSPECTIVE

The organization of home care has evolved very differently in the UK, the rest of Europe and the USA. Simplistically, the organization of home respiratory care can be divided into three main models.[9,10]

1 The discharging hospital provides home equipment and supplies and/or home care package funded by local health authority (e.g. UK, Austria).
2 Community based organizations (coordinated centrally) manage all aspects of home care (e.g. France).
3 Private sector management of equipment and care in the community with discharging hospital providing medical follow-up (e.g. USA, Italy).

The provision of respiratory support remains rudimentary in many countries worldwide. France has a well-developed home respiratory care system which may serve as a useful role model. The French system of home respiratory care and other programmes throughout Europe are discussed in detail in the following chapter. Here, the organization of home ventilation in the USA and UK is contrasted.

USA

Home ventilation has a long track record in the USA, with an estimated prevalence of 4.9 in 100,000 receiving long-term ventilatory support.[10] (This compares with 20 per 100,000 of the population using domiciliary ventilation in France.) A Consensus Report by the American College of Chest Physicians: *Mechanical Ventilation: Beyond the Intensive Care Unit* was published in 1996.[11] This established criteria for the evaluation of suitable candidates, and made recommendations on discharge policy, ventilatory aspects unique to children, and acceptable levels of home care. Despite this effort, there is no national policy, administrative structure or system for funding long-term ventilation. As a result, not all patients who warrant home ventilation receive it, and in others there are long delays before discharge from hospital can be arranged. Payment or reimbursement for equipment comes from a variety of sources – federal or state government, private insurance or the patient's own funds. It is reported that families with long-term ventilator dependent children usually exhaust their private insurance benefits and personal resources within one or two years. Nursing and home care is then covered by publicly funded Medicaid programme until the child is 21 years old, at which point most funding including nurse care ceases. The individual is then either supported by the family or can be placed in a Medicaid funded nursing home. This Medicaid policy is in conflict with the American Disabilities Act (1990) which requires that disabled individuals are cared for in the community, as far as possible. Other funding initiatives, including social security, vary from state to state. There is no centralized data collection on ventilator use, but this situation may be corrected by initiatives such as the creation of the National Centre for Mechanical Ventilation in Denver which has a responsibility for collecting information on the performance and safety of home ventilatory apparatus.

Regional information does exist, however, such as the survey of long-term respiratory support in Minnesota.[2] Between 1986 and 1992 large increases were seen in the paediatric group and in those over the age of 60 years receiving NIPPV as discussed in Chapter 15. Athough the commonest primary diagnosis in this was poliomyelitis, the number in this group was relatively static compared with a marked growth in patients with cervical trauma, motor neurone disease and muscular dystrophy. No breakdown is given as to the mode of ventilatory support. However, more patients in the USA are Grade 4 ventilator-dependent (requiring 24-hour support) than in the UK.

For the Minnesota group as a whole, the average monthly cost of ventilatory support was US$6500 (7600 Euros) per patient in the home, and US$19,351 (22,640 Euros) in a long stay institution. The projected intensive care bed cost was US$64,513 per month (75,480 Euros). It is difficult to know whether this information is representative of care packages in the USA as a whole. However in another study, Goldberg[1] describes an initial cost saving of 70% in a paediatric ventilatory home care programme compared with ICU costs.

A new growth area is the use of nocturnal bilevel pressure support ventilation. This has occurred largely as result of the rapid expansion of sleep laboratories which are identifying an increasing number of individuals with nocturnal hypoventilation secondary to obesity hypoventilation syndrome, neuromuscular disease, COPD and obstructive sleep apnoea. The relative simplicity of bilevel pressure support equipment (e.g. BiPAP, Respironics, Inc., VPAP, ResMed) has led to the creation of home respiratory support programmes in institutions which were previously unable to offer this treatment. Private home care companies are expanding to meet this need. There is little information on the number of patients receiving bilevel support and it is apparent that there is the potential for an explosion of unregulated use of this new therapy. It remains to be seen whether US managed health care reforms will make cost-effective home ventilation more accessible.

UK

Whereas long-term oxygen therapy is universally available from the National Health Service and funded centrally, there is as yet no coordinated provision of home ventilation. The Responaut programme at St Thomas' Hospital, London set up in 1965 was the earliest large scale treatment initiative.[12] Subsequently in the early 1980s two other major centres, The Royal Brompton Hospital, London, and Papworth Hospital (previously Newmarket Hospital), Cambridge began to treat patients, primarily with restrictive disorders, with negative pressure ventilation. The advent of nasal positive pressure ventilation in the mid 1980s led to a rapid increase in patient numbers, and the introduction of home respiratory support programmes in other centres in the UK. However, these are not well spead geographically and some regions have poor access to home ventilatory facilities. A UK Home Ventilator Providers Group has recently been formed with the aim of gathering data on home care provision, carrying out multicentre studies and disseminating information on effective ventilator use. It is estimated that approximately 2500–3000 adults and children are receiving home mechanical ventilation in the UK. The largest subgroups are those with chest wall and neuromuscular disease.

Department of Health guidelines (UK) exist for the prescription of LTOT (see Chapter 10). There are no guidelines for home ventilation or CPAP therapy. With the purchaser-provider system of health delivery, reimbursement for hospital care, equipment costs and the maintenance of equipment in the patient's home are sought from the referring health authority/fundholding GP/multifund groups. It is crucial that purchasers (usually health authorities) recognize the advantages and cost savings offered by home ventilation. Some providers are able to buy ventilators in bulk and offer a low-cost lease scheme which saves the purchaser excessive start-up costs. These schemes have the advantage that equipment can be substituted if it no longer meets the patient's ventilatory needs, or more advanced models become available. The cost of a nasal ventilator varies between £2000 and £6000, with an average cost of around £2800 (4592 Euros). Lease schemes which offer a range of ventilators and full service and maintenance of the equipment in the recipient's home cost about £2000 per annum. The majority of the information above concerns patients receiving non-invasive ventilation. The number of T-IPPV patients in the UK is approximately 100 and the figure remains relatively static. Some of these are managed by spinal injuries centres which have special expertise in the care of cervical cord injury patients. Other T-IPPV patients are managed by local respiratory physicians, paediatricians, or anaesthetists. It has been estimated that the cost of discharging a 24-hour T-IPPV ventilator dependent patient with a full care package in the UK is approximately £150,000 (246,000 Euros) per annum.[3] Staffing costs comprise about two-thirds of this.

REFERENCES

1   Goldberg AI, Faure EAM, Vaughan CJ. Home care for life-supported persons: an approach to programme development. *J Pediatr* 1984; **104**: 785–95.

2   Adams AB, Shapiro R, Marinii JJ. Changing prevalence of chronically ventilator-assisted individuals in Minnesota: Increases, characteristics, and the use of non-invasive ventilation. *Respir Care* 1998; **43**: 635–6.

3   Jardine E, Wallis C. Core guidelines for the discharge home of the child on long term assisted ventilation in the United Kingdom. *Thorax* 1998; **53**: 762–7.

4   Bach J. A comparison of long-term ventilatory support alternatives from the perspective of the patient and care-giver. *Chest* 1993; **104**: 1702–6.

5   Towlson S. Power cut kills man on home ventilator. *The Times* 2000; **August 14**: London.

6   British Thoracic Society Guidelines. Managing passengers with lung disease planning Air Travel. *Thorax* 2001 (in press).

7   Smeets F. Travel for technology-dependent patients with respiratory disease. *Thorax* 1994; **49**: 77–81.

8   Fraser J, Mok Q, Tasker R. Survey of occupancy of paediatric intensive care units by children who are dependent on ventilators. *BMJ* 1997; **315**: 347–8.

9   Rigaud-Bully C. Comparison of methods of organization of home mechanical ventilation in different countries. In: Robert D, Make BJ, Leger P, Goldberg AI, *et al.* (eds). *Home mechanical ventilation*, 1st edn. Paris: Arnette Blackwell, 1996: 27–40.

10 Make BJ. Epidemiology of long-term ventilatory assistance. In: Hill NS (ed.). *Long-term mechanical ventilation*, 1st edn. New York: Marcel Dekker, 2001:1–17.

11 Report on a Consesus Conference of the American College of Chest Physicians. Mechanical ventilation beyond the intensive care unit. *Chest* 1998; **113**: 292S.

12 Goldberg AI, Faure AM. Home care for life-supported persons in England. The Responaut program. *Chest* 1984; **6**: 910–14.

19

Organization of long-term mechanical ventilation in Europe

P LEGER

INTRODUCTION

Home healthcare is growing worldwide, and Europe is no exception. Our population is ageing and changing patterns of hospital care have produced a shift to home care for patients in whom specific and highly technical care in hospital is not necessary. Long-term home mechanical ventilation (LTMV), which has increased dramatically over the last 10 years, is a prime example of this movement.

Not long ago, patients using LTMV were few in number, and managed by only a handful of centres in most countries. The technique used was predominantly tracheostomy ventilation. Today the number of patients using LTMV has increased significantly, recipients are managed by a large variety of physicians and centres, and most use non-invasive techniques.

The aim of this chapter is to describe the organization and distribution of LTMV for patients with chronic respiratory insufficiency (CRI) in Europe and to analyse the evolution over the last 5 years.[1] The discussion will be limited to home mechanical ventilation and rather than describing each country individually, a global view will be provided considering the following points:

- Evolution of LTMV
- Who prescribes LTMV?
- The influence and development of home care companies
- Aetiologies managed by LTMV and how they have changed
- Home care organizations
- Caregivers: who they are and how they are paid
- Funding and breakdown of the costs of LTMV.

PROGRESSION OF LTMV

Data regarding LTMV are difficult to obtain for the majority of European countries. There is a lack of published data and few national registers exist in Europe other than in France and the Nordic countries. Therefore, the data presented here form an accumulation of information from existing data bases, published studies, individual presentations and personal interviews. The information should be considered an estimation, with a reasonable level of confidence that it is close to reality. The data from Italy[2] and from Denmark and Sweden[3] were published in 1998 and 1999. Additional information for Sweden was established using the official website (www.lung.lu.se). The data from Germany came from a survey of Dr B Schönhofer in January 1999. The data from the UK are an estimation from Dr A Simonds, although information from a census of UK home ventilator providers should soon be forthcoming. Part of the data from Switzerland were presented in a poster by Dr JP Janssens at the 2000 ERS Meeting,[4] and data from Spain were presented by Dr J Escarabill during the 2000 American College of Chest Physicians Conference.[5] The information from France was established using the Antidir Observation (www.antadir.com) and personal surveys from the non-Antadir notn-for-profit organizations and the principal private, for-profit home care companies.

Table 19.1 shows the progression of LTMV in several European countries and compares data from 1999 and 1994. As can be seen, the progression of LTMV is significant in all the European countries listed. The number of patients has doubled in six years in almost every country, and in the UK the progression is even more significant. In France, where the level of LTMV was already high, there continues to be progression from an incidence of 16–20/100,000 inhabitants. The progression of LTMV can be attributed to:

- an increasing number of prescribing physicians and indications
- the support provided by an increasing number of home care companies
- changing techniques
- the longevity of the majority of the patients treated with LTMV.

PRESCRIBING PHYSICIANS

In contrast to long-term oxygen therapy, which has specific guidelines for prescription but is prescribed by non-specialists and specialists, there are no guidelines for the prescription of LTMV in Europe, but provision is restricted to specialists in

Table 19.1 *Estimated incidence of long-term mechanical ventilation in Europe*

Country	Distribution systems	Population	No. on LTMV	No. (%) on NIPPV	No. (%) on TV	% COPD on LTMV	No. 1994	No. 1999
Belgium	H; PHC	10	1000	–	–	1	2	10
Denmark[3]	2 Centres; PHC	5.2	290	66	33	5	2	5.5
Finland	1 Centre	5.5	250	–	–	–	–	4.5
France	H; NPRA/PHC	60	12,000	75	25	25	16	20
Germany	20 Centres/PHC	82	3600	91	9	30	1	4
Holland	4 Centres/PHC	15.9	850	–	–	–	3	5
Italy[2]	PHC	57.7	1842	85	15	30	2	5
Spain	PHC	39.4	1500	90	10	8	1	4
Switzerland	PHC	7	350	95	5	11	2	5
Sweden[3]	PHC	8.9	541			4	4	6.1
UK	H	59.4	3000	99	1	30	1	5

Centre	Centre for LTMV
H	Hospital
PHC	Private Home Care Company
NPRA	Non-profit regional association
LTMV	Long-term mechanical ventilation
NIPPV	Non-invasive ventilation
TV	Tracheostomy ventilation

No. 1994 and 1999 Number of patients on LTMV for 100,000 patients.

pulmonary, intensive care and paediatric medicine (and occasionally neurologists and rehabilitation physicians). Some countries, such as Denmark and Holland, continue to restrict the prescription of LTMV to specialized centres. These centres ventilate patients with restrictive disorders almost exclusively. In some countries which have diversified away from specialized centres, to include pneumologists in private practice, the percentage of COPD patients receiving LTMV has increased dramatically. This can be seen in France and Italy where almost 25% of patients on LTMV have COPD. In Switzerland prescriptions are restricted to pneumologists and intensive care specialists and reviewed by a committee of experts which has responsibility for validating each indication.

This dramatic increase in LTMV over the last 5 years throughout Europe can be explained by the following:

- An increased knowledge and better understanding of the consequences and treatment of sleep breathing disorders. This has had an additional impact on the treatment of CRI. Nasal CPAP facilitated the development of non-invasive ventilation (NIPPV): similar interfaces are used, i.e. nasal masks, simple ventilators were developed from CPAP specifically for NIPPV (i.e. pressure support with PEEP otherwise known as bilevel ventilation), thereby making this technology easier to access.
- In intensive care practice there is a great interest in the use of NIPPV to treat many types of acute respiratory failure. Several controlled studies have shown positive results in the treatment of acute exacerbation of chronic respiratory failure in selective COPD patients, and it has been shown to help in the weaning

process after invasive ventilation. Some of these positive results have encouraged physicians to continue NIPPV in the home with the goal of increasing survival and quality of life for restrictive patients, and preventing further exacerbations in those with COPD.

- Health authorities are searching for ways to decrease, or at least to stabilize, healthcare costs. In an effort to decrease the number of days in hospital, patients are discharged home earlier and more care is being provided in the home to keep patients out of hospital. Outcome results which show a decrease in hospital days with the use of NIPPV are therefore considered in a very positive light. An increase in survival is not necessarily the prime objective.
- Vendors and home care companies are pursuing a strategy of marketing directed towards physicians. This increased awareness and familiarity with NIPPV, in addition to the home support offered by home care companies, has probably stimulated the number of prescriptions.[6]
- Finally, the life expectancy of patients with restrictive respiratory disorders, mainly non- or slowly progressive neuromuscular diseases, treated with mechanical ventilation has increased dramatically over the last 10 years. As these patients are living longer, the total number of patients on home mechanical ventilation is increasing.

WHO ARE THE PATIENTS ON LTMV? ARE THERE CHANGING PATTERNS OF DISEASE?

The classification of potential candidates for LTMV include:

- Chest wall deformities
- Slowly progressive neuromuscular diseases
- ALS (motor neurone disease)
- COPD.

In Europe, it is rarely government agencies, regulation or guidelines that limit access to LTMV, but rather pressure from the medical community, the patients themselves, patient support groups and home care companies.

Chest wall disorders and slowly progressive neuromuscular diseases are generally accepted indications for LTMV by the medical community and health authorities.

According to the data of the Antidir Observatory (National Association for Home Treatment of Respiratory Insufficiency) the number of new scoliotic patients remains stable from year to year but the number of patients suffering from pulmonary sequelae of tuberculosis has decreased slowly since 1994. This can easily be explained by the age of those patients who contracted TB before or around 1950. Similar data are reported from England and Switzerland.

In contrast the number of patients with neuromuscular disease is consistently increasing. As mentioned before, the literature shows good agreement on the efficiency of ventilation in increasing survival and quality of life for the slowly progressive diseases. These positive results coupled with the influence of some patient organizations (e.g. the associations against myopathies), have increased the availability of LTMV to this population. The annual Telethon in France, Italy,

Switzerland has also contributed to the increase in LTMV by informing patients, families and physicians of the medical progress and future therapies for these diseases. The impact of genetic research has changed perceptions of the natural evolution of neuromuscular diseases and has increased optimism about potential cures. This increase in hope has encouraged many physicians, patients and families to use life support modalities. In spite of this general tendency in Europe, some interesting national differences have been demonstrated. A study by Midgren in Sweden showed that the distribution of diagnoses treated with LTMV differs considerably between Denmark and Sweden; two countries with similar cultural and socioeconomic structure and methods of reimbursement for LTMV. In Denmark, there is a much higher priority for home mechanical ventilation in young muscular dystrophy patients than in Sweden. One explanation of this difference, is the influence of the Danish Muscular Dystrophy Group. The author explains that 'this organization acts not only as a pressure group for the benefit of patients with muscular dystrophy but also as a centre of excellence for improving competence and education of healthcare professionals'. This has almost certainly influenced Danish paediatricians and neurologists to refer their muscular dystrophy patients to centres for home mechanical ventilation as a part of the routine care offered.

LTMV in progressive neuromuscular disease, mainly amyotrophic lateral sclerosis (ALS), presents a somewhat different situation. Previously, LTMV has been rarely used to treat CRI in ALS patients. This can be partially explained by the fact that neurologists are not usually involved in long-term mechanical ventilation, especially for a progressive diseases with no known treatment. The few patients that have been ventilated (less than 1% of the ventilation population) were frequently treated as a result of an acute episode of respiratory failure. The attitude of the neurologists is changing and has been modified by the results of recent medical trials. These recent studies have given patients and physicians some hope of a potential treatment for this currently fatal disease. Today, more physicians are willing to intervene using NIPPV to treat ALS patients. An alternative valid view held by some physicians is that the use of LTMV to palliate symptoms is reasonable, providing that the benefits outweigh the disadvantages. Additional studies are necessary to clarify decision-making pathways for patients, family and physicians, and examine the impact of LTMV on quality of life.

For COPD patients, large variations in treatment with LTMV exist between countries. This variation in the number of patients on home mechanical ventilation in different countries is explained by different national systems and their regulation for LTMV in COPD, rather than by differences in the prevalence of the disease. In fact, with the exception of Belgium, which refuses to reimburse for NIPPV in COPD, regulation appears to have little influence. For example, in both Sweden and France there are no national regulations prohibiting the use of LTMV in COPD. There is however a large difference in the proportion of LTMV patients with COPD: 3–4% in Sweden versus approximately 25% in France. The enthusiasm of French physicians in providing LTMV to this patient population is attributable to several factors: the success of NIPPV in acute exacerbations of COPD; the support and encouragement of the home care organizations to ventilate these patients in the home, the absence of precise guidelines, and finally the broad interpretation of contradictory results in the literature. It is also notable that among the COPD patients ventilated in Switzerland, where a group of experts validate the indications for LTMV in each case, the number of patients using LTMV is only 10% of the ventilated population. The large discrepancies seen in LTMV use for COPD in Sweden, Switzerland and France clearly show that the absence of guidelines results in a great deal of flexibility in the interpretation of indications for NIPPV.

LTMV TECHNIQUES: NIPPV VERSUS TRACHEOSTOMY VENTILATION

Positive pressure NIPPV via a nasal or a facial mask is clearly the first-line method of choice for LTMV in Europe and probably also in the world.[7] In Italy negative pressure ventilation is still used in around 4% of the cases. Even in countries where tracheostomy was the predominant method used in the past, NIPPV is now largely prescribed, and the tendency to tracheostomy ventilation has been completely reversed. However, in France, Denmark and Holland where there is a longer track record of LTMV, there remains a significant number of tracheostomized patients, This option is practised when NIPPV fails to provide sufficient clinical benefit or in the case of recurrent exacerbations. The influence of intensivists and anaesthesiologists in these countries also explains the continued interest and support for tracheostomy. The opposite picture is seen in the UK where tracheostomy patients are in a very small minority and most have cervical spinal cord lesions or profound neuromuscular disease.

LTMV is delivered using either volume or pressure preset ventilators. For tracheostomy ventilation the majority of patients are treated using volume ventilators. For NIPPV, the general tendency today is towards pressure preset ventilation, with some variation existing between countries. Pressure preset ventilators are almost exclusively used in the UK (80% v 20%) but the reverse situation exists in Spain (20% v 80% for volumetric). In France, a recent survey on the practice of non-invasive ventilation at home shows that the use of pressure preset ventilators is increasing, but volumetric ventilators remain in use widely to ventilate restrictive patients, especially the neuromuscular group.[8] In addition to the habits and preferences of the prescribers, the choice of ventilator is governed by considerations such as the need for alarms and back-up battery during tracheostomy ventilation, and use in patients requiring support for more than 12 hours a day. Until recently only the volume ventilators could provide these requirements.

HOME CARE ORGANIZATIONS

Home care in Europe is delivered by a variety of organizations. In some countries LTMV is supported from the hospital by specialized teams which provide the equipment and follow-up for patients. Certain hospitals manage patients in a particular region, whereas others manage patients throughout the country (e.g. the UK).

Other countries have home care providers. The majority are private, for-profit organizations; however some non-profit making groups still exist. The growth of all home care companies over the last 5 years is astounding. Many for-profit companies are merging and becoming large, international organizations that are fewer in number. In addition, many are merging with major medical gas producers. The impact this will have on home care organization and costs throughout Europe is unknown.

The system of home care in France and its evolution over the past 5 years provides an excellent example of a country's adaptation to the changing face of LTMV in Europe. Ten years ago LTMV in France was almost exclusively managed by associative, non-profit organizations linked to specialized centres for LTMV. These associations were federated in the central organization Antadir.[9,10]

Today LTMV is decentralized and prescribed by a larger variety of physicians. Patients are supported by a much larger system of home care organizations in which Antadir still holds the prime place with 27 regional associations and the responsibility for approximately 50% of the ventilated patients in France. When all the non-profit organizations are combined, (Antadir and non-Antadir organizations) this combination has responsibility for 70% of the LTMV patients in France. More severe patients, and tracheostomized or severely handicapped individuals (especially those with neuromuscular disease) are still mainly managed by specialized centres and their affiliated non-profit organizations.

The for-profit companies, which were almost non-existent in LTMV 5 years ago, have in their charge approximately 30% of the French ventilated population. Currently, these companies provide non-invasive ventilation almost exclusively. The companies have had a considerable impact on changing the composition of the prescribers of LTMV in France. They are more accessible to the private pneumologists who treat a large number of COPD patients. As a result, the majority of LTMV patients supported by for-profit companies have COPD.

Following the general trend towards home care, home care companies (for-profit or not) now also provide additional health care services such as enteral and parenteral nutrition, intravenous therapy and rehabilitation, in addition to long-term oxygen therapy and CPAP. This tendency towards the use of more complex technology in the home has increased the number of medical personnel within the home care companies which may influence the overall level of competence.

RESPONSIBILITIES AND ORGANIZATION OF THE HOME CARE PROVIDERS

Regardless of the country or whether home care is provided by a hospital or home care company, the organization is similar, with all requiring administrators, technicians, nurses and/or physiotherapists. In France all non-profit organizations include physicians on the staff. In most situations, these physicians are responsible for the collection and review of patient medical data, training and education of technicians and nurses, and the selection and trial of medical equipment. The physician is not usually responsible for home visits or medical decisions regarding patient care. The administrator is responsible for establishing a relationship with the funding source (social security agency in France) in addition to managing the personnel and the finances of the organization. The role of the technician is to prepare, install and maintain all the medical equipment in the patient's home. These individuals provide 24-hour on-call support for equipment problems and repair. Nurses or physical therapists provide paramedical support in the home for the more technically dependent patients, together with follow-up supervision and education for all patients. They do not typically provide direct patient care.

The general responsibilities of home care organizations are:[10,11]

1 To establish the treatment plan for the patient, according to the physician's prescription and requirements established by the National Health authority.
2 To obtain authorization from payer source (social security in France) for payment.
3 To provide the patient with all necessary medical equipment and supplies.
4 To teach the patient and/or family how to use and maintain the equipment properly and to perform all necessary medical procedures, including changing the tracheostomy tubes, when appropriate. If the patient or family is unable to assume responsibility for this level of care, local private nurses are taught how to perform these procedures.
5 To maintain the equipment in proper working order with an organization for service and preventative maintenance depending on the type of equipment and the level of patient dependency.
6 To provide 24-hour on-call service for equipment problems.
7 To provide paramedical supervision and to ensure the patient and/or family continues to use the equipment properly. This includes checking patients, their compliance with treatment, SaO_2, fitting interfaces, dealing with side effects and equipment hygiene. In some cases services can include the monitoring of home nocturnal SaO_2 during respiratory assistance.
8 To maintain communication with the referring physicians.

Medical, paramedical and technical supervision is managed in different countries in a variety of ways:

• Systematic home visits by paramedical and/or technical staff.
• Routine visits by patients to centres or hospital responsible for establishing LTMV.
• Routine phone calls.

Documentation of both technical and paramedical intervention is usually sent to the referring physician and/or the patient's general practitioner. Any concerns arising from these visits are directly communicated.

The organization and provision of the durable medical equipment needed for LTMV is similar in Europe. There are small nuances in interpretation between countries as to exactly what is covered under the umbrella of durable medical equipment, but in general most major items are reimbursed at a reasonable replacement level.[11] Outside this general technical support for LTMV and some specific situations where nursing intervention is clear for specialized care (tracheostomy changes), patients have to manage their general care with little support from the national healthcare systems. This is not a problem for the majority of patients who are independent or gain additional independence with the use of ventilatory support. However, for the more dependent patients (paralysed, tracheostomized and/or ventilated continuously, and children in general), the situation is more complicated and help for them is extremely limited in terms of money 'allocation for dependence', or with respect to helpers in the home.[12] With the exception of some Nordic countries, there is little support in Europe for help in the home. In the Nordic countries, the public health system pays for non-professional helpers 24 hours/day. This option is clearly the preferred one for the patients, who can choose their helpers and teach them according to their needs. However, in these countries the majority of the patients treated have non-progressive or slowly progressive neuromuscular diseases. COPD or ALS patients form a minority of the total number of patients ventilated in these countries. Progress in other countries in this direction is very slow. Recently in France, following pressure from patient organizations, a law allowing the practice of tracheal suction by a non-professional helper was passed. This law requires these individuals to receive a specific competency training in validated hospitals. This law is a step in the right direction to facilitate maintenance of these dependent patients in their own environment

PAYMENT FOR LTMV

Exact costs of LTMV are difficult to establish and only the national healthcare systems which have all the information as it relates to cost, can begin to approach the question of cost breakdown and the cost-effectiveness of LTMV. To the author's knowledge there is no study in Europe which has determined the cost of LTMV, separating patient care from the durable medical equipment. One very interesting study in the US provides some idea of what the costs of different levels of care could be were they to be reimbursed.[13] Sewick et al. showed that care, provided typically by family members, would cost between US$7642–8596/month (8941–10,057 Euros) if provided by a professional nurse. Reimbursement at this level of care for patients on LTMV would certainly bring into question its cost effectiveness. In France LTMV is reimbursed by the social security. The National Health Care Financing Authority for Salaried Workers (CNAM), which works under the control of the Ministry of Health and Social Security, negotiates the rate of reimbursement that the local social security will pay for each week spent at home by a patient using LTMV. Two years ago social security decided to standardize the reimbursement and abolished the differences between non-profit and for-profit organizations. Today, several rates are defined according to the equipment provided to the patients. Rates are separated as the following:

- **Tracheostomy ventilation:** 15 Euros/day and includes ventilator with alarm and battery, humidification system, tracheal suction machine, tracheostomy tubes and suction catheters. This cost also includes safety equipment; a second ventilator for patients ventilated more than 16 hours per day and a second suction machine. Reimbursement of a set price for electricity consumption is also included in this price.
- **Non-invasive ventilation more than 12 hours/day:** 10 Euros/day including a ventilator with alarm and battery, humidification system if needed, a second ventilator for patients ventilated more than 16 hours per day, six masks/year, and a set price for electricity consumption.

- **Non-invasive ventilation less than 12 hours/day:** 9 Euros/day, including a ventilator (alarm and battery are not required), humidification system if needed, three masks/year, and a set price for electricity consumption.

Prices are increased if the patient needs supplemental O_2 in addition to ventilation.

These prices remain stable year on year, in spite of the decrease in equipment cost. By comparison, reimbursement for long-term home O_2 therapy has decreased considerably.

CONCLUSIONS

In spite of differences between countries, Europeans share some similar experiences regarding LTMV:

- The number of ventilated patients is increasing significantly each year in all the countries. LTMV has been shown to be efficient and has produced a decrease in the number of patients hospitalized unjustifiably.
- In spite of the growth in ventilated patients the total compared with the theoretical number requiring ventilatory support is low showing that even in countries where LTMV is well accepted, a significant number of patients are not treated. Conversely, LTMV may not be justifiable in some patients with COPD. There are many reasons for these variations, and in the absence of guidelines indications for use are likely to be interpreted with latitude. Controlled trials to establish precise guidelines are necessary for some groups of patients such as COPD patients. Information is also required on outcome in ALS including the impact of LTMV on quality of life. These studies are needed not only to establish indications but also to provide limits and contraindications.
- Quality of life with in patients with a tracheostomy is a another important area, and results from the past cannot be extrapolated to today's practice. A large number of the patients managed 10 years ago with tracheostomy ventilation are today ventilated non-invasively. The illness severity and level of dependency of patients needing tracheostomy ventilation today is extremely high, and therefore outcomes should be evaluated critically. From an ethical perspective, the issue of saving life versus extending life should be explored.
- Equipment provision for LTMV is not a problem in Europe. However, home care givers represent a major problem area for dependent ventilator patients. Complementary studies are necessary to show the feasibility and the generalizability of the system used in the Nordic countries. Non-professional care givers are frequently preferred by patients, the cost is cheaper for society, and their use allows professional carers to concentrate on specialized activities that cannot be done by others. Some aspects of competency training could be standardized.
- Alternative sites to home and hospital should be studied and developed when it is not possible to maintain ventilator-dependent patients at home. Cost comparisons of home versus alternative site care should be performed in Europe.
- Further exchange of information on LTMV between European countries would be of great value.

REFERENCES

1   Leger P. Non-invasive respiratory support. In: Simonds AK (ed.) *Organisation of home respiratory care in Europe*. London: Chapman and Hall, 1996.

2   Gasperini M, Clini E, Zaccaria S. Mechanical ventilation in chronic respiratory insufficiency: report on an Italian nationwide survey. *Monaldi Arch Chest Dis* 1998; **53**: 394–9.

3   Midgren B, Olofson J, Harlid R, Dellborg C, Jacobsen E, Norregaard O. Home mechanical ventilation in Sweden with reference to Danish experiences. *Respir Med* 2000 **94**: 135–8.

4   Janssens JP, Derivaz E, Breitenstein P, *et al.* Changes in prescription of home mechanical ventilation over a 7 year observation period in the Geneva lake area. Abstract 487, ERS 2000.

5   Prats E, Farrero E, Giró V, *et al.* Long-term follow-up in patients on non invasive mechanical ventilation (NIMV). Abstract 2748, ERS 2000.

6   Kellogg VA. Home respiratory care in Europe. *RT Internat* 1998; Fall: 17–19.

7   Adams AB, Shapiro R, Marini JJ. Changing prevalence of chronically ventilator-assisted individuals in Minnesota: increases, characteristics and the use of non invasive ventilation. *Respir Care* 1998; **43** (8): 643–9.

8   Guiton C, Ordronneau J, Chollet S, Veale D, Coisy-Vialettes M, Chailleux E. French National Survey on the practice of domiciliary non invasive ventilation. *Rev Fr Mal Resp* 2000; (abstract).

9   Rigaud Bully C. Organisation in different countries. In: Robert D, Make BJ, Leger P, Goldbert AI, *et al.* (eds). *Home mechanical ventilation*, Paris: Arnette Blackwell, 1994: 27–35.

10   Fauroux B, Howard P. Muir JF. Home treatment for chronic respiratory insufficiency: the situation in Europe in 1992. *Eur Respir J* 1994; **7**: 1721–6.

11   Donner CF, Zaccaria S, Braghiroli A, Carone M. Organisation of home care in patients receiving nocturnal ventilatory support. *Eur Respir Mon* 1998; **8**: 380–99.

12   Jardine E, O'Toole JY, Paton C, Wallis C. Current status of long term ventilation of children in the United Kingdom: questionnaire survey. *BMJ* 1999; **19**; 318(7179): 295–9.

13   Sewick MA, Kamlet MS, Hoffman LA, Rawson I. Economic cost of home-based care for ventilator-assisted individuals. A preliminary report. *Chest* **109**: 1597–606.

20

Ethical and medico-legal aspects of assisted ventilation

M A BRANTHWAITE

Ethics can be defined for practical purposes as the establishment of moral principles in circumstances where neither logic nor instinct provide universally acceptable solutions. The law is a framework of rules which regulate human conduct and are regarded as binding. Legal action can be used not only to enforce rules but also to develop them. One such development is the resolution of ethical conflicts created by advances in medicine, particularly those at the fringes of currently lawful behaviour. This chapter adopts a simplistic approach to the ethical principles of medical practice and considers how English law has been used to resolve ethical dilemmas and regulate professional decision-making.

FOUR ETHICAL PRINCIPLES

Widely promulgated as the foundation for good medical practice, the principles are to:

- promote beneficence
- avoid maleficence
- respect individual autonomy
- secure, so far as is possible, distributive justice.

A fifth consideration is often added, namely the scope for application of these principles.[1]

Application of ethical principles to assisted ventilation

Assisted ventilation saves lives. It does so in the short-term, for example, during anaesthesia or resuscitation. It can do so in the longer term for patients requiring intensive care. It may do so in the very long term for patients in whom spontaneous breathing cannot be restored. Saving life is instinctively perceived to be beneficent and thus a proper objective for medical practice.

Conversely, the preservation of life which is devoid of satisfaction or degraded by burdensome or undignified treatment could be regarded as maleficent. Assisted ventilation, however delivered, is likely to interfere with at least some natural functions such as speech, swallowing, touching, kissing or even moving freely while recumbent. Privacy, even for intimate personal matters, may well be lost for some periods of time at least. This may be seen as a small price to pay for survival, especially by those for whom sanctity of life transcends all other considerations. Non-invasive assisted ventilation, especially if only needed for part of each day, is likely to enhance benefit and minimize the burden of treatment.

Resolution of the conflict between beneficence and actual or potential maleficence must involve not only the practitioner but also the patient. Autonomy is defined as the ability of a sentient human being to determine how his or her own life will evolve. Society no longer accepts paternalistic medicine but demands a voice in decision-making. Autonomy is seen as a right, enshrined by law in some jurisdictions, and to be respected subject only to the need not to infringe the rights of others. Consideration of the rights of others raises immediate conflict with the fourth principle – distributive justice. Assisted ventilation is expensive in terms of both human and financial resources, whether it is provided in an intensive care unit, at home or a long-stay institution. Resources for health care are limited in all societies, some more than others, and demand is both insatiable and ever-expanding. Provision for one group necessarily limits resources available to another. Conflict is inevitable, particularly when health care is funded by the state and the public is led to believe there is 'provision for all, free at the point of delivery'. A discussion of these concerns in the context of providing domiciliary ventilation for a young child with progressive neuromuscular disease can be found in the *British Medical Journal*.[2]

LEGAL BASIS FOR ETHICAL DECISIONS

Withholding treatment

Four landmark cases provide the foundation for English law on this subject:[3–6]

Re T (1992): right of competent adults to refuse life-sustaining treatment.
Re C (1994): requirements for legal competence.
Re F (1990): consent by the court on behalf of an incompetent adult to be based upon consideration of best interests.
Re J (1992): practitioner not obliged to provide treatment (in this case to a child) if holding a sincere and reasoned belief that to do so is not in the patient's best interests.

The following analysis is based upon this caselaw.

Patients requiring mechanical ventilation often present as an emergency, too confused to give valid consent to treatment. The doctrine of necessity provides legal authority to proceed and, unless there are compelling factors to the contrary, treatment aimed at saving life must always be the preferred option. Competent adult patients can however refuse treatment, even though by so doing their lives are in jeopardy. Competence is defined at law as the ability to understand, retain and believe information given and to use it in reaching a decision about whether or not to consent. Providing treatment in the face of refusal of consent by a competent adult acting voluntarily is a civil and possibly criminal offence. Advance directives are also binding provided the author was competent, acted voluntarily, and the circumstances now pertaining were within his contemplation when the directive was made. Relatives, no matter how well-meaning, cannot give or withhold consent for an incompetent adult patient and there is no legal basis for permitting their views to over-rule an advance directive. However, legislation is anticipated which would permit the nomination of proxy medical decision-makers who could be approached if consent is required on behalf of a previously competent adult.[7] Until such legislation is in force, potentially contentious or sensitive decisions affecting such patients should be referred to the courts to ensure protection for both patient and practitioner.

Refusal of treatment by an adult is valid if the subject is:

- Legally competent
- Acts voluntarily
- Intends the decision to apply to the circumstances which now pertain

---

Legal competence requires the ability to:

- Understand
- Retain
- Believe information provided and use it in reaching a decision

---

Similar considerations apply to the more emotive and sometimes highly controversial question of withholding treatment from children. Children of 16 years and above can give but not withhold valid consent to treatment.[8,9] Children below 16 years can give valid consent, provided they are deemed of sufficient maturity and understanding to comprehend the implications of the decision.[10] Children with a chronic, life-threatening disability, often have an amazing maturity of insight and their views should always be sought, no matter what their age. Parents or legal guardians are the usual source of formal consent and they too are expected to act in the best interests of the child. If parents seek to withhold consent for treatment considered by the treating clinician to be life-saving or essential for the well-being of the child, it may be necessary to secure a care order or make the child a ward of court. Similarly, if parental wishes for treatment to be initiated or continued conflict with those of the practitioner, it may be necessary to seek adjudication by the court. The test used is to determine, on the basis of expert evidence, what is in the child's best interests. Doctors are entitled to withhold treatment including life-saving or sustaining measures such as mechanical ventilation, provided they act in the sincerely-held belief that to do so is in the best interests of the patient, and can justify this course of action by logical argument.

> - Children aged 16 years and over can give but not withhold valid consent to medical treatment
> - Children less than 16 years can also give valid consent *provided* they have sufficient maturity and understanding
> - Parents must act in the best interests of the child

Withdrawing treatment

Treatment withdrawal is the logical consequence when the burdens exceed the benefit. This too is a decision which demands respect for the autonomy of competent patients but may need to be taken vicariously when competence has been eroded by the consequences of illness or drug treatment. Often too there is at least covert concern to conserve resources or redirect them to patients deemed more likely to benefit. Finally the decision to withdraw assisted ventilation is peculiarly demanding because death is the likely and immediate consequence.

The stark proximity between cessation of assisted ventilation and death is such that 'treatment withdrawal' is usually actioned by less dramatic means. Treatment withdrawal is a misnomer. It is more accurate to state that treatment is redirected away from the preservation of life to the maintenance of comfort and dignity in dying. Discontinuing mechanical ventilation, particularly the removal of invasive equipment, can contribute to these objectives provided the patient can sustain enough respiratory effort to be comfortable, even if not breathing normally.

Occasionally sentient, physiologically stable and legally competent patients seek cessation of mechanical ventilation.[11] These rare instances are likely to reach the courts and the application is countenanced only after searching argument. More often a legal determination is sought when the decision affects a legally incompetent patient and then only when there is profound impairment of consciousness combined with protracted physiological stability. Here too the courts will seek to determine the best interests of the patient but accept there is no moral or legal obligation to provide or prolong treatment deemed to be ineffective or useless.[12]

Resource constraints

In England and Wales the Secretary of State for Health has an obligation to provide services which he deems necessary to meet all reasonable requirements for health care.[13] Occasional disaffected groups of patients have sought judicial review (an administrative remedy) on the grounds of insufficient provision but in general these attempts have failed.[14]

Individual claimants have also sought judicial review of decisions by a Health Authority to operate a blanket ban on particular types of treatment.[15] Although the provision of mechanical ventilation *per se* has not spawned case law, treatments comparable in terms of degree of specialization and small numerical need have done so and the courts have ruled such policies to be *ultra vires*, in other words, unlawful. Conversely the Court of Appeal has upheld the decision of a Health Authority to withhold treatment for recurrent leukaemia in a child.[16] Although it was accepted that the child's best interests played a dominant role in the decision, it was acknowledged that the Authority had a responsibility to determine how best to deploy its resources and was not required to give reasons for its conclusions. The ethical conflict is how to ensure distributive justice.[17] Resolution at present is being sought either through the courts[18] or by edict of administrative bodies created by statute (National Institute for Clinical Excellence). It remains to be seen how far the provisions of the Human Rights Act 1998 will be exploited to displace resource constraints as justification for failure to provide specific treatments.[19]

TRANSGRESSING THE LAW

Criminal proceedings based upon a charge of homicide could follow death occurring during or, more likely, as a result of interruption of mechanical ventilation. Civil action seeking damages to compensate for personal injury, including death, is a more probable legal consequence.

Homicide

Both murder and manslaughter are criminal offences included within the generic term homicide or unlawful killing. Conviction for either offence requires proof beyond reasonable doubt that the Defendant caused the death, both as a matter of fact and within the boundaries of law. Causation in fact is determined by the 'but for' test. But for the actions of the Defendant, would the deceased have died? Causation in law, in other words recognition of legal liability, requires not only proof of a causal factual relationship between the action and the death, but also a sufficient proximity or 'reasonable foreseeability'. Thus when two victims of assault were deemed irretrievably brain damaged and mechanical ventilation was discontinued, appeals against conviction for murder by their assailants were unsuccessful.[20] The Court of Appeal considered the original wounds had been the operating and substantial cause of death, and mechanical ventilation no more than a means of holding in abeyance the effects of the injuries. Similar reasoning is apparent in the decision of a New Zealand Court in which cessation of mechanical ventilation was authorised in a wholly-inaccessible patient with profound and long-lasting polyneuritis.[21] The cause of death was the disease, not withdrawing treatment which had by then become demonstrably futile.

Murder

A conviction for murder requires not only proof of causation in both fact and law, but also proof to the same standard that the Defendant intended either to cause death, or personal injury of a severity which he was aware could cause death. It is important to recognize the distinction between motive and intention. A physician, acting at the behest of his patient who suffered intolerable pain, injected her with potassium chloride and she died shortly afterwards. He was convicted of attempted murder, proof of causation in fact having been precluded by early cremation.[22] Despite acting at the patient's request and being moved to do so by compassion, his intention was deemed to be to kill the patient, albeit as a means of relieving her suffering.

A different approach is adopted when treatment perceived as beneficent carries with it undesirable and potentially life-threatening side effects. An obvious example is administration of opiates to the terminally ill, but similar arguments can be raised over treatment withdrawal which includes the cessation of mechanical ventilation. The practitioner will not be found guilty of homicide if deemed to have acted in the best interests of the patient, notwithstanding an awareness that some shortening of life is likely as a result.[23] Clearly the application of this comforting doctrine of double effect would be of little help were mechanical ventilation to be withdrawn from a physiologically stable, ventilator-dependent patient.

Both the legal and ethical aspects of withdrawing life-sustaining measures were explored in detail in the context of persistent vegetative state when application was made for a declaration that it would not be unlawful to discontinue hydration and nutrition.[12] The declaration was duly granted and ultimately appealed, primarily for the purpose of clarifying the law, to the House of Lords. This case, and the conviction of a medical practitioner for attempted murder referred to earlier, prompted the setting up of a House of Lords Select Committee with a remit to consider the issues surrounding the withholding of life-prolonging treatment, including euthanasia. The Committee reiterated the traditional view.[24] Both euthanasia and assisting suicide remain criminal offences, but provided clinicians act in what they sincerely and logically believe to be the best interests of their patient, acts which may or will expedite death are not necessarily to be condemned. Guidelines which incorporate these legal decisions have been published by the British Medical Association and Royal College of Paediatrics and Child Health.[25-27] In England and Wales, authority for withdrawal of life-sustaining treatment from patients in a persistent vegetative state should be sought from the courts.[28,29] In a recent judgement, it was held that such an approach did not transgress rights held under the Human Rights Act 1998.[30] The same approach should be adopted in those rare cases where consideration is given to discontinuing mechanical ventilation from a wholly ventilator dependent but otherwise stable patient, whether child or adult, sentient or incompetent.

Manslaughter by criminal negligence

A charge of manslaughter in the context of medical practice is likely to be based upon allegations of 'gross negligence', in other words negligence going beyond a mere matter of compensation between parties and so heinous that imposition of a penalty in the name of society is appropriate.[31,32] The criteria to be considered by the jury are whether the Defendant:

- displayed indifference to an obvious risk of injury to health
- foresaw the risk but determined nevertheless to run it
- appreciated the risk and intended to avoid it but displayed such a high degree of negligence in the attempted avoidance as the jury considers justifies conviction
- was inattentive or failed to advert to a serious risk, going beyond mere inadvertence in respect of an obvious and important matter which the defendant's duty demanded should be addressed.

Circumstances pertaining to mechanical ventilation can be imagined in which such criteria might apply, but in general there is a reluctance to bring criminal proceedings against medical practitioners, particularly if it is clear that system errors such as inappropriate delegation to inexperienced staff are as important or more important than individual responsibility.

Civil proceedings

Once again negligence is the likely basis for action but here the standard of proof is no more than balance of probabilities and the objective is not punishment but reparation. A claimant can only succeed if able to establish that foreseeable harm has occurred as a consequence of breach of a duty of care. The standard of care expected is that which is endorsed by a responsible body of medical practitioners, skilled and practised in that art.[33] This traditional definition has been refined more recently by a requirement that expert opinion is logical and can withstand critical analysis.[34] Difficulties are likely to arise when the subject in issue is intrinsically of high risk, undertaken infrequently and developing rapidly. These criteria all apply to long-term mechanical ventilation, particularly when maintained at home for patients incapable of spontaneous breathing. What constitutes an acceptable standard of care? First and most important, it is the standard which would have applied at the time of the events criticized.[35] Provided a practitioner can satisfy the court that reasonable measures were taken to safeguard the patient against foreseeable causes of harm, then it is unlikely that any civil action for damages would succeed.

Proof of negligence at law requires evidence of:

- A duty of care
- Breach of the duty of care
- Foreseeable harm caused by the breach of duty

Particular concern in the context of assisted ventilation is likely to focus on equipment failure, especially at home. Stringent laws of product liability apply to manufacturers of medical equipment but responsibility for failure might lie with a practitioner if, for example, recommendations for regular servicing were transgressed or the equipment was used in a manner for which it was not developed. Such restriction might curtail innovative development but clearly argued research protocols and agreed professional attitudes are likely to provide a defence to litigation, particularly in a developing field. Guidelines or protocols based on current practice are often considered to indicate proper standards of care, particularly if produced or endorsed by a widely-respected authority. They are probably better regarded as persuasive evidence of the proper standard, not strictly probative. However if guidelines do exist, it is clearly wise to conform unless there are clear, specific and well-reasoned arguments for transgressing them.

Sometimes guidelines are changed in response to an adverse incident but this does not prove the previous standards were negligent in a strictly legal sense: 'There is nothing which is so perfect that it cannot be improved by knowledge, experience and understanding'.[36] The law recognizes that medicine must advance and in its turn is developed to accommodate and respond to developments in medicine. It is comforting to conclude with a quotation from the highest court in the land:

> 'After the event even a fool is wise. But it is not the hindsight of a fool; it is the foresight of the reasonable man which alone can determine responsibility'.
> Viscount Simonds in *The Wagon Mound* (No 1).[37]

CONCLUSIONS

- Beneficence, non-maleficence, respect for autonomy and distributive justice are the ethical basis for good medical practice.
- Practitioners are not required to initiate or continue treatment considered futile.
- Competent adults can refuse life-saving or sustaining treatment.
- Children over 16 years and some below this age can consent but not withhold consent to medical treatment.
- Parents must act in the best interests of their child.
- Relatives cannot give valid consent to treatment on behalf of an incompetent adult.
- Best interests, sometimes determinable only by the courts, must form the basis for decisions on behalf of all incompetent patients.
- Euthanasia and assisted suicide are criminal offences at English law.
- English law acknowledges that some shortening of life may occur as a consequence of actions taken in the best interests of the terminally ill.
- Application to the courts should be considered when contemplating withdrawal of life-sustaining treatment from a patient who is physiologically stable.
- Practitioners are judged in the civil courts by the standards of responsible medical practice pertaining at the time of the events in question.
- Transgression of clinical guidelines is persuasive but not necessarily probative of a deficient standard of care.

REFERENCES

1   Gillon R. Medical ethics: four principles plus attention to scope. *BMJ* 1994; **309**: 184–8.
2.   Davies RH, Harvey I, Newton-John H, Ward TA. Home ventilation of a child with motor and sensory neuropathy. *BMJ* 1996; **313**: 153–5.
3   Re T. (Adult: Refusal of Medical Treatment) [1992] 3 WLR 782.

4   Re C. (Adult: Refusal of Medical Treatment) [1994] 1 WLR 290.
5   F v West Berkshire Health Authority [1990] 2 AC 1.
6   Re J. (A Minor) (Wardship: medical treatment) [1992] 4 All ER 614.
7   Dyer C. Adults will be able to appoint proxies to make health decisions. *BMJ* 1999; **319**: 1218.
8   Family Law Reform Act 1969 s8(1).
9   Re W (a minor) (medical treatment: court's jurisdiction) [1992] 4 All ER 627.
10 Gillick v West Norfolk and Wisbech Area Health Authority and Department of Health and Social Security [1986] AC 112 (and see Children Act 1989 38(6)).
11 Nancy B v Hotel Dieu de Quebec (1992) 86 DLR (4th) 385.
12 Airedale NHS Trust v Bland [1993] AC 789.
13 National Health Service Act 1977 s3(1).
14 R v Secretary of State for Social Services *ex parte* Hincks (1992) 1 BMLR 93.
15 R v North Derbyshire Health Authority *ex parte* Fisher ([1997] 8 MLR 327.
16 R v Cambridge District Health Authority *ex parte* B [1995] 2 All ER 129.
17 Ham C. Tragic choices in health care: lessons from the Child B case. *BMJ* 1999; **319**: 1258–61.
18 Stewart C. Tragic choices and the role of administrative law. *BMJ* 2000; **321**: 105–7.
19 Hewson B. Why the Human Rights Act matters to doctors. *BMJ* 2000; **321**: 780–1.
20 R v Malcherek, R v Steel [1981] 1 WLR 690.
21 Auckland Area Health Board v AG [1993] 4 Med LR 239.
22 R v Cox (1992) 12 BMLR 38.
23 Gillon R, Doyal L. Two-part commentary: Foreseeing is not necessarily the same as intending. The moral character of clinicians or the best interests of patients? *BMJ* 1999; **318**: 1431–3.
24 Report of House of Lords' Select Committee on Medical Ethics. London: HMSO, 1994.
25 British Medical Association. *Withholding or withdrawing life-prolonging medical treatment – guidance for decision making.* London: BMA Publishing, 1999.
26 British Medical Association. *Advance statements about medical treatment.* London: BMA Publishing, 1995.
27 Royal College of Paediatrics and Child Health. *Withholding or withdrawing life saving treatment in children: a framework for practice.* London: Royal College of Paediatrics and Child Health, 1997.
28 Wade DR, Johnston C. The permanent vegetative state: practical guidance on diagnosis and management. *BMJ* 1999; **319**: 841–4.
29 Oates L. The courts' role in decisions about medical treatment. *BMJ* 2000;**321**:1282–4.
30 Human Rights Act does not bar mercy killing. *The Times*, 26th October 2000.
31 Ferner RE. Medication errors that have led to manslaughter charges. *BMJ* 2000; **321**: 1212–16.
32 R v Prentice and Sullman, R v Adomako, R v Holloway [1994] QB 302.
33 Bolam v Friern Hospital Management Committee [1957] 2 All ER 118.
34 Bolitho v City and East Hackney Health Authority [1998] AC 232.
35 Roe v Minister of Health [1954] 2 All ER 131.
36 Pipe v Chambers Wharf and Cold Stores Ltd [1952] 1 Lloyd's Rep 194 at 195.
37 Overseas Tankship (UK) v Morts Dock & Engineering Co [1961] AC 388.

FURTHER READING

Branthwaite MA. *Law for doctors: principles and practicalities.* London: Royal Society of Medicine Press, 2000.

Appendix I

Suppliers of ventilatory equipment

This list is not comprehensive, but contains many of the major suppliers.

Company	Equipment
ResMed *www.resmed.com* 58 Milton Park, Abingdon Oxon, UK Tel 01235 862997	VPAP, Sullivan CPAP Autoset, Autoset CS Mirage masks, bubble masks Headgear. Humidifiers
Breas Medical Ltd *www.breas.com* 18 Lion and Lamb Yard, Farnham, Surrey GU9 7LL, UK Tel 01252 731660	PV401, PV501, PV403 Pulmonetic LTV1000 CPAP equipment masks, headgear
UK Supplier: Deva Medical Electronics 8 Jensen Court, Astmoor Industrial Estate Runcorn, Cheshire, UK Tel 01928 565836	
Respironics *www.respironics.com* 1001 Murry Ridge Lane, Murrysville Pennsylvania 15668-8550, USA	BiPAP S BiPAP S/T Harmony CPAP equipment Profile, Spectrum, Simplicity masks, headgear
UK supplier: MedicAid Hook Lane, Pagham, Sussex PO21 3PP, UK Tel 01243 276321	
B&D Electromedical 35 Shipston Road Stratford-on-Avon Warwickshire CV37 7LN, UK Tel 01789 293460	Nippy, Nippy II, Nippaed Handy mains, batteries CPAP equipment masks

Sims pneuPAC Ltd
Smithfield House
Crescent Road, Luton
Beds LU2 0AH, UK
Tel 01582 453303

brompton PAC, TransPAC
Service and maintenance
of ventilators

Mallinkrodt
www.mallinkrodt.com
www.cpapmask.com
incorporating Puritan Bennett
2800 Northwest Blvd
Minn, MN 55441, USA
Mallinkrodt Europe BV, Hambakenwetering 1
5231 DD's Hertogenbosch, The Netherlands

Shiley tracheostomy tubes
Masks, nasal plugs/pillows
Breeze SleepGear
Achieva
Companiom 2801

Weinmann
www.weinmann.de
PO Box 54 02 68 D-22502
Hamburg, Germany

Semi-customized masks
Ventilators, CO_2 monitors

UK supplier: Nuwyn Ltd
2 Gibbs Close, Wokingham
Berks RG40 4TY, UK
Tel/fax 0118 973 2564

SIMS Portex Limited
www.portex.com
Hythe, Kent CT21 6JL, UK

Endotracheal and tracheostomy
tubes. Heat and moisture
exchangers. Humidifiers

Breasy Hayel Oscillator
Breasy Medical Equipment Ltd
Breasy Place,
9 Burroughs Gardens
London NW4 4AU, UK

Hayek oscillator

JH Emerson Co
22 Cottage Park Avenue, Cambridge
MA 02140, USA
Tel (617) 864 1414

Cough In-exsufflator
Negative pressure pumps
Tank ventilator

Coppa Biella
Officine Coppa s.r.l.
Via Maglioleo
68-13051 Biella, Italy
Tel (015) 22 278

Tank ventilators

Index

Note: page numbers in italic denote tables.